D0609257

Jewish Thought
and Scientific Discovery
in Early Modern Europe

Jewish Thought
and Scientific Discovery
in Early Modern Europe

DAVID B. RUDERMAN

Yale University Press   New Haven and London

Published with assistance from the Joseph Meyerhoff Fund,
the Lucius N. Littauer Foundation, and the Frederick W.
Hilles Publication Fund of Yale University.

Designed by Sonia L. Scanlon
Set in Fournier type by Tseng Information Systems, Inc.
Printed in the United States of America by Edwards
Brothers, Inc., Ann Arbor, Michigan

Library of Congress Cataloging-in-Publication Data
Ruderman, David B.
Jewish thought and scientific discovery in early modern
Europe / David B. Ruderman.
p.   cm.
Includes bibliographical references and index.
ISBN 0-300-06112-9
1. Judaism and science.   2. Jews—Europe—Medicine—
History.   3. Jews—Europe—Intellectual life.
4. Medicine—Religious aspects—Judaism.   5. Jewish
scientists—Europe—History.   6. Jewish physicians—
Europe—History.   I. Title.
IN PROCESS
296.3′875—dc20   94-30520
CIP

A catalogue record for this book is available from the
British Library.

10 9 8 7 6 5 4 3 2 1

In memory of
Simon Robert Ruderman (1946–1992)
Jacob Ruderman (1905–1992)
Ralph Taylor (1904–1993)

CONTENTS

Photographs follow page 152

Acknowledgments ix

Introduction 1

CHAPTER ONE
Medieval Jewish Attitudes toward Nature and Scientific Activity 14

CHAPTER TWO
The Legitimation of Scientific Activity among Central and
Eastern European Jews 54

CHAPTER THREE
Padua and the Formation of a Jewish Medical Community in Italy 100

CHAPTER FOUR
Can a Scholar of the Natural Sciences Take the Kabbalah Seriously?
The Divergent Positions of Leone Modena and Joseph Delmedigo 118

CHAPTER FIVE
Science and Skepticism
Simone Luzzatto on Perceiving the Natural World 153

CHAPTER SIX
Between High and Low Cultures
*Echoes of the New Science in the Writings of Judah Del Bene
and Azariah Figo* 185

CHAPTER SEVEN

Kabbalah, Science, and Christian Polemics

*The Debate between Samson Morpurgo and
Solomon Aviad Sar Shalom Basilea 213*

CHAPTER EIGHT

On the Diffusion of Scientific Knowledge within the Jewish Community

The Medical Textbook of Tobias Cohen 229

CHAPTER NINE

Contemporary Science and Jewish Law in the Eyes of
Isaac Lampronti and His Rabbinic Interlocutors *256*

CHAPTER TEN

The Community of Converso Physicians

Race, Medicine, and the Shaping of a Cultural Identity 273

CHAPTER ELEVEN

A Jewish Thinker in Newtonian England

David Nieto and His Defense of the Jewish Faith 310

CHAPTER TWELVE

Physico-Theology and Jewish Thought
at the End of the Eighteenth Century

Mordechai Schnaber Levison and Some of His Contemporaries 332

Epilogue 369

Bibliographic Essay

The Study of Nature in Ancient Judaism *375*

Index 383

ACKNOWLEDGMENTS

I have worked intermittently on this book for more than a decade and have been encouraged by the conversations and suggestions of numerous colleagues over the years. I benefited particularly from those who read drafts of various chapters of the book and offered their critical comments. They include David Berger, Robert Bonfil, Richard Cohen, Michael Heyd, Moshe Idel, Yosef Kaplan, Y. Tzvi Langermann, Benjamin Ravid, Elhanan Reiner, Nancy Siraisi, Steven Smith, and especially Richard Popkin. The students in my "God and Nature" seminars at Yale helped me refine my arguments. I am especially indebted to Jeffrey Chajes, who read a draft of the book, and to Rabbi James Ponet, who came to study with me but taught his instructor more than he learned.

I also profited immensely from opportunities to present various aspects of the book to scholarly audiences at the Fondazione Giorgio Cini in Venice in 1983 and later at Yale University and Medical School, Ben Gurion University, Tel Aviv University, the Hebrew University, Bar Ilan University, Harvard University, the Graduate School of the City University of New York, the University of Chicago, Princeton University, Wesleyan University, the Jewish Museum, Concordia University, and the Jewish Theological Seminary. I also tried out my ideas on two gatherings of rabbis at the Southwest and New England regional conferences of the Central Conference of American Rabbis. To all of these audiences I am profoundly grateful.

I was stimulated to begin this study many years ago by browsing through the rich collections of the National Library of the History of Medicine in Washington, D.C. Additional research followed in the libraries of Yale University (especially its collection in the history of medicine), the National and University Library of the Hebrew University in Jerusalem (especially its Institute for Microfilms of Hebrew Manuscripts and the Harry Friedenwald Collection of the History of Jewish Medicine), and the library of the Jewish Theological Seminary of America.

My initial foray into the subject of this book resulted in two previous books on the sixteenth-century Jewish physician and kabbalist Abraham Yagel: *Kabbalah, Magic, and Science: The Cultural Universe of a Sixteenth-Century Jewish Physician* (Cambridge, Mass., 1988) and *A Valley of Vision: The Heavenly Journey of Abraham Ben Hananiah Yagel* (Philadelphia, 1990). These books, especially the first, are closely linked to this one and might be profitably consulted when reading it.

Several chapters of this book were previously published in preliminary form as separate articles. Chapter 3 is based on "The Impact of Science on Jewish Culture and Society in Venice (with Special Reference to Graduates of Padua's Medical School)," in G. Cozzi, ed., *Gli Ebrei e Venezia, secoli XVI–XVII* (Milan, 1987), pp. 417–48, 540–42. Chapter 6 is partially based on "Jewish Preaching and the Language of Science: The Sermons of Azariah Figo," in D. Ruderman, ed., *Preachers of the Italian Ghetto* (Berkeley and Los Angeles, 1992). Chapter 7 is based on "Philosophy, Kabbalah, and Science in the Culture of the Italian Ghetto: On the Debate between Samson Morpurgo and Aviad Sar Shalom Basilea," *Jerusalem Studies in Jewish Thought* 11 (1993): vii–xxiv. Chapter 9 is based on "Contemporary Science and Jewish Law in the Eyes of Isaac Lampronti of Ferrara and Some of His Contemporaries," *Frank Talmage Memorial Volume II, Jewish History* 6 (1992): 211–24. Chapter 11 is based on "Jewish Thought in Newtonian England: The Career and Writings of David Nieto," *Proceedings of the American Academy for Jewish Research* 58 (1992): 193–219. I thank the editor and publisher of each of these publications for permission to reprint extensive parts of these essays.

I record my sincere thanks to Charles Grench, the executive editor of Yale University Press, for his special interest in this book and for his friendship over the years. I am also grateful to Harry Haskell for his excellent editorial work on the manuscript.

As in the past, I am singularly indebted to my wife, Phyllis, and to my children, Noah and Tali, for their loving partnership in sharing my life and in helping me to create this book. The completion of this work also marks a turning point in our lives: Noah's graduation from high school and our departure from New Haven to Philadelphia, a departure filled with the mixed emotions of sadness and exhilaration in closing a valuable chapter of one's life and opening another.

INTRODUCTION

One of the most common assumptions about Jews, especially those living in modern times, is their conspicuous involvement in and propensity for scientific achievement. The assumption is based on the noticeably high percentage of Jewish scientists throughout the Western world, and particularly the high percentage of Nobel Prize recipients in physics, chemistry, and medicine who are Jews. Various writers have offered an assortment of generally impressionistic explanations of this striking phenomenon. These include a perceived openness to the sciences in Jewish religious thought, the Jewish drive to try harder in the face of prejudice and discrimination, the Jewish gene pool, and the modes of education in rabbinic Judaism that parallel those in the theoretical sciences.[1] Some remarks of C. P. Snow in a lecture delivered in 1969 are typical:

> Take any test of achievement you like—in any branch of science, mathematics, literature, music, public life. The Jewish performance has been not only disproportionate, but also ridiculously disproportionate. The record is remarkable, and quite outside any sort of statistical probabilities.

1. A good example of this kind of discussion is found in an essay by C. Domb entitled "Jewish Distinction in Science," in A. Gotfryd et al., eds., *Fusion: Absolute Standards in a World of Relativity: Science, the Arts, and Contemporary Life in the Light of the Torah* (Jerusalem, 1990), pp. 29–44. See also I. Carmin and H. Cohen, *Jews in the World of Science* (New York, 1956); R. Patai, *The Jewish Mind* (New York, 1977), pp. 315–42, especially his summaries of the views of Thorstein Veblen, Chaim Weizmann, and Lewis Feuer, pp. 331–34.

This isn't arguable. The facts are plain. But why is it? One answer is, of course, that the Jewish environment makes for the utmost use of talent. Apart from the Jewish respect for education, the very obvious truth that a Jewish person starts with two strikes against him means that he will struggle when others don't. In that case, in countries like the United States and the United Kingdom, where the environment is presumably less oppressive than at any time since the Babylonian captivity—or perhaps short interludes in Moorish Spain—one would expect this explosion of talent in due course to lose its force.

What will happen? Or is there something in the Jewish gene pool which produces talent on quite a different scale from, say, the Anglo-Saxon gene pool? I am prepared to believe that that may be so. One would like to know more about the Jewish gene pool.[2]

Even more ubiquitous is the image of the Jewish doctor, an image deeply rooted in Western culture from at least medieval times. Anatole Broyard, the former editor of the *New York Times Book Review,* writing several years ago in the *Times Magazine* about the illness that was soon to take his life, poignantly captured an impression undoubtedly drawn from the historical experience of earlier generations:

> I was also aware of a certain predisposition in myself in favor of Jewish doctors. I thought of them as the trouble-shooters—the physicians, lawyers, brokers, arbiters, and artists—of contemporary life. History had convinced them that life was a disease. My father, who was an old-fashioned Southern anti-Semite, insisted on a Jewish doctor when he developed cancer of the bladder. A Jewish doctor, he argued, had been bred in medicine. In my father's Biblical conception, a Jew's life was a story of study, repair, and reform. A Jewish doctor knew what survival was worth, because he had had to fight for his. Obliged to treat life as a business as well as a pleasure, Jews drove hard bargains. To lose a patient was bad business. In his heart, I think

2. Quoted by Domb, "Jewish Distinction in Science," p. 31.

my father believed that a Jewish doctor was closer to God and could use that connection to "Jew down" death.[3]

I cite the observations of Snow and Broyard, both non-Jews, neither to concur with nor to criticize them, but merely to illustrate how widely expressed such perceptions are. It is all the more remarkable, then, that although the relation between Jews and science and medicine is often noticed, little scholarly analysis has been devoted to exploring this perceived relation in its historical context, and particularly to elucidating the factors in the Jewish cultural experience that might have encouraged the Jewish interest in and pursuit of the sciences. There is surely no dearth of recent literature on Judaism and science, but almost all of it stems from a community of Orthodox scientists who are writing to explain, to justify, and to reconcile their simultaneous and seemingly contradictory commitments to science and traditional Jewish faith. Their numerous publications in English and Hebrew include an entire journal devoted to the subject, sponsored by the Association of Orthodox Jewish Scientists.[4] Several important religious thinkers, primarily Orthodox, have also addressed the apparent incongruity be-

3. A. Broyard, "Doctor, Talk to Me," *New York Times Magazine,* Aug. 26, 1990, p. 33 (repr. as chap. 3 of his book *Intoxicated by My Illness and Other Writings on Life and Death,* comp. and ed. Alexandra Broyard [New York, 1992], pp. 37–47).

4. I cite a representative sampling: Gotfryd et al., *Fusion: Absolute Standards;* T. Levitan, ed., *Viewpoints on Science and Judaism* (New York, 1978); S. Roth, *Science and Religion: Studies in Torah Judaism* (New York, 1966); A. Carmell and C. Domb, eds., *Challenge: Torah Views on Science and Its Problems* (London, 1976); National Conference of Synagogue Youth, *Torah and Science Reader* (New York, 1971); N. Lamm, *Torah U-Madda: The Encounter of Religious Learning and Worldly Knowledge in the Jewish Tradition* (Northvale, N.J., 1990); L. Levi, *Torah and Science: Their Interplay in the World Scheme* (Jerusalem, 1983); C. Zimmerman, *Torah and Reason: Insiders and Outsiders of Torah* (New York, 1979); *Proceedings of the Association of Orthodox Jewish Scientists* (New York, 1970–); *Emunah, Dat u-Maddah: Ha-Kinnus ha-Shenati Le-Maḥshevet ha-Yahadut 11* (Jerusalem, 1965–66). The most serious attempt to systematize and evaluate this body of material is S. Rosenberg, *Torah u-Madda be-Hagut ha-Yehudit ha-Ḥadasha* (Jerusalem, 1988). Rosenberg divides these responses into six categories (to my mind, overlapping and a bit confusing), discusses each, and offers representative readings in each category. N. J. Efron has also discussed some of this literature in "Science and the Jewish Question: The Sociologics of Science and Traditional Judaism" (paper delivered at symposium "The Interaction of Scientific and Jewish Cultures," Jewish Public Library, Montreal, June 1990).

tween the preoccupations of Jewish scientists and the demands and values of Jewish faith and practice. These writers, while assuming but not explaining the preponderance of Jews in scientific endeavors, offer a wide array of theological responses to the study of the natural sciences.[5] While generally lacking historical perspective with regard to science or Jewish attitudes, they do provide some clear notions for historians to test and refine.[6] Of a totally different sort are two recent discussions by a historian of ancient Judaism and a philosopher of modern science comparing the cognitive modes of classical rabbinic Judaism with those of premodern and modern science.[7] Although there are some truth and considerable insight in their positions, neither offers, to my mind, an adequate historical explanation of the dynamic and complex interactions between science and Judaism. Such theoretical-typological discussions tend to reduce reality to a single categorization or abstract definition, flattening the differences of specific times and places into homogeneous, immutable, and predictable entities called science and Judaism.

5. Some of this literature is cited in the previous note and discussed in Rosenberg, *Torah u-Madda.*

6. Of special importance are the positions of J. B. Soloveitchik, in *Halakhic Man,* trans. L. Kaplan (Philadelphia, 1983), and I. Leibowitz, in *Judaism, Human Values, and the Jewish State,* ed. E. Goldman (Cambridge, Mass., 1992), pp. 132–41. While Soloveitchik consistently subordinates fascination with nature to the objectives and standards of halakhic activity, Leibowitz sees science and religion as totally distinct domains. Science for Leibowitz deals exclusively with facts, religion with values. Thus they can never conflict with each other, since each functions within its distinct jurisdiction and with its own objectives.

7. I refer to the provocative essay of J. Neusner, "Why No Science in Judaism?" published by the Jewish Studies Program of Tulane University (New Orleans, 1987) and republished in a somewhat different form as chap. 7 of *The Making of the Mind of Judaism: The Formative Age,* Brown Judaic Studies, no. 133 (Atlanta, 1987), pp. 139–60, entitled "Why No Science in the Mind of Judaism?" Neusner's lecture stimulated the thinking of M. Fisch in several essays, especially "The Perpetual Covenant of Jewish Learning," in E. Spolsky, ed., *Summoning: Ideas of the Covenant in Literary Theory* (Albany, 1993), and in his book *Lada'at Ḥokhmah: Madah, Raẓionaliyut ve-Talmud Torah* (Tel Aviv, 1994). My sincere thanks to Professor Fisch for sharing his writings with me before publication. While Neusner sees the rabbinic logic of "fixed association" as generally incompatible with scientific modes of thinking and discovery, Fisch contends that the rabbis' standards of rationality were "intriguingly akin to those characteristic of the sciences as we now have come to understand them."

If the subject of Jewish culture and its relation to the sciences is to be studied historically, and not merely for contemporary and apologetic purposes,[8] it needs to be examined first within manageable historical units. Because little adequate and up-to-date historical literature on the relation exists,[9] I have chosen to focus on one period within one relatively uniform cultural landscape. From the perspective of the history of modern science, the early modern period, from the late sixteenth to the late eighteenth century, commonly referred to as the age of scientific revolution, is of critical importance. There were revolutionary scientific discoveries in astronomy, physics, and the life sciences, a far-reaching dissemination of knowledge about the natural world through printed books, a dramatic reevaluation of what constitutes knowledge and the authority it commands in European culture, and a radical transformation in the ways human beings viewed the cosmos and their place within it.[10] The impact of the new sciences on Christian cultures, both Protestant and Catholic, has given rise to an impressive and stimulating literature in recent years.[11] In contrast, the impression of science on Jewish culture of early modern Europe has hardly been examined in contemporary historical research.[12]

8. Despite the many historical insights of Norman Lamm's recent book *Torah U-Madda,* its objective is apologetics, not history, as the author admits.

9. I cite this literature throughout the book.

10. This is not the place to cite extensive bibliographical references to this vast topic. A general orientation to some standard texts can be acquired from P. Corsi and O. Weindling, eds., *Information Sources in the History of Science and Medicine* (London, 1983); from the informative essays in D. C. Lindberg and R. S. Westman, eds., *Reappraisals of the Scientific Revolution* (Cambridge, 1992); and in R. C. Olby et al., eds., *Companion to the History of Modern Science* (London, 1990). Other works are cited throughout this book.

11. See, for example, the essays of P. Corsi and M. MacDonald in *Information Sources* and the essay by J. H. Brooke in *Companion.* See also P. Dear, "The Church and the New Philosophy," in S. Pumfrey, P. Rossi, and M. Slawinski, eds., *Science, Culture and Popular Belief in Renaissance Europe* (Manchester, 1991), pp. 119–39. Another useful text with bibliographic references is D. C. Lindberg and R. L. Numbers, eds., *God and Nature: Historical Essays on the Encounter between Christianity and Science* (Berkeley, 1986). Some of this literature is also reviewed in the introduction to my *Kabbalah, Magic and Science: The Cultural Universe of a Sixteenth-Century Jewish Physician* (Cambridge, Mass., 1988).

12. I will have occasion to refer to the few studies that do exist. Cf. D. B. Ruderman, *Science, Medicine, and Jewish Culture in Early Modern Europe,* Spiegel Lectures in European Jewish

Is this dearth of interest on the part of historians of Jewish culture a reflection of their own cultural priorities and interests, or is the dialogue between science and early modern Jewish culture simply unworthy of historical scrutiny? Surely, a major part of the answer is related to the conventional ways in which the period has been depicted in contemporary historical research. As a recent scholar has pointed out, Jewish historians have usually treated the era as a mere extension of the Jewish Middle Ages.[13] Whereas the early modern period in general European history has been considered a major watershed politically, economically, socially, and culturally, it has appeared in patently dissimilar terms in Jewish historiography.[14] For the era characterized by European historians as one of momentous political and cultural changes—the Renaissance, the Reformation and the ensuing wars of religion, the consolidation of modern nation-states, the shift of political and economic power from the Mediterranean to northern Europe, the rise of capitalism, and the birth of modern science—historians of European Jewry have emphasized heightened hostility to Jews, expulsions, and political, economic, and cultural dislocation and decline. The rise of modern nation-states severely weakened and eventually undermined Jewish communal cohesiveness in the West. The hopes of Jewish-Christian rapport in the Renaissance were dashed by the renewed hostility against and oppression of Jews during the Reformation and Counter-Reformation. Denied the opportunity of sharing the political and economic boons of northern and western Europe, the majority of the Jews were obliged to settle in the eastern Mediterranean or in eastern Europe, areas of less importance for the development of European culture and society in this period. Economically, only "exceptional" Jews

---

History, no. 7, ed. L. P. Gartner (Tel Aviv, 1987), for a preliminary discussion of the issues I raise below, with bibliographic references, as well as the introduction to Ruderman, *Kabbalah, Magic, and Science.*

13. J. I. Israel, *European Jewry in the Age of Mercantilism, 1550–1750* (Oxford, 1985), p. 1.

14. I omit here unnecessary bibliographical references, but surely the reader can substantiate my generalizations by referring to the standard treatments of Jewish history from Graetz to Baer and Roth. The well-known text of R. Seltzer, *Jewish People–Jewish Thought* (New York, 1980) is typical of this approach. I hope to return to the question of periodization of early modern Jewish history in a future study. For the time being, see my review of J. I. Israel's book in the *Jewish Quarterly Review* 78 (1987): 154–59.

participated in capitalistic enterprises in the West; the majority lived far from the centers of economic growth and mercantilism. And notwithstanding occasional Jewish and converso physicians, Jewish cognizance of, and involvement in, scientific activity have appeared inconsequential.

If Jews had actually departed from the center stage of European history in the early modern period, their culture would accordingly reflect this political and economic decline. Thus, the cultural activity of Jews usually has been described as a disengagement, a retrenchment of cultural energies—from an open and symbiotic relationship with western European civilization during the Renaissance to a turning-in and estrangement from it in the late sixteenth and seventeenth centuries.[15] Most historical accounts of Jewish life in this era have focused either on the revival of Jewish mysticism and messianism surrounding the figures of Isaac Luria and Shabbatai Ẓevi, and the subsequent crisis and decline of rabbinic authority,[16] or on the rise of relatively insulated rabbinic culture

15. See, for example, Seltzer, *Jewish People,* pp. 454–55: "In contrast to the great innovative ages of the Jewish past . . . the early modern period in Jewish history was predominantly a time of intellectual and spiritual isolation." Similarly, J. Guttmann, *Philosophies of Judaism* (Philadelphia, 1964), p. 289: "The barrier which separated Judaism from the spiritual and social life of Europe was not breached until the middle of the eighteenth century. Until that time, the major European streams of thought came into only superficial contact with the world of Judaism. German and Polish Jews were not alone in rejecting any contact with foreign cultures, and occupied themselves exclusively with the Talmud and its problems. Even the broad and many-faceted culture of the Italian and Dutch Jews was rooted in the Jewish Middle Ages, and was only peripherally affected by modern culture. The eighteenth century Enlightenment was the first movement to bring about a complete and concrete social and spiritual contact with modern Europe." Cf. also M. Meyer, "Where Does the Modern Period of Jewish History Begin?" *Judaism* 24 (1975): 329–38. On the disengagement of Italian Jewry from European culture, see R. Bonfil, *Rabbis and Jewish Communities in Renaissance Italy* (Oxford, 1990), chap. 6, especially pp. 322–23: "By the end of this process Jewish cultural developments had been cut off from the wider cultural milieu, in which the foundations of modern philosophy flourished on the ruins of Renaissance philosophy without Jewish participation. . . . The enhanced sense of Jewish national uniqueness . . . isolated Jewish thought from general thought and brought about the end of fruitful co-operation between the Jewish rabbinate in Italy and Christian scholars." But see Bonfil's later view below (n. 24).

16. I refer to the dominant historical view of G. Scholem, in *Major Trends in Jewish Mysticism* (New York, 1941) and *Sabbatai Ṣevi: The Mystical Messiah* (Princeton, 1973).

and political institutions in eastern Europe.[17] The only exception to this characterization is the description of the so-called converso diaspora, which occurred
especially in Amsterdam, a primary meeting ground of Jewish and Western culture in the seventeenth century.[18] But this converso phenomenon often appears
unrelated or peripheral to the preoccupations of the major part of Jewish society
living outside western Europe in this era. Thus Jewish historians have tended to
postpone until the end of the eighteenth century and later the "reawakening"
of Jews to modern culture and their eventual reintegration into the mainstream
of European society.

This general assessment of Jewish society and culture in the early modern
period has been challenged recently on several grounds. Jonathan Israel has argued that the period between 1570 and 1713 marked the start of a reintegration
of Jews into western Europe and the positive transformation of their social and
economic status. With reentry, Jews began to exert "a most profound and pervasive impact" on western Europe in both the cultural and economic spheres.[19]
Moshe Idel has challenged several key assumptions about the evolution and dissemination of the kabbalah in this era, including the notions that the kabbalah,
especially in Italy, was a force for growing isolation from the outside world, and
that the Lurianic kabbalah was widespread in Europe and precipitated, more
than any other cause, the spread of Sabbatian messianism.[20] Yehudah Liebes has

17. See, for example, B. Weinryb, *The Jews of Poland* (Philadelphia, 1973), and, more recently, J. Elbaum, *Petihut ve-Histagrut* (Jerusalem, 1990), with its extensive bibliography.

18. On the problem of defining the culture of Amsterdam Jewry of the seventeenth century
as "traditional" or "modern," see Y. Kaplan, "The Portuguese Community in Seventeenth-
Century Amsterdam: Between Tradition and Change" (in Hebrew), *Proceedings of the Israel
Academy of Sciences and the Humanities,* vol. 7, no. 6 (Jerusalem, 1986), pp. 161–81. For further
references, see chap. 10 below.

19. Israel, *European Jewry,* esp. p. 1.

20. M. Idel, *Kabbalah: New Perspectives* (New Haven, 1988), pp. 250–71, as well as several
of his other essays, especially "Major Currents in Italian Kabbalah between 1560–1660," *Italia
Judaica,* vol. 2 (Rome, 1986), pp. 243–62 (repr. in D. B. Ruderman, ed., *Essential Papers on Jewish
Culture in Renaissance and Baroque Italy* [New York, 1992], pp. 345–68); "One from a Town,
Two from a Clan: A New Look at the Problem of the Diffusion of Lurianic Kabbalah and
Sabbatianism" (in Hebrew), *Pe'amim* 44 (1991): 5–30 (this essay has also appeared in English
in *Jewish History* 7 [1993]: 79–104).

rethought the nature and impact of Sabbatianism on Jewish culture, particularly its supposed gnostic, messianic, and political character.[21] Elhanan Reiner and Ze'ev Gries, among others, have begun to examine the impact of printing on Jewish culture in early modern Europe, along with the widening circles, and subsequent empowerment, of Jewish readers.[22] Elliott Horowitz has explored important aspects of the history of Jewish popular culture in early modern Europe.[23] Yosef Kaplan has deepened our understanding of the social and intellectual ramifications of the converso experience in Amsterdam and elsewhere in the seventeenth and eighteenth centuries.[24] Robert Bonfil has revised the view of Jewish culture in the Italian ghettos of the sixteenth and seventeenth centuries as insulated and uncreative; on the contrary, he contends, the peculiar ambiance of the ghetto was culturally vibrant and paradoxically encouraged secularizing and modernizing tendencies among Italian Jews—tendencies more potent and more significant than those of the Renaissance.[25]

21. Y. Liebes, "The Ideological Basis of the Polemic over Ḥayon" (in Hebrew), *Proceedings of the Eighth World Congress of Jewish Studies* (Jerusalem, 1982), unit 2, pp. 129–34; more expansively in his "Sabbatian Messianism" (in Hebrew), *Pe'amim* 40 (1989):4–20 (trans. B. Stein in Liebes, *Studies in Jewish Myth and Jewish Messianism* [Albany, 1993], pp. 93–106).

22. See E. Reiner, "Changes in the Yeshivot of Poland and Ashkenaz in the Sixteenth and Seventeenth Centuries and the Debate over 'Pilpul'" (in Hebrew), in I. Bartal et al., eds., *Ke-Minhag Ashkenaʐ ve-Polin: Sefer Yovel le-Chone Shmeruk* (Jerusalem, 1993), pp. 9–80, and his forthcoming Hebrew essay, "Itinerate Ashkenazic Preachers in the Early Modern Period"; Z. Gries, *Sifrut Ha-Hanhagot: Toldoteha u-Mekomah be-Ḥayye Ḥasidei Ba'al Shem Tov* (Jerusalem, 1990), and his *Sefer, Sofer ve-Sippur be-Reshit ha-Ḥasidut* (Tel Aviv, 1992).

23. See, for example, E. Horowitz, "The Eve of the Circumcision: A Chapter in the History of Jewish Nightlife," *Journal of Social History* 23 (1989): 45–70 (repr. in Ruderman, *Essential Papers,* pp. 554–88); "Coffee-Houses and the Nocturnal Rituals of Early Modern Jewry," *Association for Jewish Studies Review* 14 (1989): 17–46; and "The Way We Were: Jewish Life in the Middle Ages," *Jewish History* 1 (1986): 79–90.

24. In addition to his numerous articles, see Kaplan's *From Christianity to Judaism: The Story of Isaac Orobio de Castro* (Oxford, 1989) and his forthcoming book on social deviance in the converso community of Amsterdam. See as well chap. 10 below.

25. R. Bonfil, "Change in the Cultural Patterns of a Jewish Society in Crisis: Italian Jewry at the Close of the Sixteenth Century," *Jewish History* 3 (1988): 11–30 (repr. in Ruderman, *Essential Papers;* and see the introduction to that volume as well). See, most recently, R. Bonfil, *Jewish Life in Renaissance Italy,* trans. A. Oldcorn (Berkeley, 1994).

It is within the context of a more nuanced view of the early modern period in Jewish culture, one that is appreciative of its distinctive and autonomous character,[26] that the argument of this book should be seen. I am proposing that an important ingredient of the changing culture was an acute awareness of and positive attitude toward contemporaneous medical and scientific discoveries. This enhanced regard in turn shaped a new Jewish discourse about science.[27] That is not to suggest that medical and scientific interests were inconsequential among Jews in ancient and medieval times. Such medieval luminaries as Maimonides, ibn Ezra, and Gersonides suggest otherwise. I will summarize the evidence of this earlier involvement in chapter 1. I am arguing, however, that the interaction of medicine and science with Jewish culture was more substantial and repercussive in the early modern period than before, for intellectual and social reasons related to both internal and external factors shaping Jewish cultural development in this period.

The conditions contributing to the involvement of larger numbers of Jews in medicine and science include the growing prominence of science and technology in the political culture of western Europe; the revolutionary impact of print in publicizing and disseminating the new scientific discoveries; the unprecedented entrance of large numbers of Jews into university medical schools, first in Italy and eventually in the rest of Europe; the integration of a highly educated and scientifically sophisticated converso population into Jewish com-

26. It should be obvious from my discussion so far that despite these exciting new directions in current research, and despite the obvious strengths of Jonathan Israel's pioneering book, an overview of how these developments interface with each other and how they are integrated within the larger cultural and social landscape of early modern Europe is still to be written. That task is beyond the scope of this book. See n. 14 above.

27. By science, I mean both an appreciation and a validation of acquiring knowledge about the natural world, as well as an attempt to provide a rational explanation of it. In the early modern period, with the devaluation of the Scholastic understanding of science as *episteme,* or definitive knowledge, most Jewish thinkers, like their Christian counterparts, increasingly understood scientific rationality as contingent and hypothetical. For a useful discussion of the problem of defining science as a timelessly valid mode of inquiry or merely a social construct, see E. McMullin, "The Shaping of Scientific Rationality: Construction or Constraint," in *Construction and Constraint: The Shaping of Scientific Rationality* (Notre Dame, 1988), pp. 1–47.

munities in western and, to a lesser extent, eastern Europe; and finally, a general ideological crisis in Jewish culture—specifically, a crisis of confidence regarding the dominant place of philosophy in Jewish intellectual life, the subsequent divorce of philosophical metaphysics from science, and the consequent liberation and elevation of scientific activity within the Jewish community. When science was no longer linked to an ideology that made claims to truths challenging those of the Jewish faith but rather was viewed as a hypothetical and contingent way of describing the physical world, a new coexistence between the secular and the sacred, between scientific pursuits and Jewish religious thought, even Jewish mystical thought, could successfully emerge.

To substantiate these generalizations, I will look at three distinct but interrelated groups among early modern Jews. The first I have already mentioned: those converso physicians and other university-trained intellectuals who fled Spain and Portugal in the seventeenth century and settled in Holland, Italy, Germany, England, and even eastern Europe, serving as doctors and purveyors of scientific learning throughout the Jewish communities of Europe, while yielding considerable political and economic power. These converso physicians had a proud sense of group identity, which was heightened in turn by those who derided their conspicuous and influential position.

Besides converso doctors, certain circles of Jewish scholars in central and eastern Europe pursued scientific learning, especially astronomy, in more informal settings as a desirable supplement to rabbinic study. Jewish cultural centers such as Prague or Cracow appear to have been especially hospitable to such learning. Rabbinic luminaries like Moses Isserles and the Maharal openly encouraged the acquisition of scientific knowledge; sometimes the encouragement led their students to attain considerable expertise in astronomy, as the case of David Gans amply testifies.

The third group is of even greater significance for the history of Jewish culture in this period: the hundreds of Jews who attended Italian medical schools, primarily the University of Padua, from the late sixteenth through the eighteenth centuries. Offering talented Jewish students education in both the liberal arts and the sciences, medical facilities like Padua were more than a training ground for physicians: they offered the most intense and systematic exposure to secular culture available to Jewish intellectuals before the emancipation. Such an engagement was bound to affect the cultural values and ideals of these students, and in turn the students influenced large numbers of their coreligionists.

My purpose here, then, is to examine the interaction of Jewish culture, medicine, and science within and beyond these three subcommunities. In this effort, which is primarily a pursuit of Jewish intellectual and cultural history, I have relied chiefly on manuscripts and printed books—exegetical, philosophical, mystical, homiletical, and scientific writings in Hebrew and other languages. But I am not unaware of the so-called external history of science,[28] both the social contexts in which new attitudes toward science emerge and the use of scientific knowledge to undermine as well as bolster religious and political authority. The opportunity of a Jewish minority to acquire medical and scientific knowledge might also be seen as a significant dimension of the social and political relations between Jews and Christians in this period, of reevaluating traditional attitudes toward the "other" within the two communities. Thus my account of the Jewish dialogue with early modern science constantly intersects with this and other critical dimensions of the social and cultural world of the Jewish community in this era: the challenges to rabbinic authority, the clash between elite and nonelite groups, the debates over the place of magic and mysticism in Jewish culture, the conversionary pressures of the Counter-Reformation church and Jewish responses, expressions of anti-Semitism, especially those directed against Jewish and converso physicians, the crisis of Sabbatian messianism and converso heterodoxy, and more.

Although this book charts for the first time the interactions between Jewish and scientific cultures in the formative period of the scientific revolution, I do not argue that many Jews made significant contributions to medicine or science. On the contrary, despite widespread interest in scientific endeavor, only a handful of Jews contributed substantially to science, and even these were primarily active in the field of medicine. After presenting the evidence, I shall offer in the Epilogue an explanation for this lack of scientific achievement—a deficiency

28. For a succinct discussion of the social contexts of early modern science, see R. Porter, "The History of Science and the History of Society," in *Companion to the History of Modern Science*, pp. 32–46 and his introduction to *Science, Culture, and Popular Belief in Renaissance Europe*, pp. 1–15.

that stands in sharp contrast to the extraordinary scientific achievements of Jews in the twentieth century.

A study of Jewish responses to science invites comparison with the better-known responses of Protestants and Catholics. I often refer to the extensive literature on the Christian engagement with early modern science in order to offer some tentative observations. My primary objectives, however, are more modest: to sketch, on the basis of several case studies, a preliminary picture of Jewish engagements with science; to present that picture as evidence that scientific thought and activity were a central concern of early modern Jewish culture; and to propose that this concern was a crucial element in defining the unique features of this cultural experience. I hope that the portrait that emerges in the following pages will encourage others to look more closely at the sources of Jewish history from the perspective I have offered, to compare early modern Jewish culture with the majority Christian culture, and, finally, to consider this period and its peculiar characteristics in evaluating Jewish scientific attitudes and involvements in other settings and periods.

1

Medieval Jewish Attitudes toward Nature and Scientific Activity

Although this chapter was originally intended as a prelude to the major part of the book, it presents serious challenges in its own right regarding both content and methodology. Up-to-date overviews of Jewish involvements in the natural sciences from roughly the tenth through the fifteenth centuries hardly exist. The available surveys are primarily bibliographical or biographical, documenting specific Jewish "contributions" to science—that is, the extent to which Jews participated in the scientific activities pursued by their non-Jewish Muslim or Christian neighbors.[1] Furthermore, because most historians of Jewish culture are not

1. One of the most recent and best surveys of this kind is that of Y. T. Langermann, "Science, Jewish," in *Dictionary of the Middle Ages* (New York, 1989), 11:89–94. See also the earlier overviews of S. W. Baron, *A Social and Religious History of the Jews,* 2d ed., 18 vols. (New York, 1952–83), vol. 8; A. Marx, "The Scientific Work of Some Outstanding Medieval Scholars," in I. Davidson, ed., *Essays and Studies in Memory of Linda R. Miller* (New York, 1938); B. Z. Dinur, *Yisra'el Ba-Golah,* 10 vols., (Jerusalem, 1961–72), vol. 2, bk. 4, chap. 15; C. Singer, "Science and Judaism," in L. Finkelstein, ed., *The Jews,* 3 vols., (New York, 1960), 3: 216–65, with a postscript by B. Goldstein, "The Jewish Contribution to Astronomy in the Middle Ages," pp. 270–75. Most recently, Gad Freudenthal has written a broad survey of Jewish scientific activity in medieval Provence: "Les Sciences dans les communautés juives médiévales de Provence: Leur Appropriation, leur rôle," *Revue des études juives* 152 (1993): 29–136. (He also announces a modified version of this essay entitled "Science in the Medieval Jewish Culture of

historians of science, and vice versa, Jewish scientific activity is usually treated in a cursory and superficial manner by the first group and either ignored entirely or, in a few instances, explained in a highly technical manner by the second, who deal almost exclusively with a few well-known figures like Maimonides, Gersonides, and ibn Ezra.[2] Claiming primary affiliation with the first group, I am more interested in the history of attitudes toward nature as reflected in medieval Jewish religious thought than in the highly technical writings of Jewish astronomers and natural philosophers, although I obviously cannot ignore the latter in trying to understand the former.

By defining my subject as Jewish attitudes to nature and scientific activity, I encounter a further problem. The investigation of nature by medieval Jews—and to a great extent, by early modern Jews as well—like that of their Muslim and Christian counterparts, was usually linked to a philosophical or theological system. The physical world was not studied in isolation, and within the philosophical traditions of Muslim and Christian Europe, natural science was usually perceived as propaedeutic to the study of metaphysics.[3] Thus Maimonides' reflections on the study of nature have been seen as preliminary to and inseparable from his higher rational pursuits. Descriptions of the philosophies of individual medieval Jewish thinkers abound, and within those descriptions are occasionally embedded their reflections on nature. To attempt, then, to isolate physics from metaphysics for the purpose of this analysis might be perceived as a violation and distortion of the place of the natural world within the larger intellectual schemes of medieval Jews.

Southern France," to appear in *History of Science* in 1994.) While restricted primarily to one region, it is an important contribution to our subject and will be referred to several times below.

2. See, for example, the many references to Jews in the indexes of G. Sarton, *Introduction to the History of Science,* 5 vols. (Washington, D.C., 1927–48) and L. Thorndike, *A History of Magic and Experimental Science,* 8 vols. (New York, 1923–58).

3. See, for example, H. A. Wolfson, "The Classification of Sciences in Medieval Jewish Philosophy," in *Hebrew Union College Jubilee Volume* (Cincinnati, 1925); R. McKeon, "The Organization of Sciences and the Relations of Cultures in the Twelfth and Thirteenth Centuries," in J. E. Murdoch and E. D. Sylla, eds., *The Cultural Context of Medieval Learning,* Boston Studies in the Philosophy of Science, vol. 26 (Dordrecht, 1975), pp. 151–92.

To venture where few others have trodden is not to deny the obvious connections among theology, philosophy, and naturalistic pursuits in the medieval world but only to gain a more sharpened focus with which to view the preoccupations with nature of post-medieval Jews at a time when these same connections are increasingly becoming undone. Moreover, such an inquiry avoids the too restrictive assumption that all medieval Jewish thinkers approached the natural world exclusively or primarily within the context of their philosophical activity. For example, mystics, magicians, and judicial astrologers, three groups viewed with general suspicion and contempt by Maimonides,[4] might be perceived as outside the purview of my survey were naturalistic pursuits to be categorized as subordinate to philosophical speculation. Yet all three groups understood and deeply valued the natural world and its powerful forces. Their attitudes deserve to be studied and compared with those of the philosophers and practicing "scientists" both in their own right and as an important link with Jewish devotees of the natural world in the ancient and early modern periods.

One final hurdle requires some comment before I undertake this foray into the large subject at hand. By viewing the medieval period as a mere preview of what follows, I might distort what we are seeing, reading into the medieval period a set of issues construed from an early modern perspective. The problem is reminiscent of that raised by the pioneering work of the French historian, philosopher, and scientist Pierre Duhem (1861–1916), who approached medieval science primarily in search of precursors for Galileo and Descartes to demonstrate how medieval conceptions prefigured modern ones.[5] The focus of this book on the later period should not diminish the significance of explor-

---

4. See, for example, A. Marx, "The Correspondence between the Rabbis of Southern France and Maimonides on Astrology," *Hebrew Union College Annual* 3 (1926): 311–42; Y. T. Langermann, "Maimonides' Repudiation of Astrology," *Maimonidean Studies* 2 (1991): 123–58; and see n. 31 below.

5. See P. Duhem, *Le Système du monde: Histoire des doctrines cosmologiques de Platon à Copernic,* 10 vols. (Paris 1913–59); C. B. Schmitt, "Recent Trends in the Study of Medieval and Renaissance Science," in P. Corsi and O. Weindling, eds., *Information Sources in the History of Science and Medicine,* (London, 1983), pp. 224–29; D. C. Lindberg, "Conceptions of the Scientific Revolution from Bacon to Butterfield: A Preliminary Sketch," in D. C. Lindberg and R. S. Westman, eds., *Reappraisals of the Scientific Revolution* (Cambridge, 1992), pp. 13–26.

ing my subject in medieval times. Indeed, it provides a critical perspective to assess more clearly what is unique and what is conventional about the ways Jews living in the sixteenth century and later thought about the natural world and the scientific activity of their day.

Fully mindful of the pitfalls of arbitrarily separating physics from metaphysics and distorting one cultural world by looking through the lens of a later one, I venture forth cautiously to explore the place of nature in the consciousness of some representative medieval Jews.

Medieval Jews could draw from a reservoir of rabbinic attitudes toward the natural world, unsystematized, chaotic and even contradictory, which included an openness to most forms of spiritual and physical healing tempered only by an occasional reluctance to tamper with the supposed divine will; a more than passing knowledge of ancient cosmological schemes, astronomy, and natural philosophy; an appreciation of the power of astral forces to determine the fate of those living on earth; and an enthusiastic belief in the power of magic to transform and manipulate the physical world. Most of all, certain rabbis, interpreting and embellishing key biblical passages, assigned religious meaning to the quest to understand nature, both celestial and earthly, as a direct means of understanding God and of fulfilling his revealed commandments.[6]

The Jewish encounter with the dynamic intellectual life of medieval Islam in such centers as Baghdad, Cairo, and Cordova, and later in stimulating Christian territories such as Spain, Sicily, Italy, and Provence, provided an impetus for perpetuating the rabbinic approaches to nature while deepening their religious and intellectual significance. With the translation of the philosophical and scientific corpus of classical antiquity into Arabic, several influential Jewish figures in the Muslim world recast the Jewish tradition into a philosophic key, elevating the quest for an understanding of God and his natural creation to the ultimate ideal of Jewish religiosity. Hand in hand with this newly articulated religious aspiration went an intellectual appreciation of the intrinsic worth of understanding the cosmos, as well as an awareness of the pragmatic value such knowledge

6. I offer documentation for all of these generalizations in the appendix, which might be consulted most profitably before the rest of this chapter.

could yield in terms of social and economic status. In the relatively open intellectual and social setting of medieval Islamic cities, Jews consumed the classic texts of philosophy and science, studied the contemporary Islamic modifications and elaborations, and produced a philosophical and scientific literature of their own in Arabic and Hebrew.[7]

With the decline of the Islamic centers in Spain and the reawakening of culture in northern Europe, displaced Jewish intellectuals found themselves in the advantageous position as translators and cultural intermediaries between the Muslims and Christians. Translating of Arabic texts into Hebrew or Latin facilitated a philosophical and scientific literacy among individual Jews, and more important, fostered an abiding interest in the issues that the texts embodied. From Spain to Sicily, Italy, and Provence, the Jewish translators created more than a new library of accessible texts; they stimulated among their own co-religionists, along with the Christian patrons who encouraged their efforts, an enlargement of intellectual horizons and a rethinking of religious traditions in the light of new ideas, as well as acrimonious debate regarding the pernicious effect of such ideas on religious texts and teachings.[8]

7. The most recent survey of medieval Jewish philosophy is that of C. Sirat, *A History of Jewish Philosophy in the Middle Ages* (Cambridge, 1985). Two recent overviews of the transformation of Jewish culture under medieval Islam are B. Lewis, *The Jews of Islam* (Princeton, 1984), pp. 67–106; H. Lazarus-Yafeh, *Some Religious Aspects of Islam* (Leiden, 1981), pp. 72–89. On the place of the sciences within medieval Islam, see A. I. Sabra, "The Appropriation and Subsequent Naturalization of Greek Science in Medieval Islam: A Preliminary Statement," *History of Science* 25 (1987): 223–43.

8. The standard work on Jewish translators is M. Steinschneider, *Die hebräischen Übersetzungen des Mittelalters und die Juden als Dolmetscher* (Berlin, 1893; repr. Graz, 1956). See also J. L. Teicher, "The Latin-Hebrew School of Translators in Spain in the Twelfth Century," *Homenaje a J. M. Millas Vallicrosa*, 2 vols. (Barcelona, 1956), 2:401–44; D. Romano, "La Transmission des sciences arabes par les juifs en Languedoc," in M. Vicaire and B. Blumenkranz, eds., *Juifs et judaïsme de Languedoc XIIIe siècle–début XIVe siècle* (Toulouse, 1977), pp. 363–86; N. Roth, "Jewish Collaborators in Alfonso's Scientific Work," in R. I. Burns, ed., *Emperor of Culture* (Philadelphia, 1990), pp. 59–71. See also the entry by B. Richler, "Translation and Translators, Jewish," in *Dictionary of the Middle Ages,* 13 vols. (New York, 1982–89), 12:133–36, and esp. Freudenthal, "Sciences dans les communautés juives," pp. 41–92. A recent discussion of the so-called Maimonidean controversy with ample bibliography is found in B. Septimus,

In both the Muslim and Christian lands, Jewish involvement in science had an obvious social and economic significance. Jewish doctors in the Muslim world were not only, in the words of S. D. Goitein, "torchbearers of secular erudition and professional expounders of philosophy and the sciences";[9] they were also beneficiaries of increased social status and economic success. Their clientele included Jews and non-Jews; and in some cases, their medical careers also assured them political influence. In Spain and especially in Provence in the late Middle Ages, a sizable number of Jewish physicians were influential even though they were denied access to the new university centers as students or teachers.[10] Other Jews derived social and political advantage as astronomers and

---

Hispanic-Jewish Culture in Translation: The Career and Controversies of Ramah (Cambridge, Mass., 1982), esp. pp. 61–74.

9. S. D. Goitein, "The Medical Profession in the Light of the Cairo Genizah Documents," *Hebrew Union College Annual* 34 (1963): 177 (incorporated in his *A Mediterranean Society,* 5 vols. [Berkeley, 1967–88], 2:240–61).

10. Besides Goitein, see H. Friedenwald, *The Jews and Medicine,* 2 vols. (Baltimore, 1944; repr., 1967); C. Roth, "The Qualifications of Jewish Physicians in the Middle Ages," *Speculum* 28 (1953): 834–43; M. Meyerhoff, "Medieval Jewish Physicians in the Near East, from Arabic Sources," *Isis* 28 (1938): 432–60 (repr. in P. Johnstone, ed., *Studies in Medieval Arabic Medicine, Theory and Practice* [London, 1984]); M. Perlmann, "Notes on the Position of Jewish Physicians in Medieval Muslim Countries," *Israel Oriental Studies* 2 (1972): 315–19; I. Alteras, "Jewish Physicians in Southern France during the 13th and 14th Centuries," *Jewish Quarterly Review* 68 (1978): 209–23; idem, "Notes généalogiques sur les médecins juifs dans la Sud de la France pendant les XIIIe et XIVe siècles," *Le Moyen Age* 88 (1982): 29–47; J. Shatzmiller, "Notes sur les médecins juifs en Provence au Moyen-Age," *Revue des études juives* 128 (1969): 259–66; idem, "On Becoming a Jewish Doctor in the Middle Ages," *Sefarad* 43 (1983): 240–50.

Professor Shatzmiller has recently completed a book entitled *Doctors to Princes and Paupers: Jews, Medicine, and Medieval Society,* to be published by the University of California Press, in which he presents overwhelming evidence, especially from Provençal archives, for the participation of Jews in medicine far out of proportion to their population and place in society. He attributes this phenomenon to the medicalization of society beginning in the second half of the thirteenth century, the enormous need for doctors, exacerbated by the church's opposition to medical practice, and the inability of the universities to produce sufficient numbers of trained physicians. He notes the parallel to money lending: Jewish involvement in usury was a product of the overwhelming demand for credit in all sectors of society; so too, Jewish entry into medicine in such great numbers was related to fundamental societal needs. Shatzmiller

astrologers, employed by rich patrons or even governments valued their linguistic, scientific, and philosophic expertise. Such exceptional men represented only a small percentage of the Jewish community, but their influence on the intellectual vibrancy and political security of their own communities was far from negligible, as the careers of Isaac ibn Sid, Abraham Bar Ḥiyya, Abraham Zacuto, and others testify.[11]

From the twelfth century on, the study of the kabbalah rivaled that of philosophy and the sciences in the Jewish centers in Provence and Spain.[12] Although the kabbalists were antagonistic to the intrusion of Aristotelian philosophy into the sacred domains of Judaism, they were not oblivious of nor hostile to the natural world. Their own traditions of magic and theurgy attuned them to the powers of nature and the human potential to control and manipulate those powers for constructive or pernicious purposes. Such magic was not be defined as *scientia*, that is, knowledge for its own sake, but rather *ars* or *techne*, a skill mastered to exploit natural forces for the benefit or to the detriment of humanity.[13] And when such forms of magic as those connected with astrology or astrological medicine, for example, could be harnessed in constructive ways, they were not necessarily deemed "unscientific" at all, even by the opponents of the kabbalists. Magic as it evolved in Jewish tradition, like its Christian and Muslim counterparts, was not easily distinguished from pure scientific activity during the Middle Ages.[14] In

---

questions the notion of a long and continuous tradition of Jewish medical practice prior to this period and points out that even in Moslem countries, the numbers of qualified Jewish physicians was relatively small before the thirteenth century.

11. In addition to the surveys mentioned in n. 1 above, see B. Goldstein, "The Medieval Hebrew Tradition in Astronomy," *Journal of the American Oriental Society* 85 (1965): 145–48; idem, "The Hebrew Astronomical Tradition: New Sources," *Isis* 72 (1981): 237–51; idem, "Scientific Traditions in Late Medieval Jewish Communities," *Les juifs au regard de l'histoire: Mélanges en l'honneur de Bernard Blumenkranz* (Paris, 1985); 235–47; idem, "The Role of Science in the Jewish Community in Fourteenth-Century France," M. Pelner Cosmon and B. Chandler, eds., *Machaut's World: Science and Art in the Fourteenth Century* (New York, 1978), pp. 39–49.

12. See esp. G. Scholem, *Origins of the Kabbalah,* ed. R. J. Zwi Werblowsky, trans. A. Arkush (Philadelphia, 1987).

13. Cf. B. Hansen, "Science and Magic," in D. C. Lindberg, ed., *Science in the Middle Ages* (Chicago, 1978), p. 495.

14. See V. I. J. Flint, *The Rise of Magic in Early Medieval Europe* (Princeton, New Jersey, 1991).

fact, some Jewish thinkers even defined the occult as the highest form of a "Jewish science." Such formidable traditions of Jewish magic not only underscored the significance of understanding and controlling the forces of nature but also provided a unique perspective from which to challenge the regnant dogmas of Aristotelian metaphysics.

I have mentioned only the Jewish communities in the Muslim and Christian centers of southern Europe as the cultural settings in which Jewish involvement with nature and science took place. What about the Ashkenazic centers of northern Europe, which were relatively cut off from interaction with the Islamic traditions of philosophy and the natural sciences, and where biblical and rabbinic exegesis were the primary occupations? The record here is not clear. Our expectation of finding little science in these regions is not always supported by the evidence. Some medieval Jews in northern France and Germany revealed a passionate interest in the natural world, in the oddities of nature, and even in technical aspects of natural philosophy. A negative view of Aristotelian philosophy need not coincide with a hostile attitude toward nature, its marvelous powers, and the ability of human beings to control them. To this issue, as well as the others raised in this brief introduction, I shall return in due course.

The only way to survey the vast terrain of medieval Jewish attitudes toward nature and scientific activity is to select some representative and influential positions among Jewish thinkers and to present them against the wider landscape of Muslim and Christian scientific attitudes and involvements. Having offered this sample, I shall be in a better position to weigh its historical significance in the light of comparable approaches and activities of the two other medieval communities, as well as those of Jewish enthusiasts of nature and science living in the sixteenth century and later.

Let us begin with the Jewish philosopher, Baḥya ibn Pakuda, who lived in Muslim Spain in the second half of the eleventh century and who offers one of the most enthusiastic theological statements about the religious obligations of studying nature.[15] In his *Duties of the Heart,* he fully explicates the Jewish obligation to study nature on the basis of scripture, rabbinic tradition, and rational

15. See G. Vajda, *La Theologie ascétique de Baḥya ibn Pakuda* (Paris, 1947).

arguments. Baḥya extensively quotes biblical verses (for example Job 35:11; Isaiah 40:26; Psalm 8:4) and rabbinic statements (example B.T. Shabbat 75a, Eruvin 100b) that illustrate the connection between ruminations on nature and divine worship. He points out the "marks of divine wisdom" in nature, proceeding from the celestial world, to the earth, its elements and creatures, and human physiology.[16] For Baḥya, real religious sensibility and wonder are evoked only through cognition, through an intellectual faith armed with scientific investigation of the wonders of nature: "Contemplate, therefore, God's creatures, from the largest of them to the smallest, and reflect on those matters which are at present hidden from you . . . and because these marks of divine wisdom vary in created things, it is our duty to study them and meditate on them until the whole matter becomes established in our souls and abides in our consciousness."[17]

True spirituality cannot be attained by the light-headed and unproductive pursuits of the courtier class; neither is it attainable through the false and maleficent activities of the astrologers, who challenge the omnipotence of the Creator through their "pagan" prognostications.[18] To predict and calculate the forces of nature is a sinister act; to contemplate their wondrous activities and praise their ultimate author is the highest form of divine worship.[19]

Baḥya wrote in Arabic, and his ideas probably came from Arabic sources. In fact, for a long time his primary source was thought to be al-Ghazzali, who expresses many similar sentiments in *The Wisdom of God in His Creatures*. D. Z. Baneth later identified the actual source to be a Christian-Arab writer, from whom both the Muslim and the Jew borrowed most of their material. Given the universality of the Christian's message, al-Ghazzali and Baḥya ibn Pakuda were able to adapt it to their own religious needs, adding appropriate passages from their own sacred scriptures to Islamize or Judaize the original Christian declaration of praise for God's creation. In the case of Baḥya, the final stage

16. Baḥya ibn Pakuda, *Duties of the Heart*, trans. M. Hymanson, 2 vols. (Jerusalem, 1962), vol. 1, second treatise (sha'ar ha-beḥinah), chaps. 1–6.

17. Ibid., p. 133.

18. On Baḥya's rejection of astrology, see Langermann, "Maimonides' Repudiation of Astrology," pp. 125–26, n. 9.

19. See B. Safran, "Baḥya Ibn Pakuda's Attitude toward the Courtier Class," in I. Twersky, ed., *Studies in Medieval Jewish History and Literature* (Cambridge, Mass., 1979), pp. 154–96.

of Judaization was achieved through Judah ibn Tibbon's translation of his book into Hebrew in 1161, making the text accessible to a large Hebrew-reading audience for centuries to come. The transmission of Christian notions of nature through an Arabic idiom into a popular manual of Jewish piety offers an extraordinary example of the capacity of Jewish (and Islamic) religious thought to appropriate external cultural influences, and match them with similar sentiments located within its own tradition, thereby legitimating their usage for internal religious consumption. An eastern European Ḥasid living in the nineteenth century, inspired by his reading of Baḥya's praises of God's creation, would never have fathomed the "illegitimate" source of what he perceived to be a thoroughly Jewish sentiment! [20]

As I have mentioned, Baḥya condemned the intrusion of astrology into Judaism; the Jewish mandate to study nature firmly excluded the activity of predicting events on the basis of the movements of the stars. His consternation surely intimates his awareness that not all his Jewish contemporaries shared his point of view. By Baḥya's time and for centuries to follow, astrology was a favored preoccupation of Jewish savants despite the challenges it posed to theology. [21] One important early enthusiast of astrology was Shabbatai Donnolo, who lived in the tenth century in southern Italy, then under Byzantine rule. Fully conversant in the latest trends in Byzantine and Muslim medicine and natural philosophy, Donnolo pursued astrology as a natural outgrowth of his own cosmological views and medical training. [22] Anticipating later Jew-

20. See D. Z. Baneth, "The Common Theological Source of Baḥya ibn Pakuda and Ghazzali" (in Hebrew), in *Magnes Anniversary Volume* (Jerusalem, 1938), pp. 23–30; Lazarus-Yafeh, *Some Religious Aspects of Islam,* pp. 75–76.

21. For a succinct overview, see A. Altmann, "Astrology," in *Encyclopedia Judaica* (Jerusalem, 1971), 3:788–95; see also R. C. Keiner, "The Status of Astrology in the Early Kabbalah: From the Sefer Yeẓirah to the Zohar," *Jerusalem Studies in Jewish Thought* 6 (1986–87); English section, 1–42; R. Barkai, "Theoretical and Practical Aspects of Jewish Astrology in the Middle Ages" (in Hebrew), in his *Maddah, Magia u-Mitologia Bimai ha-Beinayim* (Jerusalem, 1987), 7–35, and his "L'Astrologie juive médiévale," *Le Moyen âge* 93 (1987): 323–48. On the debates over the place of astrology in Muslim and Christian culture, see the works listed by Langermann, "Maimonides' Repudiation of Astrology," nn. 4 and 22.

22. On Donnolo, see A. Scharf, *The Universe of Shabbetai Donnolo* (New York, 1976); S. Muntner, *R. Shabbetai Donnolo,* 2 vols. (Jerusalem, 1950); and most recently, E. Wolfson,

ish apologists, Donnolo defended astrology on two grounds. In the first place, Gentile astrology derived from Jewish sources, specifically the early medieval midrash called the *Baraita of R. Samuel,* and thus the rabbis themselves had given it their approbation. The image of a mysterious celestial dragon that Donnolo was fond of evoking pointed to Israel's lost astrological wisdom now embedded in non-Jewish sources. Second, astrology explored the analogous relationship between the universe and the human body and afforded the physician a critical tool for understanding human physiology and pathology.[23] Donnolo drew his insights primarily from the Hellenistic, Byzantine, and Muslim medicine of his day; his *Book of Mixtures,* for example, reveals few Jewish sources.[24] In stressing the connection between astral medicine and Jewish teaching, nonetheless, he was reassuring himself that his professional and intellectual concerns were a natural extension of his Jewish identity.

Abraham Bar Ḥiyya, a younger contemporary of Baḥya ibn Pakuda living in Barcelona at the beginning of the twelfth century, also felt a need to justify his interest in astrology. Having been rebuked by his colleague Judah ben Barzilai for insisting that a wedding in the Jewish community be postponed to avoid a potentially calamitous moment as prognosticated by astrologers, Bar Ḥiyya responded with a general defense of astrology from the perspective of Jewish norms and values.[25]

Bar Ḥiyya's letter to Barzilai is a valuable document, revealing much about the inroads astrology had made into Jewish culture and Bar Ḥiyya's own personal stake in the matter. Bar Ḥiyya first defends the action that precipitated

---

"The Theosophy of Shabbetai Donnolo, with Special Emphasis on the Doctrine of Sefirot in *Sefer Ḥakhmoni," Jewish History* 6 (1992): 281–316. On the temporal and geographical proximity of Donnolo to the author of *Sefer Asaf,* see the works listed in the appendix.

23. Scharf, *Universe,* pp. 14–51.

24. Ibid., pp. 94–110.

25. A. Z. Schwarz, "The Letter of Abraham Bar Ḥiyya Ha-Nasi" (in Hebrew), in *Festschrift für Adolf Schwarz* (Berlin, 1917), pp. 24–36. On Bar Ḥiyya, see also G. Vajda, "Les Idées théologiques et philosophiques d'Abraham ben Ḥiyyah," *Archives d'histoire doctrinale et littéraire du moyen âge* 15 (1946): 191–223; Abraham Bar Ḥiyya, *Megillat ha-Meggaleh,* ed. A. Poznanski, with introduction and notes by J. Guttmann (Berlin, 1924); idem, *The Meditation of the Sad Soul,* trans. G. Wigoder (Jerusalem, 1971); J. M. Millas Vallicrosa, *La Obra enciclopédica Yesode ha-Tevunah u-Migdal ha-Emuna de R. Abraham Bar Ḥiyya ha-Bargeloni* (Madrid, 1952).

Barzilai's outburst. He acted, so he claimed, as a physician acts when dissuading patients from unhealthy habits. It is legitimate from a moral point of view to avoid a situation of potential harm. Avoiding a bad constellation is analogous to avoiding harmful food.[26]

Bar Ḥiyya was aware of the dangers astrology posed to the Jewish faith. Adopting a formulation that steered clear of an astral determinism placing limits on God's omnipotence and human free will, he declared: "All those of Israel acknowledge and believe that the power bestowed from their stars is given conditionally, that it cannot work or harm by their own volition or with their own knowledge without [God's] declaration and commandment. Any God-fearing person who investigates the science of the stars believes this way, and any Jew who suspects this fact suspects that which is fully legitimate; moreover, his suspicion is illegitimate."[27]

By insisting on God's veto power over astral influences, Bar Ḥiyya successfully parried religious objections to his discipline. In doing so he was obliged to differentiate between Jewish and pagan astrology. A pagan believes in the complete power of the stars to determine events in the world; a Jew acknowledges only a partial power for the ultimate cause rests with God: "The pious sages of Israel . . . would accept this science from the holy spirit and by word of the prophets that the power of the stars and constellations is not complete. . . . At any time the Holy One, blessed be He, wishes, He can overturn their sovereignty or cancel their decree."[28] Moreover, astronomy and its "scientific" companion, natural astrology, are permissible for Jews. This form of astrology, which does not threaten Jewish religious teaching, was practiced by Abraham and championed by the rabbis. Opposed to those with "a fear of heaven" are idolatrous sects filled with a "spirit of pollution" that worship the stars and make images to serve them. Bar Ḥiyya distinguishes four different groups of this kind, distancing himself and his faith from each of them. Unlike the "science" of astrology, their activities are labeled "crafts" or "*techne*" and classified in the Bible as magical practices.[29] He closes with a confession:

26. Schwarz, "Letter," p. 24.
27. Ibid, p. 25.
28. Ibid, p. 29.
29. Ibid, pp. 31–33.

My intention was to cleanse my soul so that I could perhaps go out free. From my youth until this day, I taught myself the science of the stars and I involved myself, investigated and sought it out, considering myself an acquirer of wisdom and thought, sinless and innocent. But now when I observed that righteous and modest sages who are themselves wise and knowledgeable do not agree with my opinion, I detested my craft. Furthermore, I stated that in the days of my youth and adolescence they would judge me by the honor which I acquired before princes and queens. But now in my old age, this has become my indictment . . . perhaps the force of their words [of those who criticize him] will convince me to follow after them."[30]

Obviously Bar Ḥiyya was stunned by the criticism of his lifetime occupation, and his expression of self-doubt is a remarkable example of the debate astrology had provoked within the Jewish community. This is confirmed by Moses Maimonides' biting critique of astrology in a letter to the rabbis of southern France some years later.[31]

Despite Bar Ḥiyya's closing note of uncertainty, he had offered up to that point a spirited defense of his position, plausibly arguing that a certain type of astrology could be effectively reconciled with Jewish belief. He had defended natural astrology alone, admitting celestial influence only over larger patterns of history, while distancing himself from judicial astrology, whereby "something will happen one way and not another, and . . . the constellation under which one is born will draw him on so that he will be of such and such a kind and so that something will happen to him one way and not another," as Maimonides had put it.[32] Although Bar Ḥiyya had employed astrological calculations to predict the coming of the Messiah, he generally refrained from interpreting the biblical text, Jewish rituals, and events in the history of Judaism within an astrological

---

30. Ibid, p. 36.

31. Marx, "Correspondence"; R. Lerner, "Maimonides' Letter on Astrology," *History of Religions* 8 (1968): 143–58; Langermann, "Maimonides' Repudiation of Astrology"; G. Freudenthal, "Maimonides' Stance on Astrology in Context: Cosmology, Physics, Medicine, and Providence," in F. Rosner and S. Kottek, eds., *Moses Maimonides: Physician, Scientist, and Philosopher* (Northvale, N.J., 1993), pp. 77–90, 244–49.

32. See I. Twersky, ed., *A Maimonides Reader* (New York, 1972), p. 466.

framework. He was outspoken in his repudiation of all forms of astral magic that smacked of idolatry. His Spanish contemporary, Abraham ibn Ezra, and even more his disciples later in the fourteenth century, had fewer scruples about astrology's intrusion into the heart of Jewish belief and practice.

As Moshe Idel has pointed out, Abraham ibn Ezra was the first Jewish author to interpret a significant number of biblical events in an astrological way and to explain certain biblical commandments as defenses against the pernicious influence of the stars.[33] His most astonishing interpretations concerned the golden calf and the teraphim.[34] According to ibn Ezra, Aaron's intent was not to make an idol but to create a surrogate for the absent Moses, a calf shaped like an astral form to capture the celestial glory that would transform it into an angel to lead the tribes. Similarly, the teraphim were constructed in human form to receive emanations of higher beings. Abraham Bar Ḥiyya had pointed out similar practices involving astral magic and called them idolatrous. Abraham ibn Ezra's matter-of-fact discussion, professing no disapproval or discomfort at all, is a remarkable study in contrasts. His fourteenth-century commentators—Samuel ibn Sarza, Samuel ibn Motot, Joseph Tov Elem, Shem Tov ibn Shaprut, Joseph ibn Wakar, Solomon Franco, Solomon al-Constantini, and others—were even less inhibited in their explanation of religious precepts and commandments in terms of astrology and astral magic.[35] Bar Ḥiyya's sensitive apology and self-

33. M. Idel, "Hermeticism and Judaism," in I. Merkel and A. Debus, eds., *Hermeticism and the Renaissance* (Washington, D. C., 1988), p. 63.

34. See A. Weiser, *Ibn Ezra's Commentary on the Torah,* 3 vols. (Jerusalem, 1976), 2:204–06 (on Exodus 32) and 1:94 (on Genesis 31:19).

35. On this group, see the succinct description of M. Idel, "The Magical and Neoplatonic Interpretations of the Kabbalah in the Renaissance," in B. Cooperman, ed., *Jewish Thought in the Sixteenth Century* (Cambridge, Mass., 1983), pp. 209–11; G. Vajda, *Recherches sur la philosophie et la kabbale dans la pensée juive du moyen âge* (Paris, 1962); idem, "Recherches sur la synthèse philosophico-kabbalistique de Samuel ibn Motot," *Archives d'histoire doctrinale et littéraire du moyen âge* 27 (1960): 29–63; idem, "La Conciliation de la philosophie et de la loi religieuse de Joseph b. Abraham ibn Wakar," *Sefarad* 9 (1949): 311–50 and 10 (1950): 25–71. See also the many works of D. Schwartz, including "Mishnato ha-Pilosophit-Datit shel Shemuel ibn Zarza," Ph.D. diss., Bar Ilan University, Ramat Gan, 1989; "The Neoplatonic Movement in Fourteenth-Century Jewish Literature and Its Relationship to Theoretical and Practical Medicine" (in Hebrew with English summary), *Koroth* 9 (1989): 272–84; (with N. E. Frimer), *Hagut be-Ẓel ha-Eimah: Demuto, Ketavav ve-Haguto shel R. Shem Tov Ibn Shaprut* (Jerusalem, 1992);

doubt seem completely superfluous to their bold recasting of Jewish tradition in a magical and astrological framework.

Y. Tzvi Langermann has noted a further aspect of ibn Ezra's astrological interpretations of Judaism. In twelfth century Spain, astrology had become the favored means of interpreting religious history and theology in a naturalistic manner. By extending astrology into the realm of religious phenomena, ibn Ezra had taken an exegetical path that led ultimately to the conclusion that all peoples, religions, and cultures are alike and that diversity of nature is due merely to the varying influence of the stars. Langermann applies this insight to the disagreements between ibn Ezra and his famous contemporary Judah Ha-Levi. According to Langermann, Ha-Levi's portrayal of a typical philosopher at the opening of his *Book of the Khazars* might recall a figure like Abraham ibn Ezra. The philosopher reduces all human differences to heredity, along with "the influence of winds, countries, foods and water, spheres, stars, and constellations." If all human beings are differentiated only by these factors, then one need not be concerned "about the forms of your humility, worship, and benediction."[36] Such religious relativism renders the differences among Jews, Muslims, and Christians meaningless. The singularity of the Jewish revelation, "the fear of heaven" as Bar Ḥiyya had put it, was ultimately undermined. To claim that ibn Ezra had reached this extreme conclusion would be an overstatement. He himself had argued that Jews do not fall under the fate of the stars as long as they follow the Torah.[37] But the consequences of astrological relativism implicit in his

---

"The Doctrine of Creation in the Neoplatonic Circle of Jewish Thought in the Fourteenth Century" (in Hebrew), *Tarbiz* 60 (1991): 593–623; "Mosaic Prophecy in the Writings of a Fourteenth-Century Jewish Neoplatonist Circle," *Jewish Thought and Philosophy* 2 (1992): 97–100; "Different Forms of Magic in Spanish Jewish Thought of the Fourteenth Century" (in Hebrew), *Proceedings of the American Academy for Jewish Research* 57 (1992): 17–47; *The Speculative Philosophy of the Neoplatonic Trend in Jewish Philosophy in the Fourteenth Century* (forthcoming). See also M. Friedlander, *Essays on the Writings of Abraham ibn Ezra* (London, 1877); Y. T. Langermann, "Some Astrological Themes in the Thought of Abraham ibn Ezra," in I. Twersky and J. M. Harris, eds., *Rabbi Abraham ibn Ezra: Studies in the Writings of a Twelfth-Century Jewish Polymath* (Cambridge, Mass., 1993).

36. *Sefer ha-Kuzari* 1:1; Langermann, "Some Astrological Themes."

37. See, for example, his commentary on Exodus 33:23.

"astrological relativism"

position were apparent to Ha-Levi and Maimonides, and to Baḥya before them. Astrology was no longer the preventive medicine advocated by Bar Ḥiyya. In the provocative exegesis of Jewish texts offered by ibn Ezra and his disciples, it had the potential to undermine Jewish particularity and self-confidence while masquerading as an intellectually respectable science.

In proscribing astrology and magic, Maimonides had demonstrated his awareness of their corrosive effect on Judaism.[38] In his emphatic denial of the legitimacy of these arts, he had sought to establish barriers against the incursions of astral determinism and theurgy to insure the integrity of Judaism. But he was no less infatuated with the natural world than Baḥya, Bar Ḥiyya, or ibn Ezra. In fact, in a manner quite different from them, he allowed the authority of Jewish revelation to be severely constricted and even undermined in those areas where recent knowledge about the natural world, particularly astronomical matters, appeared to challenge the wisdom of the rabbis.

Reminiscent of Baḥya ibn Pakuda's enthusiastic outpourings about the majesty of nature and its relation to divine worship, Maimonides was no less passionate in his own pronouncements, even situating them in the beginning of his code of law as a basic principle of the Torah:

> And what is the way that will lead to the love of Him and the fear of Him? When a person contemplates His great and wondrous works and creatures and from them obtains a glimpse of His wisdom, which is incomparable and infinite, he will straightway love Him, praise Him, glorify Him, and long with an exceeding longing to know His great name; even as David said, "My soul thirsts for God, for the living God" (Psalm 42:3). And when he ponders these matters, he will recoil frightened, and realize that he is a small creature, lowly and obscure, endowed with slight and slender intelligence, standing in the presence of Him who is perfect in knowledge. And so David said: "When I consider Your heavens, the work of Your fingers—what is man that You are mindful of him?" (Psalm 8:4–5).[39]

38. In addition to the references listed in n. 31 above, see Maimonides, *Mishneh Torah*, Hilkhot Avodah Zarah, chap. 11, and I. Twersky, *Introduction to the Code of Maimonides (Mishneh Torah)*, (New Haven, 1980), pp. 479–82.

39. Maimonides, *Mishneh Torah*, Hilkhot Yesodei ha-Torah 2:2. See also 4:12.

In the introduction to his *Guide of the Perplexed,* Maimonides argues that the Torah must be grounded in reason and that divine science (metaphysics) can only be successfully undertaken after studying the natural sciences (physics).[40] Among the natural sciences, he favored medicine, as his own medical practice and extensive writings testify.[41] Unlike his contemporary Judah Ha-Levi, he refrained from claiming that all the sciences originally came from Israel, but he did believe that the rabbis once cultivated the sciences until, because of the exile, they neglected them.[42]

By recognizing that wisdom did not originate from Israel alone, Maimonides exhibited a tolerance and an appreciation for non-Jewish, especially Muslim philosophic learning as an important addition to the study of Torah.[43] It was enough to assume that philosophy and the sciences constituted an original part of the oral law, as he indicated in his famous paraphrase of the Talmudic passage in Kiddushin 30a.[44] As Isadore Twersky has shown, Maimonides was also not averse to introducing scientific knowledge into his formulations of Jewish law, not only "to integrate science, to relate a scientific vocabulary and axiology to rabbinic law, but also to recognize its autonomy and not to superimpose it on the structure and fabric of the halakha."[45]

Recognizing the legitimacy of knowledge outside Judaism is one thing; allowing it to contradict positions articulated by the rabbis is another. In one of

40. Maimonides, *Guide of the Perplexed,* trans. S. Pines (Chicago, 1963), p. 9.

41. See H. Friedenwald, *Jews and Medicine,* 1:193–216; F. Rosner, "Maimonides the Physician: A Bibliography," *Bulletin of the History of Medicine* 43 (1969): 221–35; M. Meyerhoff, "The Medical Works of Maimonides," in S. W. Baron, ed., *Essays on Maimonides* (New York, 1941), pp. 265–301; Rosner and Kottek, *Moses Maimonides;* F. Rosner, ed. and trans., *The Medical Aphorisms of Moses Maimonides* (Haifa, 1989).

42. Compare Ha-Levi, *Sefer ha-Kuzari* 2:66, with Maimonides, *Guide of the Perplexed* 1:71; and see Twersky, *Introduction,* p. 497.

43. Twersky, *Introduction,* p. 498.

44. Ibid., pp. 488–500; idem, "Some Non-Halakhic Aspects of the Mishneh Torah," in A. Altmann, ed., *Jewish Medieval and Renaissance Studies* (Cambridge, Mass., 1967), pp. 95–119.

45. See I. Twersky, "Aspects of Maimonidean Epistemology: Halakha and Science," in J. Neusner, E. S. Frerichs, and N. Sarna, eds., *From Ancient Israel to Modern Judaism, Intellect in Quest of Understanding: Essays in Honor of Marvin Fox,* 3 vols. (Atlanta, 1989), 3:3–24; the quotation is on p. 10.

the sciences, namely astronomy, Maimonides allowed the more recent knowledge of the scientists to supersede that of the rabbis. He first acknowledged this possibility in commenting on a famous incident recorded in the Talmud (Pesahim 94b) of the rabbinic sages preferring the opinion of Gentile scholars on an astronomical matter.[46] Later, commenting on astronomical distances recorded in rabbinic literature, he was even more explicit: "Do not ask of me to show that everything they [the rabbis] have said concerning astronomical matters conforms to the way things really are. For at that time mathematics was imperfect. They did not speak about this as transmitters of dicta of the prophets, but rather because in those times they were men of knowledge in these fields or because they had heard these dicta from the men of knowledge who lived in those times."[47]

He thus concluded that "whenever it is possible to interpret the words of an individual in such a manner that they conform to a being whose existence has been demonstrated"—that is, that they conform to the truth, as in the case of astronomical distances—it is fitting to do so. But if they cannot be so interpreted, rabbinic statements should be regarded as only individual opinions, not the halakha, and therefore may be rejected.[48]

Maimonides' view that contemporary astronomical knowledge was superior to that found in the Talmud and should be accepted even when it contradicted the views of the rabbis was revolutionary. That he appears to limit its applicability to astronomy should be considered together with his epistemological stance vis-à-vis celestial physics and metaphysics.[49] For Maimonides, human knowledge was limited to material things. While the truths of terrestrial physics could be known, no theory of the heavens was certain. Rational assumptions

46. Maimonides, *Guide of the Perplexed* 2:8.

47. Ibid., 3:14.

48. Ibid.

49. My own sense that Maimonides' statement about astronomy was reformulated by his son to include all the sciences has been challenged by David Berger in a note to me. Berger sees father's and son's positions as identical, claiming that the logic of Moses Maimonides' declaration implies all the sciences. He may be right but I still find it noteworthy that Abraham Maimonides made explicit what had been only implicit in his father's original comment, bringing out the full force of his father's position. See below.

about the heavens were analogous to religious beliefs: they could never be fully demonstrated by reason.[50] Might I infer from this that while neither rabbinic theories about the heavens nor contemporary scientific theories are ever certain, when we are forced to accept one against the other, the contemporary view more closely approximates the truth than the rabbinic one, although it is not synonymous with the truth itself?

Abraham Maimonides, in his treatise on the *aggadot,* appears to go one step beyond his father: "We are not obligated . . . to argue on behalf of the rabbis and uphold their views expressed in all their medical, scientific, and astronomical statements [or to believe] them the way we believe them with respect to the interpretation of the Torah, whose consummate wisdom was in their hands."[51] Note that Abraham includes all the sciences—both terrestrial and celestial— in the category of contemporary knowledge that can supersede that of the rab-

50. This is Maimonides' position as interpreted by S. Pines in "The Limits of Human Knowledge according to al-Farabi, ibn Bajja, and Maimonides," in Twersky, *Studies in Medieval Jewish History and Literature,* pp. 82–109, based especially on the statements in the *Guide of the Perplexed* 3:9; 2:22, and 2:24. J. Stern, in "Maimonides in the Skeptical Tradition" (forthcoming), n. 2, refers also to 3:23: "There is no going beyond the description of natural matters, that is, the elements, meteorological phenomena, or species, . . . [so] that our intellects do not reach the point of apprehending how these natural things that exist in the world of generation and corruption are produced in time and of conceiving how the existence of the natural force within them has originated them." See also M. Kellner, "On the Status of Astronomy and Physics in Maimonides' *Mishneh Torah* and *Guide of the Perplexed:* A Chapter in the History of Science," *British Journal of the History of Science* 24 (1991): 453–63.

For an alternative view of Maimonides' epistemology, see Y. T. Langermann, "The 'True Perplexity': The *Guide of the Perplexed,* Part 2, Chapter 24," in J. L. Kraemer, ed., *Perspectives on Maimonides: Philosophical and Historical Studies* (Oxford, 1991), pp. 159–74, which argues, on the basis of the cosmological statements in the *Mishneh Torah,* that Maimonides believed the true configuration of the heavens to be not fully beyond human comprehension. See also B. S. Kogan, "What Can We Know and When Can We Know It? Maimonides on the Active Intelligence and Human Cognition," in E. Ormsby, ed., *Moses Maimonides and His Time* (Washington, D.C., 1989), pp. 121–37 (see also the essays by J. L. Kraemer and A. Hyman in the same volume); and A. Altmann, "Maimonides on the Intellect and the Scope of Metaphysics," in his *Von der mittelalterlichen zur modernen Aufklärung* (Tübingen, 1987), pp. 60–129.

51. Abraham Maimonides, "Ma'amar al Odot Derashot Ḥazal," in *Milḥamot Adonai,* ed., R. Margulies (Jerusalem, 1953), p. 84, as translated by D. Berger, "Judaism and General Culture in Medieval and Early Modern Times" (forthcoming).

bis. The expansion is significant in allowing all sciences, both certain and less certain, to be placed above rabbinic sapience (that which was extraneous to the strict interpretation of the law) with respect to their truth value. While Moses Maimonides had safeguarded Judaism from astrological determinism, he had, at the same time, attenuated the unassailable truths of Judaism to mere interpretations of religious law while enhancing contact with and even subservience to contemporary speculations about the natural world. As we shall see later, Maimonides' position was stretched even farther in the sixteenth century by Azariah de' Rossi, who quoted Maimonides in support of the view that nonhalakhic statements of the rabbis need not be accepted as absolute truths but only as the personal opinions of the person to whom they were attributed.[52]

I have noted Judah Ha-Levi's criticism of ibn Ezra's astrology. He would probably have objected as strongly to Maimonides' assertion of the inadequacy of rabbinic sapience in astronomical matters, dismissing it as another example of the philosophers' arrogance with respect to sacred tradition. On the contrary, the Torah was perfect in itself, according to Ha-Levi, containing all wisdom and disciplines, particularly those sciences that facilitate the observance of the divine commandments. Thus one finds lore from biology, agriculture, astronomy, and even music in the Torah. Moreover, the ancient wisdom acquired by Solomon, including even the occult arts, was the font of all learning and was eventually diffused among the cultures of other peoples who copied this wisdom from Hebrew sources and then claimed it as their own.[53] Ha-Levi, unlike Maimonides, was unwilling to recognize a body of knowledge that had not been derived from the divine revelation on Mount Sinai. If the Jews didn't possess it now, one should assume that they once did or that it was not worth possessing in the first place.

When knowledge of the natural world was sanctified by Jewish pedigree, it possessed religious value for Ha-Levi. Like his colleagues, Ha-Levi extolled the beauty of nature: "For in the smallest worm there are revealed the wonders of His wisdom in a manner unfathomable to our mind."[54] But one can appreciate

52. See chaps. 2 and 9 below.
53. See Ha-Levi, *Sefer ha-Kuzari* 2:63–66, 4:24–25; and see n. 39 above.
54. Ibid., 1:68.

the beauty of an object without fully comprehending it. In fact, acknowledging one's lack of comprehension enhances one's humility and reverence for all of God's creation. And as long as one does not mistake nature for its Creator or presume to understand things that only God understands, the natural world and its splendors remain an appropriate object of human scrutiny and a valuable resource in inculcating piety and spirituality.[55]

Ha-Levi's objection to the determinism of the astrologers is thus perfectly understandable given its encroachment on divine power and interference in the religious life of the Jews. But what about the magical arts? Rather than excluding them, he considered them part of the Solomonic corpus of knowledge. Magic per se is neither moral nor immoral; it is the practitioner that renders magic bad or good. Ha-Levi's description of the difference between a true believer and an unbeliever is worth quoting in this regard:

[The person who receives divine influence requires instruction] inspired by God, detailed through sublime evidence. He who has been thus inspired, and who obeys the order with all its determinations and conditions with a pure mind, is the true believer. But an unbeliever is he who strives by specula-tion and deduction to influence conditions for the reception of this [divine] power, as revealed in the writings of the astrologers, who try to call down supernatural beings, or who manufacture talismans. He brings offering and burns incense in accordance with his own analogic deduction and conjec-tures, being in reality ignorant of that which we should do, how much, in which way, by what means, in which place, by whom, in which manner, and many other details . . . . He is like an ignorant man who enters the surgery of a physician famous for the curative power of his medicines. The physician is not at home, but people come for medicines. The ignorant man dispenses them out of the jars, knowing nothing of the contents, nor how much should be given to each person. Thus he kills with the very medicine which should have cured them. Should he by chance have effected a cure with one of the drugs, the people will turn to him and say that it helped them—till they dis-cover that he deceived them; or they note the accidental success of another drug and turn to it. . . . Men before the time of Moses, with few exceptions,

55. Ibid., 1:72, 76, 79, 2:56, 3:23.

were like these patients. They were deceived by astrological and physical doctrines; they turned from doctrine to doctrine, from god to god, or adopted a plurality [of doctrines and gods] at the same time; they forgot the guide and master of those powers.[56]

Ha-Levi employs the image of the fool in the physician's office again when describing the sin of the golden calf.[57] Similar to ibn Ezra's explanation, the passage concerns the use of magic to bring down the emanations of the heavens through the astral image of the calf. What is striking about the passage, as Shlomo Pines has explained, is that Ha-Levi does not find the calf objectionable in itself. It was a sin only because it was made by the Israelites "without the order of God."[58] In other words, astral magic is permissible to Jews when performed with God's approval. Ha-Levi applies the same distinction between good and bad astrology that Abarham Bar Ḥiyya did. If it is practiced with "the fear of heaven," it is perfectly acceptable.

For Ha-Levi, then, astral magic and its accoutrements are fully licit for Jews who know how to use talismans properly and who, through their knowledge of God's commandments and "fear of heaven," have the correct attitude. The difference between pagan and Jewish magic is illustrated by the difference between the fool dispensing medicine and the wise physician. One kind of magic is bad because it is not effective; the other is good because it works. In failing to categorize all magic as evil, but rather offering his tacit approval of magic sanctioned by ancient Jewish traditions, Ha-Levi adumbrated a notion of the "spiritual sciences" that would appear in Jewish thought throughout the Middle Ages and well beyond.[59]

Among the Spanish Jewish thinkers after Ha-Levi, Moses Naḥmanides appears to have been profoundly influenced by him, particularly with respect to

56. Ibid., 1:79 (trans. of I. Heinemann, in *Three Jewish Philosophers* [New York, 1969], pp. 40–41).

57. Ibid., 1:97.

58. S. Pines, "On the Term 'Ruḥaniyut' and Its Origin and on Judah Ha-Levi's Doctrine" (in Hebrew), *Tarbiz* 57 (1988): 511–40.

59. On the magical meaning of the term *spiritual sciences* in Jewish sources, see M. Idel, "The Study Program of Yohanan Alemanno" (in Hebrew), *Tarbiz* 48 (1979): 310–11; 319–20.

the idea of "spiritual sciences" stemming from Jewish ancestry.[60] Naḥmanides was one of the most complex representatives of medieval Jewry. A physician and "gentleman" who studied Aristotelian philosophy and the natural sciences, he was a moderate supporter of Maimonides in the controversy that erupted in the thirteenth century. At the same time, he was firmly associated with the introduction of the kabbalah into Spain; he was deeply committed to rabbinic traditions of study that had flourished in the north; he was occasionally critical of the excesses of Maimonidean rationalism and naturalism; and he threw himself passionately into the religious and cultural battle with Christianity, defending his proud ancestry against a new Christian assault in the city of his residence, Barcelona.[61]

Langermann has described Naḥmanides' approach to the natural sciences as "an acceptance and devaluation of science within the framework of Jewish thought."[62] Attempting to define a middle ground between hostility to the sciences on the one hand and an enthusiastic embrace of them on the other, Naḥmanides felt comfortable, according to Langermann, with this moderate position, which was adopted by other traditional thinkers in the following centuries.

See also his "Perceptions of Kabbalah in the Second Half of the Eighteenth Century," *Jewish Thought and Philosophy* 1 (1991): 83–104.

60. See M. Nehorai, "The Doctrine of Miracle and Nature for Naḥmanides and its Relation to R. Yehudah Ha-Levi" (in Hebrew), *Da'at* 17 (1986): 23–31.

61. On Naḥmanides, see I. Twersky, ed., *Rabbi Moses Naḥmanides (Ramban): Explorations in his Religious and Literary Virtuosity* (Cambridge, Mass., 1983), esp. B. Septimus, "Open Rebuke and Concealed Love: Naḥmanides and the Andalusian Tradition," pp. 11–34; M. Idel, "We Have No Kabbalistic Tradition on This," pp. 51–73; D. Berger, "Miracles and the Natural Order," pp. 107–28. See also D. Berger, "Naḥmanides' Attitude toward Secular Learning and Its Bearing upon His Stance in the Maimonidean Controversy," M.A. thesis, Columbia University, 1966; B. Septimus, "Piety and Power in Thirteenth-Century Catalonia," in Twersky, ed., *Studies in Medieval Jewish History and Literature*, pp. 197–230; M. Idel, "Kabbalah, Halakhah and Spiritual Leadership" (typescript); E. R. Wolfson, "By Way of Truth: Aspects of Naḥmanides' Kabbalistic Hermeneutic," *Association for Jewish Studies Review* 14 (1989): 103–78; Y. T. Langermann, "Acceptance and Devaluation: Naḥmanides' Attitude towards Science," *Jewish Thought and Philosophy* 1 (1992): 223–45.

62. Langermann, "Acceptance and Devaluation," p. 223.

At first glance, however, the middle ground chosen by Naḥmanides is not so apparent. His famous sermons on Psalm 19:8 (entitled *The Law of the Lord Is Perfect*) and on Ecclesiastes (*Kohelet*) include a zealous contradiction of the position of Maimonides regarding nature as the source of knowing God. Naḥmanides categorically declares: "One who believes in the Torah may not believe in the existence of nature at all."[63] His doctrine of hidden miracles in nature seems to challenge Maimonides' naturalistic explanation of supernatural phenomena.[64] But other statements take a more moderate position regarding nature. Although he criticizes Maimonidean naturalism in his commentary on the Torah, he offers naturalistic interpretations of his own. Commenting on the rainbow, he seems aware of the conflict within him: "*Against our will* [my emphasis], we must believe the words of the Greeks that the rainbow comes about as a result of the sun's burning in the moist air, for the rainbow appears in a vessel of water placed in the sun."[65] He also defends philosophical and scientific studies in a letter written to a correspondent in northern France, expressing reservations about the cultivation of Greek wisdom only when a Jew is obliged to acquire this knowledge from foreign books. He adds, however, that Maimonides offers a protective shield against this danger.[66] And as David Berger has shown, he recognizes that the universe functions almost always in a naturalistic way for both Jews and non-Jews. Consistently upholding the belief that God may intervene in the natural order whenever he pleases, so that Judaism's doctrine of reward and punishment is not violated, Naḥmanides is neither an occasionalist nor a denier of the natural order.[67]

The Law of the Lord Is Perfect offers a further exposition of Naḥmanides' views, linking him directly to Ha-Levi. In a revealing passage, Naḥmanides lambasts Aristotle and his myopic conception of science:

63. Naḥmanides, *Sermon on Kohelet,* in C. Chavel, *Kitvei Ramban,* 2 vols. (Jerusalem, 1962), 1:192; see also his *Torat Adonai Temimah,* 1:153, and his commentary on Exodus 13:16.

64. See Berger, "Miracles and the Natural Order."

65. See Naḥmanides' commentary on Genesis 9:12 and *Torat Adonai Temimah* 1:174; for other examples, see his commentary on Genesis 8:11 and Leviticus 13:3.

66. See Chavel, *Kitvei Ramban* 1:339; Septimus, "Open Rebuke," p. 24.

67. Berger, "Miracles and the Natural Order."

Hence you see the stubbornness of the leader of the philosophers, may his name be erased, for he denies a number of things that many have seen, whose truth we ourselves have witnessed, and which have become famous in the world. In those ancient times, for example, in the days of our master Moses of blessed memory, they were known to all, because in that generation all the sciences were spiritual, such as the subjects of demons, sorcery, and the varieties of incense that are offered to the heavenly host. For on account of their closeness to the creation of the world and to the flood, there was no one who denied creation [out of nothing] or who rebelled against God. Rather they used to seek some advantage by worshiping the sun, moon, and constellations. They made forms in order to receive a higher power. Even among the philosophers, as written in the *Book of Talismans,* it was possible for a person by way of forms to bring [down] inspiration and speech. When the Greeks arose—and they are a new nation who had not received wisdom as an inheritance, as the author of the *Book of the Khazars* [Judah Ha-Levi] has explained [I:63–65; 3:29],—the well-known man arose and denied everything other than sensibilia. He sought out science based [only] on the senses while denying the spiritual ones. He claimed that the subject of demons and the art of sorcery were worthless and all activity in the world is due to "natures."[68]

Naḥmanides' argument is similar to that of Ha-Levi, who contrasted the unbeliever, striving for divine influence through his useless deductions and speculation, with the Jewish believer, achieving immediate success in bringing down the divine effluvia through the secret wisdom of the Jewish people. Deductions and speculation recall Naḥmanides' characterization of the "leader of the philosophers." In both accounts, the contrast is between the myopic and ineffectual endeavors of the pagan philosopher (the fool in the doctor's office or Aristotle himself) and successful endeavors of the Jewish people, the heirs of a secret wisdom originating from the time of Moses. But Naḥmanides adds several details to sharpen the contrast. For him, the difference is not merely inept pagan versus effective Jewish magic. It is rather a cultural conflict between Greek and

68. Naḥmanides, *Torat Adonai Temimah,* 1: 147. (I consulted Langermann's translations of Naḥmanides, pp. 230–31 for this and the following passage in rendering my own.)

Jewish science.[69] And I might add, given the centrality of Aristotle in Christian scholasticism, and given Naḥmanides' public stance against Christianity, that he might have also perceived the contrast between a Christian science and a Jewish science. Furthermore, the contest is not between two types of magical activity, as it was for Ha-Levi. In Naḥmanides' version, Greek science knows only what it superficially smells, hears, sees, feels, or touches, in contrast to a more subtle and profound science, a spiritual one, that discerns and manipulates natural phenomena unexposed to the natural eye. While Ha-Levi had placed the pagans and Jews in two opposing camps, Naḥmanides sees them in a kind of spiritual alliance. Both Moses and his coreligionists and the ancient astrologers and sorcerers had a clearer vision of the created world because they lived at a time closer to creation; both were also more "spiritual" because they did not rebel against God. In contrast, the Greek philosophers inherited no such vision or wisdom, and thus they were incapable of penetrating the surface of creation, as both the Israelites and the ancient pagans had done.

Naḥmanides later concludes: "All these things and those like them [the occult arts] are old and true sciences, passed on in a tradition by those who received the Torah. When we were lost [exiled], these sciences were lost along with us. A few still retain a distorted recollection of them but the philosophers have [subsequently] come and denied them."[70]

Naḥmanides thus accepted Ha-Levi's notion of a tradition of the occult originating among the Jews in ancient times. He not only confirmed that it works; he elevated it to the status of a spiritual science, superior to the science practiced in thirteenth-century Christian Spain by the scholastic naturalists, whose chief representative among the Jews was Maimonides. Naḥmanides did not develop his notion any further; he conceded that this superior science had been mostly forgotten, and what was still remembered by a few was inaccurate. Although it does not explain this kind of science, his remark is still significant for two

69. Note that Ha-Levi, in the passage referred to by Naḥmanides, also contrasts the Greeks, who lack an inheritance, with the Jews, "the progeny of Shem," and adds that the former are incapable of anything more than "abstract speculation." But Naḥmanides goes farther with the contrast, focusing on the difference between two kinds of science, sensory and spiritual, the first Greek, the second Jewish.

70. Naḥmanides, *Torat Adonai Temimah* 1:162.

reasons. First, he affirmed, like Ha-Levi, his belief in the legitimacy of the occult arts as a means of penetrating the secrets of the natural world. More important, he offered a perspective wedded to the ancient traditions of the Jews that resisted defining the real world according to the principles of Aristotelian physics and offered encouragement to those seeking alternative ways of comprehending nature. Naḥmanides' Jewish pride would not allow him to follow his mentor Maimonides in accepting uncritically the Greek philosopher's ideas about the sublunar world.

The notion of two magics, an effective and edifying one practiced by Jews and a destructive black magic associated with sin and idolatry, has a long career in the traditions of Jewish mystics beginning in the thirteenth century, formulated notably by the author of the *Sefer ha-Zohar (Book of Splendor)*.[71] In a way not unlike that of medieval Christianity's appropriation of certain forms of magic and simultaneous disapproval of other non-Christian varieties,[72] the *Zohar* associated evil magic with original sin as a rebellion against God's sovereignty, while approving the positive theurgic function of observing the commandments, studying the Torah, and praying. Accompanying the positive magic was a tradition of ancient magical-medical wisdom among the Jews, lost but still faintly recalled, based on the exegesis of Genesis 5:1: "This is the book of the generations of Adam." The books of Enoch and Jubilees both recalled a tradition of men receiving secret books from angels.[73] Noah received secret recipes from the angel Raphael, according to the Jewish physician Asaf in the sixth or seventh century. Here the secrets were cast in a medical context, introducing Asaf's own herbal recipes.[74] The early medieval *Book of Secrets* mentioned a similar tradi-

71. See D. Cohen-Aloro, "The Zohar's View of Magic as a Consequence of Original Sin" (in Hebrew), *Da'at* 19 (1987): 31–66.

72. See Flint, *The Rise of Magic in Early Medieval Europe;* R. Kieckhefer, *Magic in the Middle Ages* (Cambridge, 1990), pp. 8–14; P. Brown, "Sorcery, Demons, and the Rise of Christianity: From Late Antiquity into the Middle Ages," in M. Douglas, ed., *Witchcraft Confessions and Accusations* (London, 1970), pp. 17–45; repr. in P. Brown, *Religion and Society in the Age of St. Augustine* (London, 1972), pp. 119–46.

73. Cohen-Aloro, "Zohar's View," pp. 50–52.

74. S. Muntner, Introduction to *Sefer Asaf ha-Rofe* (Jerusalem, 1958), pp. 147–49. For further discussion of this motif and additional references, see the appendix.

tion[75] and the motif reappeared in the *Sefer ha-Zohar*.[76] The notion of an ancient Jewish book of magic and medical wisdom complemented Naḥmanides' idea of a Jewish spiritual science opposed to a Greek sensory one. Both traditions—the lost book of medicine and Naḥmanides' spiritual sciences—would be recalled by Jewish thinkers well into the early modern period.[77]

Four years before Naḥmanides' death, Levi ben Gerson, known as Gersonides, was born in the district of Orange in Provence.[78] Naḥmanides' profound influence on thirteenth-century Jewry would have been felt by the young philosopher and astronomer, but there is every reason to doubt that the rabbi's notion of a Jewish spiritual science met with his approval. Gersonides, to a greater extent than even Maimonides, was an adherent of Aristotelian physics. His scientific corpus, together with his philosophical and exegetical writings, established him as an imposing figure in the history of Jewish thought in general and Jewish scientific thought in particular.

Seymour Feldman calls Gersonides a backward-looking philosopher, in the Aristotelian-Averroistic tradition. His philosophical optimism, his rigorous defense of the integration of reason and revelation, and his belief that Judaism could be understood philosophically placed him at odds with the growing nominalist tendencies of Christian scholastic thought beginning to establish rigorous dividing lines between religion and reason, divorcing philosophy from the-

75. M. Margoliouth, ed., *Sefer ha-Raẓim* (Jerusalem, 1967), pp. 56–57.

76. Cohen-Aloro, "The Zohar's View," p. 52.

77. See D. B. Ruderman, *Kabbalah, Magic, and Science: The Cultural Universe of a Sixteenth-Century Jewish Physician* (Cambridge, Mass., 1988), pp. 40–41 and 183, n. 83.

78. On Gersonides, see J. Shatzmiller, "Gersonides and the Jewish Community of Orange in His Day" and "Some Further Information about Gersonides and the Orange Jewish Community in His Day" (in Hebrew), in B. Oded et al., eds., *Studies in the History of the Jewish People and the Land of Israel*, vol. 2 (Haifa, 1972), pp. 111–126; and vol. 3 (Haifa, 1974), pp. 139–43; C. Touati, *La Pensée philosophique et théologique de Gersonide* (Paris, 1973); and especially two recent anthologies: G. Dahan, ed., *Gersonide en son temps* (Louvain, 1991) and G. Freudenthal, ed., *Studies on Gersonides: A Fourteenth-Century Jewish Philosopher-Scientist* (Leiden, 1992). Especially useful is M. Kellner's essay "Bibliographia Gersonideana" in the Freudenthal volume, pp. 367–416.

ology and from the natural sciences.[79] Writing at a time when the recently translated commentaries of Averroes had revolutionized the study of philosophy in Europe, Gersonides upheld the value of a philosophically sound and self-consistent Jewish theology.[80]

Although Gersonides was committed to an approach to understanding the cosmos that Naḥmanides would have labeled disparagingly as "sensory," it would be misleading to view him as merely backward-looking. The key to understanding his novel position in Jewish thought, as Gad Freudenthal has argued, is the relation between his theology and astronomy. Freudenthal calls Gersonides "an epistemological realist," by which he means that knowledge of the universe represented for Gersonides the ultimate goal of humankind, the attaining of immortality. Knowledge of the natural world was not merely preliminary to metaphysics, nor was its purpose to "save the appearances" of ancient assumptions about the way the heavens operate.[81] Furthermore, there were no limits to what human beings could learn.[82] Maimonides had written that "it is impossible for us to accede to the points starting from which conclusions may be drawn about the heavens; for the latter are too far away from us and too high in place and in rank. And even the general conclusion that may be drawn from them, namely, that they prove the existence of their Mover, is a matter the knowledge of which cannot be reached by human intellects. And to fatigue the minds with notions that cannot be grasped by them and for the grasp of which they have no instrument, is a defect in one's inborn disposition

---

79. But note S. Möbuss, *Die Intellektlehre des Levi ben Gerson in ihrer Beziehung zur christlichen Scholastik* (Frankfurt am Main, 1991), who suggests an Ockhamist influence on Gersonides' notion of the intellect.

80. S. Feldman, ed. and trans., *Levi Ben Gershom: The Wars of the Lord*, 2 vols. (Philadelphia, 1984–87), 1:49–52.

81. On this notion, see P. Duhem, *To Save the Phenomena,* trans. E. Doland and C. Machler (Chicago, 1969).

82. G. Freudenthal, "Spiritual Success and Astronomy: Gersonides' War against Ptolemy" (in Hebrew), *Da'at* 22(1989): 55–72. See also his "Cosmogonie et physique chez Gersonide," *Revue des études juives* 145 (1986): 295–314; his critical review of Feldman in *Revue des études juives* 148 (1989): 379–84; and his "Sauver son âme ou sauver les phénomènes: Sotériologie, épistémologie et astronomie chez Gersonide," in Freudenthal, *Studies on Gersonides,* pp. 317–52.

or some sort of temptation. Let us then stop at a point that is within our capacity . . . ."[83] Gersonides strongly disagreed. The progressive accumulation of knowledge had no limits whatsoever and provided the only guarantee of the immortality of the soul.[84]

For Gersonides, astronomy was the highest science. In the opening of a long discourse on astronomy in the *Wars of the Lord,* he offered apologetic arguments for the study of astronomy based on its nobility, its applications to the other sciences and philosophy, and its political and practical utility.[85] He also cited biblical passages praising it as a means of understanding God.[86] Gersonides insisted that astronomical theory be philosophically sound and conform to observation. Openly critical of the Ptolemaic models of planetary motion, he denied that they could represent the true structure of the heavens unless verified through observation. Departing from the traditional explanations of medieval astronomy, he invented his own instruments—the Jacob's staff, the camera obscura, a tool to measure the moon's elongation from the sun, and a modified astrolabe— to offer new models previously not considered, and then to verify them on the basis of his own observations.[87]

Whether one interprets Gersonides' philosophical optimism and search for divine truth through the stars as a "step backward" or as "creating a new scientific discourse examining the real universe rather than transcending it,"[88] his originality as an astronomer, his commitment to the study of the heavens for its own sake and as a means of understanding the Divine, his extraordinary confidence in the ability of the rational faculties of human beings to fathom all of creation, and the fusion of his scientific quest with his Jewish identity are indisputable. That he had little influence on later Jewish thinkers suggests that

83. Maimonides, *Guide of the Perplexed* 2:25 (Pines trans., p. 327).

84. See also M. Kellner, "Maimonides and Gersonides on Astronomy and Metaphysics," in Rosner and Kottek, *Moses Maimonides,* pp. 91–96.

85. See B. R. Goldstein, *The Astronomy of Levi Ben Gerson (1288–1344)* (Berlin, 1985), p. 24. See also Goldstein, "Levi Ben Gerson's Contributions to Astronomy," in Freudenthal, *Studies on Gersonides,* pp. 3–19.

86. Goldstein, *Astronomy,* p. 24.

87. Ibid., pp. 7–9.

88. Freudenthal, "Spiritual Success," p. 71.

his position was anomalous.[89] In sensing the limits of the human capacity to know the heavens, Maimonides was closer to the Christian nominalists of the fourteenth century who had severed the relation between theology and science, allowing each an autonomy of its own.[90] Whether, in the final analysis, Gersonides' reintegration of the two liberated or limited his empirical investigation, it is clear that later Jewish thought was more in line with Christian theology. Ironically, although Gersonides was the greatest Jewish scientist of the Middle Ages, he had the least influence on later Jewish thinkers, at least with respect to his scientific writings. His originality was constrained by a metaphysics going out of fashion steadily among both Jews and Christians.

To what extent do the views of the few discussed so far reflect those of the many? Are we entitled to speak about interest in the natural world through a wider spectrum of Jews than the elites of Spain and southern France here surveyed? Only a tentative answer is possible, based on the inroads of Maimonideanism and the study of Aristotelian philosophy in medieval Jewish culture. To the extent that physics was an essential feature of the curriculum leading to "the divine science," the study of it was encouraged. Thus, there were a significant number of Hebrew encyclopedias designed for more popular consumption, generally following the curriculum of natural scientific and theological studies advocated by the reigning philosophical school. This output is particularly noticeable in Provence and Spain during the thirteenth and fourteenth centuries. It includes such works as Judah ben Solomon Cohen's *Midrash ha-Ḥokhmah,* Shem Tov ben Joseph Falaquera's *De'ot ha-Pilosophim,* or *Sefer ha-Mevakesh,* Gershom ben Solomon of Arles' *Sha'ar ha-Shamayim,* and Meir ben

89. On his lack of influence, see Freudenthal, "Spiritual Success," pp. 71–72; Goldstein, *Astronomy,* pp. 9–15.

90. On the nominalist revolt, see E. Grant, *Physical Science in the Middle Ages* (New York, 1971), pp. 24–35; idem, "The Condemnation of 1277, God's Absolute Power, and Physical Thought in the Late Middle Ages," *Viator* 10 (1979): 211–44; H. Oberman, "Reformation and Revolution: Copernicus' Discovery in an Era of Change," in Murdoch and Sylla, *Cultural Context,* pp. 397–435. Nominalism and Jewish thought in eastern Europe are also discussed in chap. 2 below.

Isaac Aldabi's *Shevilei Emunah*.[91] Few of these books have been studied systematically for their essential themes, their sources, the extent of their readership, or their relation to similar compendiums of knowledge in the Christian world, and thus it is hard to assess their significance and influence within the culture of medieval Judaism.

One final and important question alluded to above has not yet been addressed in this cursory overview. Was a positive attitude to the natural world primarily the product of southern European culture, which was closest geographically and intellectually to the traditions of Islamic philosophy and science? The conventional portrait of northern European Jewish culture as one devoted exclusively to biblical and rabbinic exegesis has been challenged in recent years. Ashkenazic Jews, according to this revision, were not insulated from either philosophy or the natural sciences but rather showed an awareness and an appreciation of both. This "rationalistic" tradition of Ashkenazic Jews was then passed down to their eastern European descendants, who fostered similar interests while simultaneously devoting themselves to Torah study.[92]

Leaving aside the question of philosophy, the evidence for nature study among Ashkenazic Jews is partial and sporadic. Scientific texts recently discovered by Y. Tzvi Langermann and Israel Ta-Shema suggest the possibility that some Ashkenazic Jews acquired considerable knowledge of the natural world.[93]

91. On Falaquera, see R. Jospe, *Torah and Sophia: The Life and Thought of Shem Tov ibn Falaquera* (Cincinnati, 1988), and S. Harvey's translation of *Sefer ha-Mevakesh* (Cambridge, Mass., 1988). On Gershom of Arles, see *The Gate of Heaven*, trans. F. S. Bodenheimer (Jerusalem, 1953). On the others, see F. S. Bodenheimer, "On Some Hebrew Encyclopedias of the Middle Ages," *Archives internationales d'histoire des sciences* 6 (1953): 3–13; Marx, "Scientific Work"; and see esp. Freudenthal's recent analysis in "Les Sciences dans les communautés juives," pp. 53–60. J. Shatzmiller, in his forthcoming book, stresses the pragmatic dimension of these compendiums, which, along with Hebrew translations of Avicenna's *Canon*, were designed to introduce Jewish students to the sciences in preparation for careers in medicine.

92. See esp. E. Kupfer, "Concerning the Cultural Image of Ashkenazic Jewry and Its Sages in the Fourteenth and Fifteenth Centuries" (in Hebrew), *Tarbiz* 42 (1972–73): 113–47. The implications of this essay for the study of science among eastern European Jews will be considered in chap. 2 below.

93. Y. T. Langermann, "An Unknown Ashkenazic Composition on the Natural Sciences" (in Hebrew), *Kiryat Sefer* 62 (1988–89): 448–49; idem, "A Hebrew Version of the Encyclo-

This limited evidence indicates that some were impressed by the natural land-scape while still engrossed in their legal commentaries and codes. Moreover, rabbinic study could often spawn an interest in nature. Perhaps David Berger is right in differentiating between philosophic and nature study among Ashkenazic Jews; while they were resistant to the first, the second raised few theological problems for them.[94]

One unusual approach to nature emanating from the circle of German piet-ists during the thirteenth and fourteenth centuries has been described by Israel Ta-Shema and Joseph Dan. A remarkable manuscript from the hand of Judah the Pious, the primary figure in this circle, entitled *God's Conversation Concerning All His Wonders,* offers examples ranging from the credible (a dog finding his prey, a magnet), to the incredible (animals speaking Hebrew, the rays on Moses's face, and the activity of demons). Some of the wonders, as Ta-Shema points out, are indeed based on observation and assume a sophisticated understanding of natural processes. Others stretch the imagination beyond all limits.[95] Such compendiums of fact and fancy need to be compared with similar Christian works to establish the degree of their originality and their importance.

What is most interesting about Judah's discourse is not the subject itself but rather the theological perspective. According to Judah, God establishes wonders in nature to reflect his divine presence. In the ordinary course of nature, contrary to the views of the thinkers I have discussed so far, God's presence is

---

pedia of Guillaume de Conches" (in Hebrew), *Kiryat Sefer* 60 (1985): 328–29; I. Ta-Shema, "Sefer ha-Maskil: An Unknown French-Jewish Book from the End of the Thirteenth Century" (in Hebrew), *Jerusalem Studies in Jewish Thought* 2, no. 3 (1982–83): 416–38; G. Freudenthal, "Blessed Is the Air and Blessed Is Its Name in *Sefer ha-Maskil* of R. Solomon Simhah of Troyes: Toward a Portrait of Scientific-Midrashic Cosmology under Stoic Influence from the Thirteenth Century" (in Hebrew), *Da'at* 32–33 (1994): 182–234.

94. I refer to Berger's discussion of Ashkenazic Jewish culture in "Judaism and General Culture in Medieval and Early Modern Times."

95. Y. Dan, *Torat Ha-Sod shel Ḥasidei Ashkenaz* (Jerusalem, 1968), pp. 88–94; idem, *Iyyunim be-Sifrut Ḥasidei Ashkenaz* (Ramat Gan, 1975), pp. 142–45. I am indebted to Professor Ta-Shema for his reflections on this subject in a letter he sent me on Nov. 20, 1990. See also J. Shatzmiller, "Doctors and Medical Practice in Germany around 1200: The Evidence of Sefer Ḥasidim," *Journal of Jewish Studies: Essays in Honour of Yigael Yadin* 33 (1982): 583–93.

not reflected. Only the pietist can look with his sensitive lens beyond the ordinary, attaining insights not available to the uninitiated. Ostensibly adopting an antinaturalist position by denying a value to the study of ordinary nature, the pietist finds ultimate meaning in the unusual, the miraculous, which is nonetheless within the world of nature as well. And conceivably, one has to recognize the ordinary in order to define and describe the extraordinary. Thus Judah's manuscript offers an alternative mystical model for studying nature from that of the dominant physics of medieval scholasticism. Both Judah the Pious and, to a lesser extent, Naḥmanides studied and explained nature out of a religious and cultural orientation that was at odds with the norms of Aristotelian natural philosophy.

My survey of medieval attitudes to the natural world from Baḥya ibn Pakuda to Judah the Pious has included an appreciation of nature as valuable in itself and as a source of religious meaning (Baḥya, Ha-Levi, Maimonides, and others); a full range of attitudes toward astrology and astral magic, from open hostility (Baḥya, Maimonides) to restrained acceptance (Bar Ḥiyya), to uninhibited enthusiasm for all its manifestations, including the reinterpretation of precepts and rites and the leveling of apparent differences among religions (ibn Ezra and his commentators); a tendency to dissociate scientific knowledge from the sacred dicta of the rabbis and to consider knowledge of celestial physics speculative and never fully attainable (Maimonides); an argument that the Torah is the font of all wisdom, including the sciences, and that the wisdom of other cultures is also ultimately derived the Torah (Ha-Levi and others); an assumption that ancient Jewish magic and medicine constitute a spiritual science superior to that of the Greeks and medieval philosophers (Ha-Levi, Naḥmanides, and the kabbalists); reinvigorated Aristotelian philosophy committed to understanding all of creation, with astronomy as the highest science and fueled by a critical and empiricist temper (Gersonides); the diffusion of scientific information in popular compendiums throughout the Jewish world and the occasional evidence of nature study and appreciation on the part of Ashkenazic Jews, even those far removed from the centers of philosophical and scientific investigation.

As one might expect, Jews' reflections on nature often closely resemble those of their Muslim and Christian neighbors. The dissemination of classical philosophy and science in higher medieval culture is the most obvious reason for these shared views.[96] The study of physics as the first stage of the philosophical curriculum;[97] the preoccupation with astronomy and with the more scientific forms of astrology (compare, for example, the notions of good and bad astrology in Isidore of Seville[98] and Abraham Bar Ḥiyya); and the promotion of medicine and the biological sciences[99] all stem from this collective body of knowledge inherited from antiquity, which was enlarged and transformed during the Middle Ages.

A second area of common interests involves the intersection of religion, magic, and science. The permeability of boundaries between magic and experimental science in both the ancient and medieval worlds has long been noted.[100] The transformation of condemned magic, sometimes through experimental science, into friendly magic often appears to cross religious and cultural boundaries. The early medieval church's appropriation of magical systems of pagan antiquity is reminiscent of tendencies in early rabbinic and medieval Judaism, such as the *Sefer ha-Zohar*'s distinction between destructive magic and creative theurgy and the invoking of astrological magic and medicine as opposed to

96. See B. Stock, "Science, Technology, and Economic Progress in the Early Middle Ages," and D. C. Lindberg, "The Transmission of Greek and Arabic Learning in the West," in Lindberg, *Science in the Middle Ages*, pp. 1–90; Grant, *Physical Science in the Middle Ages*, pp. 1–22; and S. H. Nasr, *Science and Civilization in Islam* (Cambridge, Mass., 1968).

97. See J. A. Weisheipl, "The Nature, Scope, and Classification of the Sciences," in Lindberg, *Science in the Middle Ages*, pp. 461–482; idem, "Classification of the Sciences in Medieval Thought," *Medieval Studies* 27 (1965): 54–90. See also W. A. Wallace, "The Philosophical Setting of Medieval Science," in Lindberg, *Science in the Middle Ages*, pp. 91–119.

98. On "good" Christian astrology, see Flint, *Rise of Magic*, pp. 128–46; (for Isidore, see p. 130); and H. C. Kee, *Medicine, Miracle, and Magic in New Testament Times* (Cambridge, 1986).

99. See the surveys of medieval medicine and natural history by C. H. Talbot and J. Stannard in Lindberg, *Science in the Middle Ages*, pp. 391–428 and 429–60; N. G. Siraisi, *Medieval and Early Renaissance Medicine* (Chicago, 1990); and M. Ullmann, *Islamic Medicine* (Edinburgh, 1978).

100. See the works listed in n. 72 above as well as G. E. R. Lloyd, *Magic, Reason and Experience* (Cambridge, 1979); Hansen, "Science and Magic"; and P. Zambelli, ed., *Scienze, credenze occulte, liveli di cultura* (Florence, 1982). On the ancient period, see the appendix.

"more menacing forms of supernatural intercession."[101] But one should also note the dissimilarities between the Christians and Jews. The initial polemic against magic in the church is not found among the rabbis, whose ability to tolerate most forms of magic remained constant.[102] Whereas much medieval Christian magic flowed naturally "into the streambed of Aristotelian thought," as Bert Hanson has noted[103] certain forms of Jewish magic were markedly anti-Aristotelian and even anti-Christian, as we have seen.[104] The assertion of Jewish magic or science as an act of self-differentiation from the dominant culture appears to be a unique development within Jewish medieval thought.

Much has been written about the assault on Aristotelian naturalism by Christian theologians in the late thirteenth and fourteenth centuries. Rejecting the deterministic causality of the philosophers, they maintained that God was free to create what he willed in nature. Science became conditional and hypothetical, and alternative theories about the radically contingent universe could now be proposed.[105] This nominalist and empiricist revolution has no exact parallel in Jewish thought.[106] I have mentioned Maimonides' hypothetical approach to the study of celestial physics; but he was no nominalist with respect to the terres-

101. Flint, *Rise of Magic*, p. 145. See also the recent critique of Flint's work by R. Kleckhefer, "The Specific Rationality of Medieval Magic," *American Historical Review* 99 (1994): 813–36.

102. See the appendix.

103. Hansen, "Science and Magic," p. 490.

104. The most extreme example is the 15th-century *Sefer ha-Meshiv,* On this work, see M. Idel, "Investigations in the Method of the Author of *Sefer ha-Meshiv,* (in Hebrew), *Sefunot* 17 (1983): 185–266; and idem, "The Attitude to Christianity in the *Sefer ha-Meshiv*" (in Hebrew), *Zion* 46 (1981): 77–91.

105. See the references in n. 90, along with E. Grant, "Scientific Thought in Fourteenth-Century Paris: Jean Buridan and Nicole Oresme," in Cosman and Chandler, *Machaut's World,* pp. 105–24; and compare the recent treatment by A. Funkenstein, *Theology and the Scientific Imagination from the Middle Ages to the Seventeenth Century* (Princeton, 1986). See also chap. 2 below.

106. The subject deserves more study. See W. Z. Harvey, "Nissim of Gerona and William of Ockham on Prime Matter, "*Jewish History* 6 (*Frank Talmage Memorial Volume* 2) (1992): 87–98.

trial sciences. Gersonides' philosophy, as we have seen, was radically different from that of the nominalists.[107] Ḥasdai Crescas's elaborate critique of Aristotelian philosophy at the beginning of the fifteenth century appears to be the first Jewish assault on scholastic naturalism, but its precise connection to the work of the nominalists Ockham, Oresme, and Buridan, if any, is still to be determined.[108] The real break with Aristotelian philosophy by Jewish thinkers took place still later, in the period that I describe in the subsequent chapters.

Beyond the obvious similarities and differences of approach I have mentioned, there remains the larger social context, especially the new universities such as Paris, Oxford, Montpellier, and Bologna. Preceded by the cathedral schools, the university drew together all those concerned with Aristotelian natural philosophy, astronomy, astrology, and medicine. It also was the only institution that could promote under one roof the unitary character of learning. All university students, from the faculties of law, theology or medicine, were required to pass through the faculty of arts, and thus they shared a common basis for scholarship.[109]

With few exceptions, Jews were barred from university study. Despite the legends regarding Jewish involvement in the founding of such universities as Salerno or Montpellier, almost no Jews studied formally at any medieval university before the fourteenth century, and regularized admission did not occur until the late sixteenth century at even the most tolerant institutions, such as Padua.[110] Even then, Jews could study only in the faculty of medicine for obvious

107. But compare n. 79.

108. See H. Wolfson, *Crescas' Critique of Aristotle: Problems of Aristotle's Physics in Jewish and Arabic Philosophy* (Cambridge, Mass., 1929); and A. Ravitzky, *Crescas's Sermon on the Passover and Studies in His Philosophy* (in Hebrew) (Jerusalem, 1988).

109. See the overview by P. Kibre and N. Siraisi, "The Institutional Setting: The Universities," in Lindberg, *Science in the Middle Ages,* pp. 120–44; J. Murdoch, "From Social into Intellectual Factors: An Aspect of the Unitary Character of Medieval Learning," in Murdoch and Sylla, *Cultural Context of Medieval Learning,* pp. 271–348; H. Rashdall, *The Universities of Europe in the Middle Ages,* 3 vols. (Oxford, 1936); G. Leff, *Paris and Oxford Universities in the Thirteenth and Fourteenth Centuries: An Institutional and Intellectual History* (New York, 1968); N. Siraisi, *Arts and Sciences at Padua* (Toronto, 1973).

110. On this later development, see below. J. Shatzmiller discusses the medieval situation thoroughly in his forthcoming book.

theological reasons. Gad Freudenthal maintains that the greatest impediment to the study of the sciences among medieval Jews was their lack of institutional support. The philosopher-savant, with leisure for systematic study and reflection, could not exist within the Jewish community. Jewish education revolved around the study of religious law, and lacking access to universities, Jews had no place to pursue autonomous research in philosophy and the sciences. Thus the Jewish community, at least in Christian Europe, could produce no major scientific figures; Gersonides is the sole exception that proves the rule.[111]

The lack of access to universities was a major factor in Jewish intellectual life in the Middle Ages and diminished Jewish involvement in the sciences. Yet Freudenthal's assertion needs to be modified in at least two respects. First, there was at least one social context in which Jews could pursue scientific interests: the medical profession. The conspicuous success of Jews in this profession in the medieval Islamic world is well known.[112] Through strong kinship ties and a network of apprenticeships, the quality and quantity of trained Jewish physicians remained high. Through their medical practice, they attained not only considerable economic success and political power, but knowledge and practical experience in the natural sciences. Medicine's connection with astrology also facilitated their mastery of physics, mathematics, and astronomy. Their involvement in medicine was as extensive in Christian Europe. In some places, like Languedoc between the twelfth and fifteenth centuries, more than a third of the licensed doctors were Jews. Although excluded officially from the University of Montpellier, many Jewish physicians maintained close ties with the faculty of medicine. Many Jewish physicians were regularly examined and licensed by the local authorities in the rest of southern France, Aragon, and Italy.[113] Thus the Jewish community partially filled the educational void in the sciences through

111. G. Freudenthal, "The Place of Science in Medieval Hebrew-writing Jewish Communities: A Sociological Perspective" (paper delivered at the symposium "The Interaction of Scientific and Jewish Cultures," Jewish Public Library, Montreal, June 3–5, 1990). My thanks to Professor Freudenthal for sharing a copy of his paper with me. His position is considerably expanded in "Les Sciences dans les communautés juives," esp. pp. 92–134.

112. See the references in nn. 9 and 10.

113. This situation is documented in Professor Shatzmiller's book.

support of a high level of medical training among some of its most privileged members.

The second modification of Freudenthal's view arises from the fact that individual Jews were supported, sometimes handsomely, in their pursuit of astrology and medicine and especially in their translation of scientific texts by Christian governments and private patrons. Some of these individuals acquired vast learning in the natural sciences through their privileged status. The percentage of such Jewish savants was small in comparison to the percentage of Christian university students, but surely not negligible.[114] Moreover, systematic rabbinic learning, especially in Spain and southern France, did not discourage scientific and philosophic pursuits among other Jewish students.[115] Indeed, it spawned both a technical philosophical literature in Arabic and Hebrew and a more popular literature of scientific knowledge gathered in compendiums, as we have seen.

Many of the attitudes described in this chapter reappear in various guises later on: the appreciation of nature study as a religious ideal, for example, as well as the belief in the ancient Jewish provenance of magic and medicine, astrology and astronomy, accompanied by a feeling of superiority. In the early modern period, we also notice exceptional Jewish physicians, magicians, and astrologers frequenting the homes of Christian nobility and statesmen.

But important differences are also notable. The study of medicine and the sciences was revolutionized by two major factors: the growing numbers of Jews gaining admission to university faculties of medicine and the introduction of the printing press. Hebrew books were produced and books in other languages were increasingly read by Jews. Ironically, the medieval Hebrew encyclopedias had their widest distribution after the printing press rather than before. Important intellectual changes also distinguish the two periods. We need only mention at this stage the changing intellectual context of the Renaissance and

114. On the translators, see the works cited in nn. 1 and 8.

115. See, for example, I. Ta-Shema, "Philosophical Considerations for Halakhic Decision Making in Spain" (in Hebrew), *Sefunot,* n.s., 3 [=18] (1985): 99–110. Compare Freudenthal, "Les Sciences dans les communautés juives," pp. 92–134.

post-Renaissance as a nurturing ground and further stimulant for the coadunation of magical and scientific mentalities. The breakdown of the Aristotelian worldview, the divorce of physics from metaphysics, produced a major epistemological and methodological breakthrough in the sciences and a transformed relation with Jewish religious thought.

Despite these major differences, medieval Jewish attitudes toward nature and scientific activity helped shape Jewish attitudes in the early modern period. Most important, early modern Jews saw their scientific studies as a cultural legacy and a badge of honor. They reveled in Jewish medical and scientific genealogies. They were the proud heirs of Maimonides, ibn Ezra, and Gersonides, and that recollection sustained and legitimated their cultural endeavors. The Jewish astrologers, physicians, and occultists whom they honored in this medieval hall of fame had successfully integrated their Jewish identities with their scientific ones, and they believed that they could do so too.

2

The Legitimation of Scientific Activity among Central and Eastern European Jews

To the historian of Jewish-Christian relations in early modern western Europe, the terrain of central and eastern Europe appears bland and stolid in comparison. From the perspective of the West, Jewish intellectual life seems relatively isolated and inner-directed; on the surface, Jewish writing displays little of the current thinking and literary tastes of the outside world; and the primary dialogue of Jewish thinkers with ideas outside their own culture is with those stemming from earlier Jewish cultures of the ancient and medieval worlds. While Jews of the West were generally conversant in all the major languages of their host civilizations, listened to sermons in those languages, and even published books in them, their counterparts to the East were comfortable, for the most part, only in Hebrew and Yiddish. Thus the homeland of Copernicus, at least at first glance, seems an unlikely setting for a serious interest in scientific matters, even on the part of Jews living near the University of Cracow.[1]

The picture of Jewish culture in this region is certainly more complex than so facile a description might suggest. To an outsider, it seems to require especially intense scrutiny in light of

1. One easily gains this impression by comparing M. A. Shulvass's account of eastern European Jews in *Jewish Culture in Eastern Europe: The Classical Period* (New York, 1975) with his account of Italian Jews in *The Jews in the World of the Renaissance* (Leiden, 1973). Shulvass devotes only one chapter in the first book to the liberal arts and other disciplines, while in the second book his treatment of the topic is extensive.

the apparently conflicting interpretations of this cultural world in recent scholarly writing. By all accounts, the study of the natural world, especially astronomy, seems to have played some role in the intellectual life of this Jewish community in the sixteenth and seventeenth centuries. The challenge, then, is twofold: first, to describe its origin and diffusion and to evaluate its significance within the larger cultural space of central and eastern European Jewry, a task already undertaken in part by others; and second, to place this scientific activity in a broader European context, compare it with activity in other Jewish communities of the same era, and assess its impact on contemporary and later Jewish cultural life both in the East and beyond. In order to accomplish both tasks, we must first confront the broader issue of defining the cultural experience of this Jewish community in the sixteenth and seventeenth centuries in the light of contemporary historical treatments of the subject.

In recent years, scholarly depictions of the intellectual and cultural world of central and eastern European Jewry have revolved around two contentious issues of interpretation, each with a different focus but ultimately related to each other. The first concerns the place of rationalism and antirationalism in Ashkenazic culture. The terms of reference have not been carefully defined by the scholars. Rationalism is taken to be loosely synonymous with philosophical study, which in its medieval sense includes speculation on the sublunar world (physics) and what is beyond that world (metaphysics). There is little awareness of the possible shifts in meaning that rationalism might have undergone from the early Middle Ages through the seventeenth century; what one age might consider rational might appear irrational to another. Nor has there been much discussion of the epistemological crisis in the Christian world in the early modern period regarding truth and the limits of reason.

In 1972, Ephraim Kupfer published an essay in which he attempted to demonstrate a strong current of rationalist culture and philosophical activity among certain circles of German Jews from the late fourteenth to early fifteenth centuries.[2] Kupfer claimed that this learning was transported to the East and stimu-

2. E. Kupfer, "Concerning the Cultural Image of Ashkenazic Jewry and Its Sages in the Fourteenth and Fifteenth Centuries" (in Hebrew), *Tarbiz* 42 (1972–73): 113–47. For a recent critique, see I. Yuval, *Ḥakhamim be-Doram* (Jerusalem, 1989), pp. 286–311.

lated the resurgence of rationalist pursuits among eastern European Jews in the latter half of the sixteenth century. Several years later, Lawrence Kaplan championed the so-called Kupfer thesis in a study of Rabbi Mordecai Yaffe and sixteenth-century Polish Jewish culture.[3] The issues both scholars confronted were whether "the rational tinge"[4] of Ashkenazic culture in this later period was indigenous or an import from Italy or Spain, whether it reflected a tradition of Ashkenazic culture or rather constituted a novelty reflecting the specific social and cultural circumstances of the late sixteenth century, and whether its decline by the early seventeenth century signaled a return to the usual norm of Ashkenazic culture—an indifference and even antagonism to philosophical concerns—or, on the contrary, reflected a critical rupture with the past, an aberration from what had been perceived as a traditionally licit and honorable pursuit.

Kaplan noted that philosophical study had been so integrated into Ashkenazic rabbinic culture by the late sixteenth century that Moses Isserles could refer to it as "a legacy of our fathers."[5] Indeed, the novel component of Ashkenazic culture in this era, "paradoxical as it may seem," was not philosophy but kabbalah that originated in Italy and eventually became a part of Ashkenazic traditions, even displacing speculative rationalism altogether.[6]

The revisionism of Kupfer and Kaplan challenged the earlier views of Ḥayyim Hillel Ben Sasson and Salo W. Baron regarding the origin of philosophical study among eastern European Jews. In his broad surveys of Jewish history, Ben Sasson had assumed that a new rationalism had been stimulated by Sephardic and Italian influences.[7] Baron did not live to complete his own synthesis

---

3. L. Kaplan, "Rationalism and Rabbinic Culture in Sixteenth-Century Eastern Europe: Rabbi Mordecai Jaffe's *Levush Pinat Yikrat,*" Ph.D. diss., Harvard University, 1975; idem, "Rabbi Mordecai Jaffe and the Evolution of Jewish Culture in Poland in the Sixteenth Century," in B. Cooperman, ed., *Jewish Thought in the Sixteenth Century* (Cambridge, Mass., 1983), pp. 266–82.

4. The phrase is from Kaplan, "Rationalism and Rabbinic Culture," p. 268.

5. Ibid., p. 267, quoting Moses Isserles, *Responsa* no. 6, ed. A. Siev (Jerusalem, 1971).

6. Ibid., p. 268.

7. H. H. Ben Sasson, *Perakim be-Toledot ha-Yehudim bi-mai ha-Beinayim* (Jerusalem, 1962), pp. 205–6; idem, *Trial and Achievement: Currents in Jewish History* (Jerusalem, 1974), p. 155.

of the intellectual life of Polish-Lithuanian Jewry. However, in an early chapter of his multivolume history of the Jews, he offered some tantalizing suggestions about the impact of Polish humanism on Jewish intellectual life. According to Baron, Jewish culture flourished in sixteenth-century Poland because of the positive influence of the Italian Renaissance, the growing diversity of the region's population, and the subsequent religious toleration.[8] For both Ben Sasson and Baron, the primary impetus to rationalistic pursuits in Ashkenazic culture came from outside—either from another more enlightened, Jewish community or from the Christian majority.

The most ambitious elaboration of Kupfer's thesis is that of Joseph Davis.[9] Although Davis has reservations about the existence of a continuous thread of rationalism in Ashkenazic culture, he nevertheless attempts to construct a history of Ashkenazic rationalism from the twelfth century until the seventeenth century, from northern France to Bohemia and Poland. Davis identifies rationalistic pursuits among the students of Rashi with a reactionary decline between 1200 and 1350, followed by an upsurge between 1350 and 1450. He refers in this latter period to the circle of philosophical enthusiasts in Prague identified by Kupfer, as well as to the writing of another German author, Simeon ben Samuel. Davis acknowledges a subsequent indifference to philosophical study between 1450 and 1550, followed by an efflorescence of intellectual life around the time of Moses Isserles, between 1550 and 1620.[10] He cautiously accepts Kaplan's formulation of an Ashkenazic tradition of moderate rationalism culminating in Isserles, but he adds two qualifications. In the first place, the integration of kabbalah with philosophy in rabbinic culture was not, as Kaplan maintained, a novelty, contra Kaplan, but a tradition going back as far as the fourteenth century among German Jewry. Indeed, despite its earlier roots among Ashkenazic Jews, rationalism remained "intrinsically insecure" in Poland while kabbalah thrived. The harmonization of rabbinics, philosophy, and kabbalah achieved

8. S. W. Baron, *A Social and Religious History of the Jews,* 2d ed., vol. 16 (New York, 1976), pp. 52–53, 309.

9. J. M. Davis, "Rabbi Yom Tov Lipman Heller, Joseph ben Isaac ha-Levi, and Rationalism in Ashkenazic Culture, 1550–1650," Ph.D. diss., Harvard University, 1990.

10. Ibid., pp. 11–113.

by Isserles and his students disintegrated in subsequent generations.[11] Second, Davis admits that there are gaping holes in the tradition of Ashkenazic rationalism, particularly in the hundred year period preceding Isserles. Given the lack of substantial evidence, it is difficult to assume facilely a direct link between the rational rabbis of fourteenth century Prague and their successors in the late sixteenth-century.[12] The evidence adduced by Davis can be reformulated in the following way: Although there were precedents for rationalistic activity in Ashkenazic culture from the twelfth century, no continuous tradition existed. Rather, an oscillation between rationalistic and antirationalistic pursuits describes more precisely the "legacy of our fathers."

The most recent phase of the debate about rationalism in Ashkenazic culture surrounds the publication of Jacob Elbaum's massive Hebrew study of Jewish cultural development between 1550 and 1620, whose title can be translated as "Openness and Insularity: Late Sixteenth-Century Jewish Ashkenazic Literature in Poland and Ashkenaz."[13] Despite the book's obvious value as an encyclopedic survey, Elbaum's interpretation of Jewish culture in this period, particularly in its rational elements, has encountered vigorous criticism. Most relevant to my subject is the unpublished review by Israel Ta-Shema,[14] which examines Elbaum's explanation of the blossoming of rabbinic and rational culture and its decline by 1620. Elbaum had attributed the blossoming to the impact of printed books, especially from Italy and the Ottoman Empire; the vital connections of Poland and Prague with Italy—both the presence of Italian Jews in Ashkenazic lands and the exposure of Polish and German Jews to Italy, especially through the study of medicine at universities; spiritual trends emanating from the land of Israel; and improved economic and physical conditions in central and eastern

11. Ibid., pp. 177–78.

12. Ibid., pp. 104–5.

13. J. Elbaum, *Petiḥut ve-Histagrut: Ha-Yeẓirah ha-Ruḥanit ha-Sifrutit be-Folin u-ve-Arẓot Ashkenaẓ be-Shalhe ha-Me'ah ha-Shesh Esreh* (Jerusalem, 1990). See also his "The Cultural Connections between Polish and Ashkenazic Jewry and Italian Jewry in the Sixteenth Century" (in Hebrew), *Galed* 7–8 (1985): 11–40.

14. My thanks to Professor Ta-Shema for allowing me to read a typescript of this unpublished review. See also M. J. Rosman, "Culture in the Book" (in Hebrew), *Zion* 56 (1991): 321–44.

Europe in the second half of the sixteenth century. In positing external stimuli as the primary reason for this cultural renaissance, Elbaum was expanding upon the thesis of Ben Sasson. His explanation for the transformation from "openness" to "insularity" was the diffusion of kabbalistic spirituality from the school of Isaac Luria of Safed, which produced a radical shift in cultural priorities.

Ta-Shema questions Elbaum's argument on several grounds. In the first place, most of the elements in the blossoming of Ashkenazic culture, such as printed books and contacts with Italy and the land of Israel, were present during and after its supposed decline. Ta-Shema acknowledges the deterioration of physical conditions in eastern Europe but questions its importance for cultural change. He also challenges the assumption that the diffusion of Lurianic kabbalah in Poland caused the region's cultural closure. In recent years, the assumption of Gershom Scholem that Luria "conquered" Poland has been questioned by several scholars.[15] Moreover, why should the kabbalah of the school of Luria precipitate closure, whereas the previous kabbalistic school of Moses Cordovero had sustained openness?

The ultimate issue for Ta-Shema, as it was for Kupfer and Kaplan, is defining the Ashkenazic cultural experience. Is insularity or openness the normal situation of Ashkenazic Jews? For Elbaum, Ta-Shema believes, the Ashkenazic norm was closure; thus the sixteenth-century renaissance was an anomaly stimulated by external factors. For Ta-Shema, despite his reservations about Kupfer's thesis, the situation is the opposite. Ashkenazic Jewry in the Middle Ages was open to external influences; despite a temporary decline in the late fourteenth century, Moses Isserles and his colleagues brought about a return to the creativity of an earlier period. The only differences between the sixteenth century and the Middle Ages were the greater size of the Jewish population and the availability of printed books. Ta-Shema acknowledges a shift in the seventeenth century to rabbinic commentary and spirituality, but he claims that insularity never pre-

15. See M. Idel, "One from a Town, Two from a Clan: A New Look at the Problem of the Diffusion of Lurianic Kabbalah and Sabbatianism" (in Hebrew), *Pe'amim* 44 (1991): 5–30 (in English in *Jewish History* 7 [1993]: 79–104); Y. Barnai, "Christian Messianism and the Portuguese Marranos: The Emergence of Sabbateanism in Smyrna," *Jewish History* 7 (1993): 19–26; Ze'ev Greis, *Sifrut ha-Hanhagot: Toldoteha u-Mekomah be-Ḥayye Ḥaside R. Yisrael Ba'al Shem Tov* (Jerusalem, 1990).

vailed. The broad cultural interests of the eighteenth-century rabbis Jonathan Eybeshitz and Jacob Emden confirm this impression for Ta-Shema.

The second scholarly debate took place before the one on rationalism, but for reasons that will become clear as this chapter unfolds, I have chosen to present it out of sequence. In 1958, Jacob Katz published the original Hebrew version of his classic book *Tradition and Crisis,* a study of the transformation of Jewish society in central and eastern Europe in the early modern period.[16] The work elicited strong reactions from several of Katz's colleagues.[17] I shall discuss Ḥayyim Hillel Ben Sasson's criticism of the book's depiction of cultural relations between Jews and Christians. Ben Sasson published his criticism as a long review essay; Katz uncharacteristically published a response to which Ben Sasson appended a final rejoinder.[18] Katz mentioned in his reply to Ben Sasson the imminent appearance of his book *Exclusiveness and Tolerance.*[19] With the publication of this volume, Katz presented a fuller exposition of his original themes.

In a chapter entitled "Ghetto Segregation," Katz describes relations between Jews and Christians in central and eastern Europe in the sixteenth and seventeenth centuries as dominated by Jewish exclusiveness and indifference to events in the outside world.[20] According to Katz, polemics against Christianity had virtually ceased by the sixteenth century, references to Jewish-Christian relations were increasingly rare in Jewish literature, and "Judaism now became, more than ever, a closed system of thought."[21] In this new environment, "Judaism

16. J. Katz, *Masoret u-Mashber: Ha-Ḥevra ha-Yehudit be-Moẓei Yemei ha-Beinayim* (Jerusalem, 1958) (trans. B. D. Cooperman, *Tradition and Crisis: Jewish Society at the End of the Middle Ages* [New York, 1993]).

17. See esp. the Hebrew review by S. Ettinger in *Kiryat Sefer* 35 (1959–60): 12–18; and H. H. Ben Sasson, "Concepts and Reality in Jewish History at the End of the Middle Ages" (in Hebrew), *Tarbiẓ* 29 (1959–60): 297–312.

18. J. Katz, " On the Halakha and the Derush as Historical Sources" (in Hebrew), *Tarbiẓ* 30 (1960–61): 62–68, followed by Ben Sasson's rejoinder, pp. 69–72.

19. Katz, "On the Halakha," p. 62; idem, *Exclusiveness and Tolerance: Studies in Jewish-Gentile Relations in Medieval and Modern Times* (Oxford, 1961).

20. Katz, *Exclusiveness and Tolerance,* pp. 131–42.

21. Ibid., p. 136.

sank into the lethargy of a mental attitude which accepted Jewish fundamental beliefs as uncontested truth. . . . The question which posed itself to the Jew of that time was not why, and in what, the Jewish and Christian religions differed. If any such question arose, it took the form: What are the special features and qualities of the Jew, and why is his destiny unique?"[22] In other words, Jews referred to non-Jewish beliefs as if they were abstractions; their adversary was more fictitious than real. Katz was astonished that such indifference prevailed at the height of the Reformation. Nevertheless, when the initial commotion over Luther had passed, Jews for the most part ceased to interest themselves in the religious differences plaguing the Christian world.[23]

The best example of this changed attitude, according to Katz, is found in the writings of the Maharal (Judah Loew ben Bezalel) of Prague. Although the Maharal mentions incidental encounters with Christians, the primary focus of his extensive writings is on the ancient dichotomy between Israel and the nations as a whole. The Maharal was concerned not with the doctrinal differences that separated Judaism from Christianity, but rather with the Jewish religion in its own right and the destiny of the Jewish people. Katz compares the Maharal's attitude with that of Judah Ha-Levi, claiming that the Maharal outdid his medieval predecessor in eliminating all historical and theological criteria from the definition of Judaism. No other thinker went as far as the Maharal in proclaiming the unique essence of Jewish peoplehood.[24] Katz concludes, "It is safe to assume that it was the isolation of Jewish life from that of the outside world which made such theories possible and acceptable."[25]

Later in the book, Katz discusses another characteristic of this period: the evaluation of Christianity as a nonidolatrous religion by a number of Jewish homily writers and legal commentators.[26] He quotes the opinion of Moses Rivkes, a Lithuanian rabbi who left Vilna for the West after the massacres of 1648. "But the peoples in whose shade we, the people of Israel, are exiled and amongst whom we are dispersed do in fact believe in *creatio ex nihilo* and in

22. Ibid., pp. 136–37.
23. Ibid., p. 138.
24. Ibid., pp. 138–42.
25. Ibid., p. 142.
26. Ibid., pp. 162–68.

the Exodus and in the main principles of religion, and their whole aim and intent is to the Maker of heaven and earth, as the codifiers have written."[27] Rivkes adds that Christians also share Jewish beliefs in prophecy and revelation and in the truth of the Hebrew Bible. Katz finally mentions similar sentiments regarding the shared traditions of Jews and Christians in the writings of the eighteenth-century rabbis Yair Bacharach and Jacob Emden.[28]

Katz's argument is flawed in two ways. In the first place, the comparison between the Maharal and Ha-Levi seems to undermine rather than confirm his impression about the theology of the former being shaped in isolation. As Ben Sasson pointed out,[29] Ha-Levi assaulted philosophy armed with an intimate knowledge of contemporary philosophy, science, and comparative religion. He composed his antiphilosophical work in the language of philosophers, Arabic. His advocacy of the unique destiny of Jews was prompted by engagement with the outside world, not by isolation.

Even more damaging to Katz's argument is the statement of Moses Rivkes, which suggests why Christian polemics and doctrinal disagreements between Judaism and Christianity had receded by the sixteenth century. Jews were not unaware of or indifferent to the struggles between the warring Christian camps, which had distracted Christian theologians from the "Jewish heresy." Christians of all persuasions were busy defining their faith and religious priorities. The Jewish minority in their midst was of little consequence to their debates. Some Jews perceived that Christianity, in its new guise, was less threatening as a religious faith to Jewish doctrine and belief. They even came to appreciate the similarities between the two faiths. In this new climate of religious upheaval, Jews like Rivkes regarded polemics as outdated and inappropriate. In cultural centers such as the cities of Italy or Amsterdam, polemical encounters on doctrinal matters had also receded in number and intensity.

If Jews and Christians hold similar doctrinal positions, their differences must be defined along social and ethnic lines: Jews have a different life-style, a dif-

27. Ibid., p. 165.

28. Ibid., pp. 166–67.

29. Ben Sasson, "Concepts and Reality," p. 307. For a discussion of the influence of philosophy in Arabic on Ha-Levi, see S. Pines, "Shi'ite Terms and Conceptions in Judah Ha-Levi's *Kuzari,*" *Jerusalem Studies in Arabic and Islam* 2 (1980): 165–251.

ferent psychological makeup, and a different spiritual destiny. The Maharal's formulations represent a realistic assessment of the new relations between Jews and Christians rather than an abstract theology conceived in isolation. For the Maharal, the Jew functions simultaneously on two levels: on a sphere of shared values and intellectual interest, and on a plane that differentiates him and his spiritual destiny from the rest of the world. This view, as I shall demonstrate below in reference to science, takes full cognizance of the world Jews share with Christians.

Ben Sasson questioned how Katz could portray a dynamic social and economic world existing simultaneously with an isolated intellectual world. His method of rebuttal was to offer literary evidence that Jews and Christians were fully aware of each other, such as observations on the Reformation by R. Ḥayyim ben Beẓalel, the brother of the Maharal;[30] debates between Christians and the Maharsha and Isaac Troki;[31] and especially David Gans's chronicle *Ẓemaḥ David,* which refers to the invention of the printing press, describes the landscape of Prague, displays pride in Bohemian traditions, and presents portraits of Hus and Luther and the Reformation, all from the perspective not only of a Jew but of an urban European.[32] Ben Sasson objected to Katz's characterization of the Maharal's theology as shaped in disengagement from the surrounding world. Moreover, he noted an Ashkenazic tradition of pride in the cultural environment flourishing from the twelfth century to the generation of Gans and the Maharal.[33]

Ben Sasson later wrote a pioneering essay on Jewish responses to the Reformation in which he quoted a number of long passages from the Maharal's writings that suggest beyond a doubt the influence of reformist attitudes such as biblicism and fundamentalism. The Maharal's notion of nationality as a kind of natural organism, while rooted in a specific Jewish reality, is expressed in terms suggesting the broader nationalistic context of Bohemia and Moravia from which

30. Ibid., pp. 302–3.
31. Ibid., pp. 303–4.
32. Ibid., pp. 305–7.
33. Ibid., pp. 307–10.

they resonate. The Maharal's denunciation of censorship and support for the free expression of ideas transcends Jewish particularistic concerns. For Ben Sasson, such declarations reflect the ideas of tolerance emanating from the enlightened court circles of Prague. There is no doubt in his mind about the profound impact religious and nationalistic ideas from Maharal's urban environment were having on the development of his thinking.[34]

Over the thirty years since the appearance of *Exclusiveness and Tolerance,* a large scholarly literature has focused on the three central figures of Jewish intellectual life in central and eastern Europe: Isserles, Gans, and the Maharal. Several authors have implicitly adopted Katz's position by treating Jewish cultural life in relative isolation from its surroundings. This is especially true of several studies of the Maharal and Isserles.[35] Gans, by virtue of his interest in history, geography, and astronomy, has been viewed as more fully attuned to his environment.[36] Whether Gans's case is the exception that proves the rule, or

34. H. H. Ben Sasson, "The Reformation in Contemporary Jewish Eyes" (in Hebrew with English translation), *Proceedings of the Israel Academy of Science and Humanities* 4, no. 5(1970–71): 62–166, esp. 68–73.

35. See, for example, B. Z. Bokser, *From the World of the Cabbala: The Philosophy of Rabbi Judah Loew of Prague* (New York, 1954); F. Thieberger, *Great Rabbi Loew of Prague* (London, 1955); A. Mauskopf, *The Religious Philosophy of the Maharal of Prague* (Brooklyn, 1949); B. L. Sherwin, *Mystical Theology and Social Dissent: The Life and Works of Judah Loew of Prague* (London and Toronto, 1982); R. Shatz, "The Doctrine of the Maharal: Between Existence and Eschatology" (in Hebrew), *Meshihi'ut ve-Eskatologia,* ed. Z. Baras (Jerusalem, 1984), pp. 167–85; idem, "The Legal Approach of the Maharal: Antithesis of Natural Law" (in Hebrew), *Da'at* 2–3 (1978–79): 147–57; A. Neher, *Le Puits de l'exil: La Théologie dialectique du Maharal de Prague* (Paris, 1966); B. Gross, *Nezah Yisra'el: Hashkafato ha-Meshihit shel ha-Maharal mi-Prag al ha-Galut ve-ha-Ge'ulah* (Tel Aviv, 1974); Y. Ben Sasson, *Mishnato ha-Iyyunit shel ha-Ramah* (Jerusalem, 1984); Elbaum, *Petihut ve-Histagrut;* and A. Siev, *R. Moses Isserles* (Jerusalem, 1957).

36. See, for example, G. Alter, "Two Renaissance Astronomers (Gans, Delmedigo)," *Rozpravy Československí Akademie Věda* 68 (1958): 9–14; M. Breuer, "The Characteristics of *Zemah David* of R. David Gans" (in Hebrew), *Ha-Ma'ayan* 5 (1965): 15–27; idem, "An Outline of R. David Gans' Image" (in Hebrew), *Bar Ilan* 11 (1973): 97–118; idem, "Modernism and Traditionalism in Sixteenth-Century Jewish Historiography: A Study of David Gans' *Tsemah David,*" in B. Cooperman, ed., *Jewish Thought in the Sixteenth Century* (Cambridge, Mass., 1983), pp. 49–88; idem, David Gans' *Zemah David* (Jerusalem, 1983); J. Sedinova, "Non-Jewish

whether his interaction with the outside was typical of many Jews, is a question to which we shall return later.

Two other studies of the Maharal take Ben Sasson's position. The first is Aharon Kleinberger's extensive comparison of the Maharal's pedagogic views with those of the Bohemian reformer J. A. Comenius. Kleinberger observes a parallelism between the two men, without claiming that they influenced each other.[37] The second study, by Otto Dov Kulka, sheds important new light on Jewish intellectual life in the Maharal's environment.[38] Kulka examines the Maharal's accounts of his engagements with Christian disputants, persuasively confirming Ben Sasson's assertion that in light of the Reformation controversies, a proper understanding of the Torah for Jews was uppermost in the Maharal's mind.

Ben Sasson referred to the Reformation as a general context for the Maharal's thinking,[39] while Martin Buber compared him with Calvin.[40] Kulka, however, argues that the Maharal's understanding of Jewish peoplehood was forged against the specific backdrop of intense nationalist ideologies in Moravia, Bohemia, and Posen from the age of Hus to that of Comenius. Competition between Germans and Czechs was particularly keen in Prague, where Jews lived among a Czech majority, a strong German minority, and a smaller Italian minority. Kulka singles out the Maharal's contemporary Jan Brahoslav, the leader of the Unitas Fratrum, as a potential influence.[41] The Czech followers of the Bohemian

Sources in the Chronicle by David Gans' Tsemaḥ David," *Judaica Bohemiae* 8 (1972): 3–15; A. Neher, *Jewish Thought and the Scientific Revolution of the Sixteenth Century: David Gans (1541–1613) and His Times,* translated from the French by D. Maisel (Oxford, 1986).

37. A. F. Kleinberger, *Ha-Maḥshava ha-Pedagogit shel ha-Maharal mi-Prag* (Jerusalem, 1962)

38. O. D. Kulka, "The Historical Background of the National and Educational Teaching of the Maharal of Prague" (in Hebrew), *Zion* 50 (1985): 277–320. See also M. Breuer, "The Maharal's Debate with the Christians: A New Look at *Sefer Be'er ha-Golah,*" *Tarbiz* 55 (1985): 253–60.

39. See works cited in nn. 17 and 34 above.

40. M. Buber, *Bein Am le-Arzo* (Jerusalem, 1985), pp. 86–99.

41. In addition to the references cited by Kulka, see M. S. Fousek, "The Ethos of the Unitas Fratrum," in M. Rechcigl, Jr., ed., *Czechoslovakia Past and Present,* vol. 2 (The Hague, 1968),

confession held strikingly similar views on educational reform to those of the Maharal and several of his disciples. Kulka plausibly suggests how the Maharal might have encountered the Brethren, convincingly undermining Katz's notion that his theology reflected an isolation from Prague's intellectual and religious life. Thus, Kulka has both buttressed the insights of Ben Sasson and offered an exemplary reexamination of Jewish culture in central and eastern Europe.

Nevertheless, Kulka's promising approach elicits two caveats. Anyone who has read R. J. W. Evans's masterful portrait of Rudolfine Prague cannot help sensing a certain incompleteness in Kulka's reconstruction.[42] Evans's Prague is more complex and multifaceted than the clerical circles of the Czech brethren. It is a world teeming with Lutherans, Calvinists, Old and New Utraquists, and Jesuits. Most important from the perspective of Jewish (and scientific) culture, it is a magnet for panosophic, eirenical, alchemical, Hermetic, and Rosicrucian influences, a culture "where science and art, experiment and speculation were still homogenous."[43] In the court of Rudolf II the occult arts reigned supreme, offering their practitioners a means of penetrating a higher reality. A universe traversed by the likes of Johann Pistorius, the Christian kabbalist, his colleagues John Dee, Michael Maier, Oswall Croll, and many others could hardly have gone unnoticed by a large and well-connected Jewish community within walking distance of the palace. Could Mordecai Maisel, the most affluent citizen of Prague, have avoided such company? Gans offers evidence that Rudolf toured the Jewish quarter in 1592 and even held a highly secret meeting with the Maharal.[44] In addition to Pistorius's kabbalistic tome, Evans mentions a tantalizing

---

pp. 1221–31; M. Strupl, "John Brahoslav: Father and Charioteer of the Lord's People in the Unitas Fratrum," ibid., 1232–246; and P. Brock, *The Political and Social Doctrines of the Unity of Czech Brethren in the Fifteenth and Early Sixteenth Centuries* (Mouton and The Hague, 1957).

42. R. J. W. Evans, *Rudolf II and His World: A Study in Intellectual History, 1576–1612* (Oxford, 1973). See also F. A. Yates, "Imperial Mysteries," *New Statesman,* May 18, 1973, pp. 734–35 (review of Evans); idem, *The Rosicrucian Enlightenment* (London and Boston, 1972); and T. Dacosta Kaufmann, *The Mastery of Nature: Aspects of Art, Science, and Humanism in the Renaissance* (Princeton, 1993).

43. Evans, *Rudolf II,* p. 161.

44. See Neher, *David Gans,* pt. 1, chaps. 1 and 5.

manuscript featuring a Czech translation of the *Sefer Raziel*,[45] leading him to ask: "What is the relevance of the world of Loew [the Maharal] to the world of Rudolf?"[46] No answer has been forthcoming in the more than twenty years since the publication of Evans's work. Given the mood of confessional reconciliation through philosophical and occult studies that marked Christian intellectual life in Rudolf's Prague, the passionate interest in kabbalah and Jewish magic on the part of some of Prague's leading intellectuals and political elite, and the intricate comingling of occultist, magical, and "scientific" pursuits in this era, it is difficult to assume that Kulka has given us the last word on the intellectual ambience invigorating some of the reflections of the Maharal and his colleagues or, for that matter, on the contemporaneous influence of Jewish thought on Christian thinking.

My second caveat concerns the difficulty of treating central and eastern European Jewish culture as one distinct entity.[47] Most of the scholarly treatments cited above (including those of Katz and Ben Sasson) assume a continuous landscape linking Poland and Lithuania with Bohemia and Germany. Elbaum's survey, for example, makes no distinctions at all between the different regions. It is certainly true that the links between Poland and Bohemia were significant: key Jewish intellectuals seem to have moved easily between Cracow, Posen, Prague, and other cities. And the influence of the Maharal and Isserles clearly transcends their local neighborhoods. The potential influence of the Czech Brethren on Jewish thought can be felt in both Poland and Bohemia, as Kulka has demonstrated. Nevertheless, regional variations may also be decisive in considering the possible dialogue between Jewish and Christian cultures, as illustrated by two small examples. Gans's chronicle was based on several contemporary histo-

---

45. Evans, *Rudolf II*, p. 237.

46. Ibid., p. 241.

47. This point has been raised recently in David Fishman's paper "R. Moses Isserles and the Study of Science among Polish Rabbis," pp. 19–20, to be published in the proceedings of a conference on Jacob Katz's book *Tradition and Crisis* by the Harvard Center for Jewish Studies. My thanks to Professor Fishman for providing me with a copy of his paper, a revised version of the first chapter of his doctoral dissertation "Science, Enlightenment, and Rabbinic Culture in Belorussian Jewry, 1772–1804," Harvard University, 1985.

ries composed in German.[48] In other words, the German coloring of Rudolfine Prague facilitated his entrance into the intellectual life of his city, including his well-publicized meetings with the astronomers Brahe and Kepler. On the other hand, a lack of competence in either Latin or Polish may have been among the factors hindering Jewish students in Isserles' circle from establishing meaningful links with the Christian intellectual community of Cracow. Furthermore, Christian Hebraism played a lesser role in Polish than in Czech culture. The only learned Hebraist at the University of Cracow in the sixteenth century was an immigrant from Mantua named Francesco Stancaro, who was accused of heresy.[49] The different cultural ambiances of Prague and Cracow naturally affected the quantity and quality of Jewish-Christian relationships in the two cities.

What does all of this have to do with the place of scientific activity in the culture of central and eastern European Jewry? The two aforementioned debates provide a springboard for a more focused examination of the subject. The major weakness of works that discuss the "Kupfer thesis" about rationalism in Ashkenazic culture is their failure to distinguish clearly between physics and metaphysics. This critical distinction, as we shall see, defines Ashkenazic rationalism in this period and represents the most important contribution of late sixteenth-century Ashkenazic thought to discussions of scientific activity in Jewish culture. Following the argument of Ben Sasson and others that Jewish culture should be linked more closely to its immediate intellectual context, I will argue that Jewish discussions about demarcating the spheres of physics and metaphysics did not take place in a vacuum, nor did they simply reiterate the positions of earlier Jewish thinkers. Instead, they probably reflected an emerging consensus of Protestant (and Catholic) thinkers about the appropriate structural relationship between scientific learning and Christian faith in the early modern era.

In order to fully substantiate these hypotheses, I now turn to some of the key Ashkenazic thinkers and texts that address the place of the natural sciences in Jewish culture. I am not the first to summarize this material. Jacob Elbaum

48. See Sedinova, "Non-Jewish Sources."
49. See Baron, *Social and Religious History,* pp. 53–58.

devoted an entire chapter of his book to the subject.[50] More recently, David Fishman has presented a cogent summary of the topic based on his doctoral dissertation.[51] I will rely heavily on both expositions, along with other recent work on individual thinkers, in offering my own interpretation.

Although isolated references suggest that Jews in eastern Europe were engaged in scientific learning prior to the second half of the sixteenth century, the first substantial evidence relates to the rabbinic luminary Moses Isserles of Cracow (1525–1572).[52] Fishman correctly emphasizes that his learning (and that of his disciples) was concerned almost exclusively with astronomy and was clearly a byproduct of Talmudic scholarship. Moses Maimonides' medieval treatise on the laws of the sanctification of the new moon had encouraged the study of the heavens on purely halakhic grounds, and thus commentaries and elaborations on his work constituted an independent area of halakhic specialization within Talmudic studies.[53] Two of Isserles' works are concerned with astronomical issues: *Torat ha-Olah* (Prague, 1570), the first eleven chapters of which correlate the measurements of the Temple in Jerusalem and the meaning of the sacrifices with astronomical and cosmological processes; and his unpublished commentary on George Peurbach's *Theoricae Novae Planetarum,* based on the Hebrew translation of Ephraim Mizraḥi entitled *Mahalakh ha-Kokhavim* (The course of the stars).[54]

Isserles' astronomical knowledge was based entirely on an indigenous tradition of Hebrew sources: he had access to Peurbach's standard textbook only through a Hebrew translation and, in his famous reply to his antagonistic col-

50. Elbaum, *Petiḥut ve-Histagrut,* pp. 248–279.

51. See n. 47 above.

52. See the works of Y. Ben Sasson and A. Siev listed in n. 35 above, as well as H. Davidson, "Medieval Jewish Philosophy in the Sixteenth Century," in Cooperman, *Jewish Thought,* pp. 132–36.

53. See Fishman, "R. Moses Isserles," pp. 12–14.

54. The introduction to the commentary was published by Siev, *R. Moshe Isserles,* pp. 177–178. See Ms. Oxford Bodleian Opp. 1673 [Neubauer n. 2033], fols. 149a-194b. See esp. Y. Tzvi Langermann, "The Astronomy of Rabbi Moses Isserles," in S. Unguru, ed., *Physics, Cosmology, and Astronomy, 1300–1700* (The Netherlands, 1991), pp. 83–98. On Peurbach, see C. Doris Hellman and N. M. Swerdlow, "Peurbach, Georg," *Dictionary of Scientific Biography* 15 (1978): 473–79; and E. J. Aiton, "Peubach's *Theoricae novae planentarum:* A Translation with Commentary," *Osiris,* 2d ser., 3 (1987): 5–43.

league Solomon Luria, he sanctioned the study of the sciences among Jews only with respect to works written in Hebrew. Nevertheless, one might ponder the origin of his fascination with astronomy. His knowledge of the subject, and particularly of contemporary developments, is hardly impressive. Herbert Davidson is unquestionably right in characterizing his efforts, like those of the Maharal's, as harmonizing disparate texts rather than addressing real problems.[55] He displays little intellectual curiosity, approaching astronomy like a Talmudist preoccupied with reconciling conflicting interpretations.

On the other hand, can Isserles' genuine interest in the heavenly movements be reduced to rabbinic concerns alone? Although the laws on the sanctification of the new moon were studied in different times and places, Jewish intellectuals were particularly drawn to this subject in settings that generally valued astronomy as a discipline of value in its own right. As we have seen, Maimonides, Abraham Bar Ḥiyya, Abraham ibn Ezra, and others were surely inspired by the philosophical and scientific ambiance of medieval Spain. Is it sufficient to say that Isserles was a faithful student of the Maimonidean tradition of integrating astronomical and rabbinic learning, that he was merely following the tradition of his Ashkenazic forebears, and that his ardent disciples walked in his footsteps out of respect for their teacher? Does this explain why a preoccupation with astronomy arose in Isserles' generation and not before? Does it explain the anti-Maimonidean deemphasizing of medicine and natural philosophy, the thunderous opposition of Solomon Luria and before him Joseph Ashkenazi,[56] and the precipitous decline and virtual disappearance of astronomical study by the third decade of the seventeenth century? Can we ignore the larger intellectual context of Cracow? Was it merely a coincidence that Isserles lived in the same city where Copernicus had written his revolutionary work? Fishman

---

55. Davidson, "Medieval Jewish Philosophy," p. 139.

56. On Ashkenazi's opposition to philosophy and astronomy, see P. Bloch, "Der Streit um den Moreh des Maimonides in der Gemeinde Posen um die Mitte des XVI Jahrhunderts," *Monatsschrift für Geschichte und Wissenschaft des Judentums* 47 (1903): 153–169, 263–279, 346–356; G. Scholem, "New Information on R. Joseph Ashkenazi, 'The Tanna of Safed'" (in Hebrew), *Tarbiẓ* 28 (1959–60): 59–89, 201–35; I. Twersky, "R. Joseph Ashkenazi and the Mishneh Torah of Maimonides" (in Hebrew), *Salo Baron Jubilee Volume* (Jerusalem, 1975), pp. 182–194.

himself muses that "it may not be too imaginative to suggest that Isserles was aware of the study of astronomy at the University of Cracow."[57]

The only scholar who has seriously studied Isserles' astronomical speculations, Y. Tzvi Langermann, can point to no evidence linking Isserles to his immediate surroundings.[58] Albertus de Brudzewo's commentary on Peurbach (Cracow, 1495) appears to be unrelated to Isserles' work.[59] More relevant are the Hebrew commentaries of Moses Almosnino and Mattathias Delacrut that preceded Isserles.[60] Yet, at the very least, Isserles' choice to comment on a standard astronomical textbook based on traditional but still current Aristotelian and Ptolemaic notions of the universe is more than an act of rabbinic piety. Granted, examining the laws of the sanctification of the new moon or reconciling rabbinic and Greek notions of the universe constitute nothing more than extensions of Talmudic scholarship. But by writing a commentary on a general astronomical work, had Isserles not taken the rabbinic mandate a major step forward? Surely he had in mind the introduction of a systematic curriculum of astronomical study, far beyond any meaningful digressions on the subject that might have evolved haphazardly from Talmudic studies. And could such a bold pedagogic move for a scholar so preoccupied with halakhic issues be solely an echo of past traditions rather than a tentative acknowledgment of the dramatically new focus on astronomical study in his own immediate environment? Was it sheer coincidence that in Isserles' day the Cracow school of astronomy had underscored the importance of detaching observational and mathematical astronomy from philosophical study, perceiving it as worthy of investigation in its own right?[61]

57. Fishman, "R. Moses Isserles." p. 15.

58. See n. 54 above.

59. Langermann, "Astronomy," p. 85.

60. See M. Steinschneider, *Die hebraeischen Uebersetzungen des Mittelalters und die Juden als Dolmetscher* (Berlin, 1893), pp. 639–41, 645–46.

61. See A. Wroblewski, "The Cracovian Background of Nicholas Copernicus," in S. Fishman, ed., *The Polish Renaissance in Its European Context* (Bloomington and Indianapolis, 1988), pp. 147–60; P. W. Knoll, "The Arts Faculty at the University of Cracow at the End of the Fifteenth Century," in R. Westman, ed., *The Copernican Achievement* (Berkeley and Los Angeles, 1975), pp. 137–56; C. Morawski, *Histoire de l'Université de Cracovie* (Paris, 1905), 3:173–203.

To be sure, nothing in Langermann's study of the Peurbach commentary suggests genuine intellectual curiosity on Isserles' part. He refuses to open himself up to any cosmological speculation; he follows unswervingly the principle of circular heavenly motion; and he remains conservative in explicating the standard medieval views on cosmology. This is in striking contrast to his more imaginative positions in *Torat ha-Olah*. Langermann singles out Isserles' spirited defense of the traditional view of *creatio ex nihilo,* challenging the Aristotelian notion that the heavenly motions are eternal and unchanging.[62] Since the moon's motion is neither uniform nor circular but rather spiral and wobbly, Isserles argues, it is perhaps desirable to assert that the heavenly bodies undergo generation and corruption. Some individual orbs of the moon are characterized by *hipukh* (contrariety) and manifestly violate the basic principle that each body is supposed to have only one uniform motion. Langermann points out that in his general philosophical work Isserles proves to be more open to alternative cosmological schemes, particularly in the service of defending and reconciling theological principles. But in his commentary written "for pedagogic rather than investigative purposes," he is rigidly conservative and unimaginative.[63] We might add that in transitional periods, as Robert Bonfil has argued, an overt conservatism often masks novelty and independence.[64] Despite the precedents Isserles vigorously invokes to obscure the novelty, teaching Peurbach to a classroom of rabbinic students in Cracow is undoubtedly an audacious act, which we might expect to be introduced with caution and in the most conservative manner possible.

Only if one views Isserles' commentary as a bold pedagogic innovation, albeit tentative and conservative in its formulation—as an accommodation to and recognition of the privileged place of astronomy within the larger cultural world of Cracow, and not merely as a pious fidelity to previous Jewish traditions—can the controversy between Isserles and Luria be fully appreciated. Luria's charge that Isserles' students had composed a prayer in honor of Aris-

62. *Torat ha-Olah* (Lemberg, 1858), 3:49.

63. Langermann, "Astronomy," p. 95.

64. R. Bonfil, "Preaching as Mediation between Elite and Popular Cultures: The Case of Judah Del Bene," in D. B. Ruderman, ed., *Preachers of the Italian Ghetto* (Berkeley and Los Angeles, 1992), pp. 67–88.

totle is made within the context of his general objection to mixing rabbinic studies and philosophy.[65] Isserles opens his response by deflating the seriousness of Luria's concern, indicating that his opponent's worry is no more than "an old debate among the sages which doesn't require an answer from me" since the Rashba [Solomon ibn Adret (ca. 1235–ca. 1310)] had fully addressed the issue of philosophy several hundred years earlier.[66] The Rashba had specifically prohibited young students alone from the study of astronomy. Isserles also recalls the responsum of the Ribash [Isaac ben Sheshet Perfet (1326–408)], who limited the meaning of the "Greek sciences" to riddles hidden from the masses. The Ribash explicitly permitted "*the famous books on nature*" [my emphasis] and only cautioned restraint when reading works that might damage faith in divine providence and creation.[67]

Having summarized the position of the earlier respondents, Isserles proceeds to respond directly to his critic. In the first place, he claims, the rabbis "only feared the study of the cursed Greeks like the book of physics together with the metaphysics as they are mentioned there in the aforementioned responsum. And they are surely justified in this since they feared lest someone be led to follow some [false] belief or be charmed by their wine, which is the venom of asps [68] and false opinions. However, they did not forbid the study of the *words of the scholars and their investigations on the essence of reality and its natures. On the contrary, through this [study], the greatness of the Creator of the world, may He be blessed, is made known* [my emphasis], which is the true meaning of *shi'ur komah* [the measurement of God's stature]. Our sages declared concerning this: 'He who knows [how to calculate the cycles and planetary courses but does not do so, of him Scripture states: "But they regard not works of God, neither have they considered the work of His hand" (Isaiah 5:12)].'"[69]

---

65. Isserles, *Responsa*, no. 6, pp. 23–29.

66. Isserles, *Responsa*, no. 7, p.29–30, where A. Siev provides the appropriate citation in his notes.

67. Ibid., no. 11, p. 31.

68. Based on Deut. 32:33.

69. Isserles, *Responsa*, p. 31, quoting B. T. Shabbat 75a. As Fishman points out ("R. Moses Isserles," p. 12), although he speaks in general about nature study, he quotes a rabbinic passage on astronomy.

Isserles' third and final point is to emphasize that even if all non-Jewish books had been prohibited because of the pernicious ideas they contained, the rabbis would never have forbidden works "of our own sages from whose waters we drink, and especially the great rabbi Maimonides."[70] He concludes: "Therefore I also state that I am innocent of this iniquity, for although I have quoted occasionally from Aristotle's words, I swear by heaven and earth that I have never consulted any of his works except what I found in the *Guide [of the Perplexed]*, in which I toiled and found praise of God and in the other *works on nature* [my emphasis], such as the *The Gate of Heaven* and the like composed by the rabbis. From these alone I copied the words of Aristotle."[71] He cites Maimonides as saying that all that Aristotle understood in the sublunary world, and even beyond, is considered true, with the exception of some beliefs "dependent on God, his angels, and spheres," in which he deviated from the truth.[72]

A common thread links these three answers: That part of philosophy which concerns itself with metaphysical speculation undermines the cardinal principles of the Jewish belief, is dangerous, and should be prohibited. However, that part which concerns itself with knowledge about the processes of the natural world is not only religiously permitted but is praiseworthy. By first referring to the Ribash's responsum upholding this position, by stating explicitly his approval of the study of the "essence of reality and its natures," and by placing the *Guide of the Perplexed* in the category of nature books and quoting Maimonides on the truth value of Aristotle's words on the natural world, Isserles consistently differentiates the study of metaphysics from that of physics. To be sure, some confusion remains in this answer. Maimonides' philosophy treats both physics and metaphysics together. Yet Isserles juxtaposes Maimonides' composition with that of Gershom of Arles, an actual encyclopedia of nature, calling them both works of nature. Then he immediately underscores this point by quoting Maimonides' acknowledgment of Aristotle's reliability with reference to the natural sublunary world alone. It is as if he is saying that even when metaphysics is

70. Isserles, *Responsa*, p. 32.

71. Ibid. Isserles refers to the thirteenth-century writer Gershom ben Solomon of Arles, author of *The Gate of Heaven* (ed. and trans. F. S. Bodenheimer [Jerusalem, 1953]).

72. Ibid.

treated by Maimonides, the philosophical views have been sanitized by the Jewish pedigree of the author. They are safe theologically to study; however, their real importance to Jewish students is their focus on the natural world per se.

Isserles does not single out astronomy in his answer to Luria but speaks generally about the study of nature, since initially their controversy had focused on a halakhic issue related to mineralogy and biology.[73] Throughout the responsum he deems it important to justify himself by constant recourse to his mentor, Maimonides. If Maimonides had successfully integrated the study of nature with the Jewish faith, Isserles was merely following in his footsteps in "the way of our ancestors." But one should not fail to appreciate the obvious disagreement between Isserles and Maimonides on astronomy, and by extension on all naturalistic pursuits—a disagreement that Isserles seemingly had no desire to expose in his apologetic response. However, in *Torat ha-Olah,* Isserles again quotes Maimonides' statement about Aristotle possessing the truth about the sublunary world. This time, however, he is less vague on the human ability to grasp reality beyond the moon. Instead of admitting that Aristotelian metaphysics may have some validity, he offers the full force of Maimonides' argument that all statements about the superlunary world are only hypothetical.[74] But then he strenuously objects to Maimonides' position regarding rabbinic speculations on astronomy. For Maimonides had written "that the field of astronomy was not complete during the time of the prophets and early sages, but the observer should be appalled to think that the rabbis didn't know what they were saying."[75] To admit Maimonides' position would have undermined Isserles' assumption that the rabbis' knowledge could and should be harmonized with current astronomical information.[76] It would have shattered his belief in

73. Isserles, *Responsa,* no. 5, pp. 18–23, esp. p. 19 on the definition of "tinara" in rabbinic texts.

74. *Torat ha-Olah,* p. 22a.

75. Ibid., p. 22b, quoting *Guide of the Perplexed,* 3:14; and see my discussion in chap. 1.

76. Azariah de' Rossi expands Maimonides' position to include all rabbinic non-halakhic statements and thus provokes the wrath of the Maharal. Note his reaction to Isserles' harmonization as translated by Fishman, "R. Moses Isserles," p. 30, from *Me'or Einayim,* Imre Binah 11:179–80 (Vilna, 1866; repr. Jerusalem, 1970): "One cannot believe that our sages were of his opinion. And if they intended to say what he says, then they did not fully comprehend these

the infallibility of rabbinic sapience and ultimately subverted the defense of his position against Luria. It was better to conceal their differences, to becloud both Maimonides' skepticism regarding astronomical knowledge, especially with regard to the rabbis, and his scholastic belief that metaphysics and physics were still firmly connected.

Despite the obscurity of his answer to his rabbinic colleague, and despite the seeming traditionalism of his astronomical commentary, the pedagogical and theological novelty of Isserles' position should not be overlooked. In the first case, he had effectively championed the autonomous study of nature within the Ashkenazic curriculum; in the second, he had tentatively severed the medieval link between physics and metaphysics—something which the Maharal would do even more boldly and decisively.[77]

In most accounts of the study of the natural world among eastern European Jewry, the Maharal is cited for his approval of the discipline and for his support of the investigations of others, especially his student David Gans, but he is generally thought to have remained on the sidelines, preoccupied with general theological and pedagogic concerns and producing no original work of his own.[78] André Neher notes a seeming correlation between the Maharal's com-

---

matters. And I say regarding him: if you wish to bring a burnt-offering [*Olah*] to the Lord, offer it unto the truth. But it is preferable to be silent than to justify the righteous ones with impossible arguments."

77. In private communications, Y. Tzvi Langermann and David Berger question my interpretation of Isserles as an advocate of the autonomous study of nature and its separation from metaphysics. Langermann points out that Isserles' general tendency was to obfuscate rather than delineate boundaries, so that Luria could never pin him down. He accordingly mentions in one breath "the essence of reality" [is this physics or metaphysics?] and the *shi'ur komah* [a kabbalistic notion], and then cites a rabbinic statement about astronomy. In the *Torat ha-Olah,* he freely harmonizes physics with metaphysics, kabbalah with philosophy. I recognize the veiled obscurity of Isserles' reply to Luria and the harmonizing tendencies of his other writing. However, I still maintain that one can detect a tentative acknowledgment of the integrity of nature study in Isserles' answer and even an attempt, albeit unsuccessful, to separate physics from metaphysics. In this sense, Isserles was moving in the direction of the Maharal's decisive delineation.

78. Fishman's comment ("R. Moses Isserles," p. 20) is typical in this regard: "As for the Maharal, he did not write any original astronomical treatises himself. His favorable comments

ments on the sun and those of Brahe, as if to regain for him a central place in astronomical speculation among Ashkenazic Jewry.[79] The supposed parallel between the two is interesting but unconvincing: the focus of the Maharal's intellectual activity lay elsewhere than in theorizing about the heavens.

It is perplexing to underscore the novelty and currency of astronomical study among Ashkenazic Jewry at the end of the sixteenth century, while relegating its most important and systematic thinker to the periphery. Fishman handles this problem by seeing Isserles as the real pioneer in this discipline and by arguing that Poland, not Prague, was the center of Jewish astronomical writing in this era. Although three of Isserles' major students in this discipline—Mordecai Yaffe, Yom Tov Lipmann Heller, and David Gans—spent part of their careers in Prague, Fishman points out that each had initiated his study in Poland.[80] Such a distinction appears to me to be arbitrary, especially in the case of Gans, whose critical transformation obviously took place in Prague in the company of Brahe and Kepler. But it does explain why the Maharal of Prague had little to contribute to a subject of great importance to his closest colleagues.

I believe that the Maharal's specific contribution to the study of the sciences is much greater than Fishman and others have acknowledged. Although he left no scientific writing per se, the Maharal's discussions of the theory of knowledge, the criteria of establishing truth, and the relation between religious belief and scientific investigation have had a critical impact on Jewish thinkers throughout the modern period. As I have already suggested, the Maharal's most important clarification was to disentangle natural philosophy from the assumptions and restraints of Jewish theology and Aristotelian metaphysics, and in so doing to provide an autonomous realm in which scientific pursuit could legitimately flourish.

The Maharal's appreciation of the study of nature as a religious obligation is reminiscent of Isserles. He too paraphrases Maimonides' statement about Aristotle, but less tentatively and ambiguously than Isserles: "We should pay

---

about the discipline indicate that he was a beneficiary and supporter of the Polish tradition established by Isserles." See also Kleinberger, *Ha-Maḥshava ha-Pedagogit*, pp. 80–81.

79. Neher, *Jewish Thought*, pp. 245–50.

80. Fishman, "R. Moses Isserles," pp. 19–20, taking issue with both Breuer and Neher (see nn. 35 and 36 above).

attention to what the scholars of the nations have said about what is below the sphere of the moon because they were *scholars of the natural world* [my emphasis] . . . but we should not pay any attention to what they say regarding what is beyond nature."[81] He is open to learning from non-Jews, because they also acquired their knowledge through divine agency. Like Isserles, he asserts that "Greek wisdom" is not synonymous with the study of nature. Study of the the former is not permitted, "but study of the sciences that focus on reality and the order of the world is certainly permitted. . . . They are like a ladder to ascend to the science of the Torah."[82] And like Isserles, the Maharal privileges astronomy among all the sciences: "But one is surely required to study the science of the movement of the stars and spheres."[83] He even notes explicitly the dynamic quality of the sciences of his day, mentions the master "of the new astronomy," and seems fully aware of the alternative account of astronomical motion Copernicus had proposed.[84] While noticing the scientific progress of his day, he boldly affirms that "one should and is required to learn everything that focuses on the essence of the world, because everything is the work of God. So one should focus on it and recognize his Creator through it."[85] The sentiment is merely a paraphrase of Maimonidean piety; the context, however, is surely the exciting world of post-Copernican astronomical discovery at the end of the sixteenth century.

It is in the Maharal's discussion of the place of miracles in Jewish thought, as Tamar Ross has demonstrated,[86] that the uniqueness of his position is most clearly observed. In opposition to the medieval rationalistic tradition, the Maharal is generally unwilling to reconcile the natural order with the miraculous. They reflect different realities, and neither undermines the other. As Ross points out, the Maharal formulates an original position in arguing that each domain of reality is legitimate and truthful in its own right. The difference between view-

81. *Netivot Olam,* Netiv ha-Torah 14 (Jerusalem, 1980), p. 59.

82. Ibid., p. 60.

83. Ibid.

84. Ibid., pp. 60–61.

85. Ibid., p. 61.

86. T. Ross, "The Miracle as an Additional Dimension in the Thought of the Maharal of Prague" (in Hebrew), *Da'at* 17 (1986): 81–96.

ing a phenomenon of nature as a miracle and as an integral part of the natural order is a matter of perspective.[87] Objecting to Gersonides' understanding of the miracle of the sun standing still in the book of Joshua, the Maharal questions the philosopher's working assumption that "two opposites cannot exist with respect to the same subject simultaneously." On the contrary, he argues, "it is possible that the sun follows its accustomed course while [at the same time] it stands still as a miracle. For it is possible for one subject to possess two opposite conditions because of two perspectives—the course of nature being one unique subject and the unnatural, the other. . . . Thus for Joshua and his people who needed the unnatural miracle, [the sun] stood still, but for the rest of the world who did not require the miracle, they experienced the natural course [of the sun]."[88]

Given the separation between the two realms, a person who operates exclusively within one can never comprehend the other: "Since man, who is natural, can only understand the natural, the supernatural will always be hidden from him. He cannot conceive it on the basis of his knowledge. Thus all miracles are impossible from [the vantage point] of nature, but from [the vantage point] of the separate [that is, miraculous] world beyond nature, they are possible."[89] As Ross points out, the distinction between the world of nature and a higher world is ultimately a Platonic notion, one that can be located in the writing of medieval Jewish thinkers like Ha-Levi and Naḥmanides.[90] As we have seen, Naḥmanides' idea of the "hidden miracle" is close to that of the Maharal's in allowing for the theoretical coexistence of the natural order and the miraculous.[91] But the Maharal differs in his insistence that each domain is legitimate in its own right and that neither contradicts the other. Drawing an analogy from the nature of rabbinic disagreements, where "these and these are the words of the living God,"[92] the Maharal views the naturalist and the believer in miracles

87. Ibid., esp. pp. 89–92.

88. *Sefer Gevurot ha-Shem* (New York, 1969), pp. 15–16.

89. Ibid., p. 16.

90. Ross, "Miracle," p. 90.

91. See chap. 1 above.

92. For a full discussion of this rabbinic paradox, see Kleinberger, *Ha-Maḥshava ha-Pedagogit,* pp. 64–66, and Ross, "The Miracle," p. 93, n. 64.

as each grasping a single aspect of reality. Each must listen to the other to gain a complete understanding of the truth. While the Torah offers a deeper insight into creation, it undermines neither the autonomy of the natural order nor the naturalist's understanding of that order.

The Maharal presents the clearest exposition of his position in his well-publicized critique of Azariah de' Rossi's *Me'or Einayim*.[93] The Mantuan Jewish scholar had attempted to justify the extraordinary liberties he had taken in correcting apparently mistaken rabbinic chronologies and facts by adducing Maimonides' stance vis-à-vis rabbinic astronomy.[94] Maimonides did not regard rabbinic statements on the heavens as fact, and especially not as divine truths. When the rabbis spoke on such matters, they merely voiced personal opinions and reflected the cultural and intellectual assumptions of their times. Since these statements were not Torah, they could be rejected in favor of more informed opinion from contemporary astronomers. Abraham Maimonides had reiterated the same stance but had extended it to include all rabbinic statements about the natural world, including medicine. De' Rossi went even farther. For him, rabbinic statements about chronology or homilies relating information about the natural and social world were not necessarily divine revelation. They were personal opinions that could be corrected, revised, or even rejected when contradicted by contemporary scholarship. For de' Rossi, rabbinic *aggadot* should be read and evaluated like any other literary works and were subject to the same criteria of truth. When rabbinic dicta were compared with Greek and Latin historical sources, the former's standards could be proved deficient and ultimately rejected. For this reason, the forced efforts of Isserles to uphold the opinions of the sages in the face of contradictory scientific truth were ludicrous to de' Rossi.[95]

In mixing the words of the "separate world" of the Torah with the "natural world" of historical scholarship, de' Rossi (and ironically Isserles as well) deeply

93. *Be'er ha-Golah,* be'er 6 (New York, 1969), pp. 105–41; the critique of de' Rossi begins on p. 126. For a recent discussion of this controversy, see L. Segal, *Historical Consciousness and Religious Tradition in Azariah de' Rossi's "Me'or Einayim"* (Philadelphia, 1989), pp. 133–61.

94. See chap. 1 above.

95. See the discussion in Segal, *Historical Consciousness.* De' Rossi's reaction to Isserles' work is quoted in n. 76 above.

offended the Maharal's sensibility. As he constantly states, one should judge "the words of Torah alone and the words of their science alone."[96] Although de' Rossi did not refer to astronomy per se, the Maharal linked his approach to that of the astronomers who had conceivably contradicted rabbinic sapience. In his long chapter on defending the integrity of a large selection of rabbinic homilies, he begins with those dealing with astronomy before taking up his assault against his Italian colleague.[97] In essence, the astronomer and the historian share the same methodological fallacy. They reduce the truths of the Torah to a naturalistic understanding, thereby confusing the understanding appropriate to one realm of cognition with that of the other. The astronomers, like de' Rossi the chronologist, can relate only to the visible and perceivable; they can never comprehend the essence of creation. This is why de' Rossi's attempt to evaluate rabbinic sapience by the standards of the naturalist is a total misreading of rabbinic tradition: "The rabbis don't comment from the perspective of the natural cause, since it is small and inferior. This is appropriate for naturalists or doctors but not for rabbis, who speak from the perspective of the [final] cause which compels nature."[98] To read their words superficially and literally, one misses the secret meaning they impart.

What is significant about the Maharal's answer is not solely its defense of the integrity, relevance, and authority of rabbinic knowledge against the contemporary assaults of scientific and historical scholarship. More crucial is his consistent understanding of the appropriate relationship between science and faith and their differing perspectives and methodologies; his appreciation of the intrinsic value of exploring the natural world along with a recognition of its epistemological limitations; and his strategy of demarcating God's word and human reason, of removing the competition between the two, and thus allowing each to function separately and, paradoxically, harmoniously.

Despite the Maharal's respect for Maimonides, he is no Maimonidean. Rationalism in its medieval sense as a priori metaphysics is anathema to him. As we have seen, it is only a posteriori physics which he deems permissible and desirable. Why physics and not metaphysics? Because the former does not claim to

96. *Be'er ha-Golah,* p. 118, but the sentiment is expressed constantly throughout the chapter.
97. Ibid., pp. 105–126.
98. Ibid., p. 106.

be truth; it should not even be considered a science in the sense of yielding an absolute truth: "It is not even appropriate to call the science of astronomy a science because science is only attainable by one who actually knows something as it is, and that condition you will never find in their [so-called] science, for no one can verify its truth, and what is the difference if one lies a great deal or lies a little? In the final analysis, he can never know the truth of a thing . . . he can never know its essence. He will only know that it existed in such a way, but this can never be called science."[99] Because the only true science is that of the Torah, which alone can penetrate the essence of a thing, only its knowledge is certain and indubitable. The naturalist functions in a world of appearances; he knows only what his finite senses allow him to know. Rational pursuit, having been cut down to size, can now be valued. Its findings are tentative and contingent; it can never grasp complete reality. It can never be confident in its conclusions without the aid and intervention of divine sapience as revealed at Sinai. At the same time, it is liberated from a closed rational system that postulates how the world originated and how it is supposed to run. In its newly formulated domain, it is free to roam where it pleases, to experiment, to imagine new possibilities and fresh insights. The Maharal was no scientist, but he had formulated a theological structure whereby Jewish faith was safeguarded from science and science was protected from the unwarranted intrusions of Jewish faith.

David Gans, Isserles' and the Maharal's most outstanding student in the sciences, has been the subject of recent studies by André Neher, who devoted an entire book to his scientific interests and especially to his astronomical text *Neḥmad ve-Na'im,* and Mordecai Breuer, who edited and studied his historical chronicle *Ẓemaḥ David.*[100] As with Isserles and the Maharal, I shall restrict myself to making a few observations about Gans's thought which are relevant to the central issues raised in this chapter.

Three features strike the reader of Gans's two works. First, he appears to be a more knowledgeable and up-to-date student of the sciences, particularly cosmology and astronomy, than any of his Jewish contemporaries. His primary

99. Ibid., p. 119.
100. See n. 36 above.

exposure to the Rudolfine observatory and his contact with Brahe and Kepler obviously inspired his enthusiasm for and knowledge of contemporary astronomy. At the same time, his learning and tentativeness as a student did not allow him to progress beyond the level of his teachers. Despite his awareness of the Copernican view, he ultimately retreated to a safe geocentric position, reflecting, as Neher plausibly argues, the positions of Brahe and Kepler as of 1600.[101]

Second, Gans is eclectic, sends conflicting messages, and consciously avoids taking strong, controversial stands. Although fully aware of the differences between his two Jewish teachers, he respectfully presents their positions without attempting to reconcile them. Thus he cites *Torat ha-Olah* on the need to explain rationally the sages' understanding of nature,[102] and at the same time refers to the Maharal's emphatic separation of rabbinic and scientific knowledge in his *Be'er ha-Golah*.[103] Untidier still are his references to de' Rossi and Eliezer Ashkenazi,[104] his silence concerning their disagreements with the Maharal, and his seeming acceptance of the Maimonidean position that the rabbis' opinions on astronomy need not be deemed authoritative.[105] There is, in contrast, his remarkable account of a conversation with Brahe, who vindicates rabbinic opinion against the regnant and ultimately fallacious position of medieval astronomy.[106] For Neher, this lovely anecdote is the culmination of Gans's book.[107] It is probably an exaggeration, although there is no doubt that Gans, like Tobias Cohen and others after him, was motivated to write his astronomy by a sense of inadequacy and a desire to bolster Jewish pride. The approbation of so illustrious a Christian astronomer was bound to leave a positive and dramatic imprint on Gans's Jewish readers. Yet despite Brahe's gesture, whether real or imagined, the book can hardly be seen as advocating Jewish superiority in science. On the contrary, by putting together a conventional handbook on the subject, includ-

101. Neher, *Jewish Thought*, pp. 216–50.

102. *Neḥmad ve-Na'im* (Jesnitz, 1743), p. 8a.

103. Ibid.

104. Ibid., pp. 9a–9b. On the Maharal's disagreement with Ashkenazi, see Sherwin, *Mystical Theology*, pp. 58–62.

105. Ibid., p. 7b, where he even quotes the *Guide* 3:14.

106. Ibid., p. 82b.

107. Neher, *Jewish Thought*, pp. 216–28.

ing a smattering of up-to-date information from Prague, Gans left the distinct impression that Jews may have once been proficient in the field but now lagged painfully behind their Christian contemporaries.[108]

The third striking feature of Gans's work is that notwithstanding his limited knowledge of both astronomy and history and his unspectacular conclusions, his efforts in both areas are still quite unconventional from a Jewish point of view. Although incapable of taking a definite position with respect to the conflicting views of his mentors, both Jewish and Christian, he is still decisive in choosing to write in secular disciplines and in eschewing rabbinic pursuits. He stands virtually alone as a chronicler of Bohemian Jewry[109] and, with the exception of the brilliant but complex Joseph Delmedigo, is the only Jewish author of his generation to write an original treatise on theoretical astronomy, as opposed to works devoted to the laws on the sanctification of the new moon.[110] Even his teacher's commentary on Peurbach pales in significance in comparison with Gans's systematic and unique presentation.

While both Isserles and the Maharal had singled out astronomy as the science deserving special honor and attention on the part of Jewish students, Gans goes beyond both in actually composing a "Jewish" astronomy, reflecting the latest knowledge and standing on its own as a textbook. Gans's elaborate introduction—both his genealogies of Jewish and Gentile astronomers and his five justifications for placing the subject within the Jewish curriculum—testify to the novelty of his work and to his recognition that it was bound to incur opposition. Despite the explicit approval of astronomy by both Isserles and the Maharal, which Gans conspicuously displays in support of his effort, he is clearly insecure about the entire enterprise. Having presented the list of Jewish luminaries of science to demonstrate that astronomical study was hardly a novelty in Jewish intellectual life, and having underscored the Jewish roots of the discipline now practiced by non-Jews, following the well-trodden apologetic strategies of Maimonides, Bivago, and de' Rossi,[111] he nevertheless acknowledges the virtual disappearance of this learned tradition among his contemporaries: "Thus the

108. See the fifth reason he gives for studying astronomy (p. 10a), quoted at n. 116 below.

109. See A. David, ed., *Kronika Ivrit Mi-Prag Me-Reshit ha-Ma'ah ha-17* (Jerusalem, 1984).

110. Fishman provides an ample list ("R. Moses Isserles," pp. 19–20), with full annotation.

111. *Neḥmad ve-Na'im,* pp. 7b–9a.

exalted sciences were depleted among us to the point that their memory was almost completely lost. Only occasionally in a city or two in a state does one find someone who knows something of this science. Moreover, books in our possession that treat astronomical matters at this time are scarce."[112] Accordingly, he continues, "if Jews are obliged to master this discipline from Gentile books, they should not consider themselves inferior or at fault."[113] He refers to two camps hostile to this project: ignoramuses who know no better and "true scholars who believe in the veracity of this discipline and acknowledge that all its ways are based on reason, but who nevertheless speak evil of this science and its students, claiming that it is inappropriate for a person to waste his time on this subject and at the same time questioning its utility."[114]

The second group is particularly distressing to Gans, since it includes those who apparently know better but still remain in the opposition camp. His response to it is both thorough and energetic, yet it was probably ineffectual in changing the mind of his knowledgeable critics. He begins by repeating the response of Isserles that the forbidden Greek disciplines do not include the natural sciences. On the contrary, the study of natural science enhances religious faith, as thinkers from Baḥya ibn Pakuda to Eliezer Ashkenazi acknowledge; and it enhances ritualistic practice by facilitating the calculation of the new moon.[115] His most telling justification is the last, revealing his deeply felt inferiority and the need to counter the charges of non-Jews regarding Jewish boorishness: "What should we do at a time when the wise Gentiles speak to us, asking us the reason for the order of intercalation, and our tradition is insufficient [to respond] to them? Is it appropriate for us to put our hands to our mouths, appearing as a mute incapable of opening his mouth? Is this not [a matter] of our honor or that of our Maker?"[116]

The Maharal was equally concerned with fortifying Jewish cultural pride, but he did not make the study of astronomy a critical precondition. Rather, as we have seen, he chose to preserve the integrity of the rabbinic tradition by

112. Ibid., p. 9a.
113. Ibid., p. 9b.
114. Ibid.
115. Ibid., pp. 9b–10a.
116. Ibid., p. 10a.

demarcating it from human knowledge in general, and subsequently to elevate it. The above quotation suggests that Gans would not have been satisfied with this strategy. Yet he seems to have imbibed his master's teaching in another way. The sense of separating a Jewish divine realm from a Gentile secular one is the essential organizing principle of his historical chronicle as well as his briefer histories of astronomy in *Nehmad ve-Na'im*. Was it merely a coincidence that Gans divided his composition into two distinct but parallel parts: a history of the nations and a history of the Jews? Was it merely his own way of dealing with the relationship of the Jew to the other, an acknowledgment that mediating their two histories would not work, as Joseph Ha-Cohen had tried earlier? "Rather than mixing two stories of different natures, better to tell them separately," as Robert Bonfil puts it.[117]

Another reason for his division might be a recognition of the Maharal's insight that *historia divina* and *historia naturalis* were both licit in their own right as long as neither intruded upon the other.[118] Gans may have learned his most profound lesson from his teacher in Prague. Despite his vacillations between his two prominent mentors, in the final analysis the Maharal's voice spoke most decisively through the pages of Gans's work. Astronomy was a legitimate undertaking for Jewish students, and so was secular history, but only if they remained securely within their own hermetically sealed dominions. Distinct and above them were a sacred Jewish metaphysics and a sacred Jewish history. By severing the connection between them, Gans sought to preserve the integrity of the secular and the sacred, to legitimate the pursuit of each, and forcefully to avoid the entanglement which had once proved so damaging to both faith and science.

In the end, Gans was remembered for his chronicle rather than for his denser astronomy published in its final version only once after his death in 1743. His writings in astronomy, geography, and history far surpassed any of his contemporaries' achievements. In the changing cultural climate of the seventeenth century, as Fishman has pointed out, his impact on the study of the sciences

117. R. Bonfil, "How Golden Was the Age of the Renaissance in Jewish Historiography?" *History and Theory* 27 (1988): 94.

118. Breuer, in "Modernism and Traditionalism," p. 77, notes Gans's approach and even compares it with Luther's, without mentioning the Maharal's possible influence.

among eastern European Jewry was almost nil.[119] Nevertheless, the singularity of his intellectual profile should not obscure his clear connection to his cultural surroundings, both Jewish and Christian. He was an enthusiastic student of Christian chroniclers and astronomers, yet he also followed a pattern established by his Jewish teachers in valuing the study of the sciences, especially astronomy, while accentuating its divorce from both Jewish sacred writing and Aristotelian metaphysics.

Both Neher and Breuer have spoken of a Jewish circle of scientific enthusiasts surrounding Gans; others have placed the Maharal or Isserles, or both, at the center of this circle.[120] What is clear is the emergence of a community of interest in scientific pursuits, primarily astronomy, both in Poland and in Bohemia in the second half of the sixteenth century and the early seventeenth century. By all accounts, interest in science among the intellectual leadership of these regions waned by the 1630s. Fishman and Davis have offered a general profile of the group, which included Abraham Horowitz, Mordecai Yaffe, Yom Tov Lipman Heller, Manoah Hendl b. Shmarya, Chaim Lisker, Jacob Kopelman, and Joseph b. Isaac Ha-Levi.[121] It is not my intention to survey all or even most of their writings. I wish only to highlight certain features of their thought, particularly those continuities that appear to derive from the three thinkers considered above.

Mordecai Yaffe's "moderate rationalist" interests have received due attention in Lawrence Kaplan's dissertation.[122] As Kaplan has shown, Yaffe's positions on science and its relation to rabbinic teaching closely mirror those of his teachers, the Maharal and Isserles. Kaplan calls Yaffe's *Levush Malkhut* a *summa* of rabbinic Judaism of his day, integrating both halakhic and "meta-halakhic" study into a broad curriculum of Jewish learning. The introduction to the work reveals Yaffe's pedagogic goals and his notion of the organization of knowledge. He first mentions that he has composed a commentary on Maimonides' *Guide of the Perplexed,* a commentary on the *Laws of the Sanctification of the New Moon,* and finally

119. Fishman, "R. Moses Isserles," pp. 20–21.

120. See nn. 35 and 36 above.

121. Both Fishman, "R. Moses Isserles," and Davis, "Rabbi Yom Tov Lipman Heller" list complete references to these writers, so I will not reproduce them here.

122. Kaplan, "Rationalism and Rabbinic Culture."

a commentary on the kabbalistic Torah commentary of Menaḥem Recanati.[123] Then he continues: "For every student of 'The angels of God' [Genesis 28:12] who desires to enter into the *pardes* [pleasure garden, i.e. the divine secrets] and to ascend the rungs of that ladder which is set erect upon the ground but whose head reaches the heavens, knows that he must start at the very bottom. . . . And the order of study that I have set forth corresponds precisely to the order of the rungs of the ladder,[124] i.e., the levels of reality from bottom up. First, one studies the speculative sciences dealing with nature that encompass all the sciences of this, our lowly [sublunar] world, all of which are treated in the *Guide of the Perplexed*. Afterwards, one ascends and studies the science of astronomy that deals with the intermediate world, i.e., the world of the celestial spheres, which contain all of the stars, with the sun at their head as a king leading his troops, the moon as his deputy, and the rest of the stars as his hosts. And after that he will ascend even higher on the rungs of the ladder and will enter into the *pardes* of wisdom onto the road that leads straight away unto the house of the Lord, i.e., he will study the science of kabbalah. Then he will merit attaining the apprehension of the First Cause, may He be blessed, who stands over them to maintain their existence and to guard them."[125]

Yaffe's classification reflects the influence of his teachers, especially the Maharal. He singles out the study of the natural world as the critical and preliminary stage of religious education; he distinguishes it from astronomy, which he elevates above all the sciences; and then he defines the divine science of kabbalah as the highest and ultimate level of spiritual illumination. Yaffe's division is reminiscent of Isserles' similar one.[126] What is puzzling for Kaplan is

123. Introduction to *Levush Malkhut* (New York, 1962), unpaginated.

124. On this motif in medieval philosophy, see A. Altmann, "The Ladder of Ascension," *Studies in Mysticism and Religion Presented to Gershom G. Scholem* (Jerusalem, 1967), pp. 1–32 (English section); M. Idel, "The Ladder of Ascension: The Reverberations of a Medieval Motif in the Renaissance," in I. Twersky, ed., *Studies in Jewish Medieval History and Literature* (Cambridge, Mass., 1983), pp. 83–93.

125. Translated by Kaplan in "Rationalism and Rabbinic Culture," pp. 397–99.

126. Isserles had also referred to this threefold division in *Torat ha-Olah*, p. 22a and later on p. 85b, where the division is broken down into three types of magical activity. Moshe Idel has plausibly speculated that this passage is influenced by the tripartite division of Agrippa in

Yaffe's equating naturalistic study with the contents of Maimonides' *Guide,* a work that begins with sublunary physics but naturally continues to the subject of metaphysics along the lines of the scholastic curriculum. Like Isserles and the Maharal, Yaffe had no place in his Jewish curriculum for philosophical metaphysics despite his appreciation of Maimonides' work. His strategy for using and commenting on the *Guide* was to redefine its nature by reducing it to a work which dealt exclusively with physics. In this, as we have seen, he adopts a position that Isserles had articulated in a similarly awkward manner in his response to Solomon Luria. Isserles had described the *Guide* as a book of nature, obscuring the metaphysical dimension of the work just as Yaffe did.

Yaffe, however, deviated from Isserles' position on the relation of the sciences to kabbalah. While Yaffe followed his teacher up to a point in treating the *sefirot* philosophically in the early part of his work, ultimately he opted for a clear-cut division between the two realms. In his commentary on Recanati, as Kaplan points out, the unity of the divine realm is not reducible to philosophical explanation.[127] In the final analysis, divine truths are distinct from naturalistic ones. Having vacillated between Isserles' harmonizing and the Maharal's segregationist approaches, Yaffe comes down on the side of the Maharal. The natural sciences are given a firm and honored place in the Jewish curriculum; astronomy is singled out for special esteem; and kabbalistic metaphysics is elevated and safeguarded from the potential intrusion of the other disciplines. Kaplan has shown how Yaffe smoothed over the more radical interpretation of Maimonidean philosophy, offering a safe, tame, and unexciting "moderate rationalism."[128] I would add that Yaffe not only blunted the radical sting of Maimonidean philosophy; he attenuated its scope by redefining it as the study of the natural world alone, arrested its metaphysical thrust into areas of Jewish belief such

---

his *De Occulta Philosophia.* If this is indeed the case (Agrippa's book might have reached him through the Cologne edition of 1533), then the conventional view that he read, as he claims, non-Jewish philosophy and science only through Hebrew books has to be reevaluated. See M. Idel, "Differing Conceptions of Kabbalah in the Early Seventeenth Century," in I. Twersky and B. Septimus, eds., *Jewish Thought in the Seventeenth Century* (Cambridge, Mass., 1987), pp. 168–69, n. 155.

127. Kaplan, "Rationalism and Rabbinic Culture," pp. 98–100.

128. This is the theme of chap. 3 of Kaplan's dissertation.

as prophecy and divine providence, and simultaneously isolated and raised to the highest prominence the study of kabbalistic metaphysics. In so doing, he systematically erected an educational program that shunted medieval philosophy aside while highlighting scientific and kabbalistic studies as separate but legitimate fields. Kaplan may be right that his vision had little staying power in the new cultural landscape of eastern Europe in the later seventeenth century; this was not the case, however, for other Jewish communities, especially Italy. Several Jewish thinkers of the eighteenth century and beyond would find Yaffe's system perfectly compatible with their own.[129]

Joseph Davis has recently studied the thought of Joseph b. Isaac Ha-Levi and Yom Tov Lipman Heller, both profoundly influenced by the Maharal and his epistemological restructuring of knowledge.[130] Of the two, Ha-Levi is the more interesting because of his radical shift from one view of rationalism to another and because of his reevaluation of the relationship between reason and faith. Ha-Levi's first work, the *Givat ha-Moreh,* is "a throw-back to Jewish philosophy of the fourteenth and fifteenth centuries,"[131] in Davis's words, a kind of Neo-Aristotelianism, supremely confident in the ability of reason to grapple with metaphysical problems impinging upon religious faith, and bold enough, in striking contrast to other contemporary views, to consult and cite philosophical works of non-Jewish authors. The work is a fish out of water with respect to the Jewish cultural ambiance in which it emerged. One wonders, however, whether it might be possible to locate any other intellectual context for Ha-Levi's proclivities in Prague or elsewhere, such as the lingering Averroistic currents of late sixteenth-century Italy.

Be that as it may, Ha-Levi's philosophical passion was short-lived. Apparently wounded by the controversy over his book, he disavowed most of his previous positions in his second work, *Ketonet Passim,* apparently adopting positions favored by the rabbinic establishment of his day—essentially the theological views of the Maharal. The Maharal's influence is especially notable in his pious affirmation of the superiority of Torah knowledge; in his recitation

129. See esp. chap. 7 below.
130. Davis, "Rabbi Yom Tov Lipman Heller."
131. Ibid., p. 265.

of the same threefold division of learning we have seen in Yaffe's work; in his distaste for Aristotelian metaphysics and his embrace of physics; in his distinct sense of the contingency of nature; and in his reiteration of the legitimacy of scientific pursuits, separate from and inferior to kabbalistic metaphysics.[132] His magical and alchemical interests faintly recall the Prague ambiance of his Christian contemporaries.[133] Davis is right in calling his final position a text-based kabbalistic science, thoroughly devoid of empirical aspirations and caught in a limbo between increasingly obsolete Aristotelianism and the new kabbalistic spirituality. Nevertheless, Ha-Levi's strategic retreat from medieval philosophy was ultimately a reassessment of what was rational and what was worth knowing, not a total renunciation of the human striving to understand. While hardly an empiricist, he had at least left open the possibility of a new reconciliation between naturalistic pursuits and mystical theology among Jewish thinkers.

Heller's intellectual profile conforms quite well to that of contemporary followers of the Maharal. Like the Maharal, he valued non-Jewish thought nearly exclusively for its information about the natural sciences. His approbation of Gans's *Magen David,* the first edition of the astronomy, displays his positive and enthusiastic evaluation of astronomy and mathematics. Despite his limited knowledge, he refers occasionally to natural phenomena and even quotes naturalists to confirm a halakhic opinion. Unlike Ha-Levi and Yaffe, he is less comfortable with kabbalistic metaphysics and appears increasingly unhappy with the cultural turn in that direction among his contemporaries. There is little innovative or systematic thought in his well-known commentary on the Mishnah and other writings. Nevertheless, he provides another telling example of how the Maharal's students closely aligned themselves to both his theological and pedagogical ideals.[134]

By Heller's death in the middle of the seventeenth century, the modest inroads scientific pursuits had made within eastern European culture had virtually disappeared. Contemporary scholars have variously attributed this cultural shift

132. Ibid., pp. 288–338.
133. Ibid., p. 323.
134. Ibid., pp. 339–516.

to the intrusion of Lurianic kabbalah and the Sabbatian aftermath,[135] to the decline of the Polish Renaissance,[136] and to the emergence of a populist revolt of preachers and nonelites jockeying for power and influence through the mediums of the popular sermon and printed book.[137] The issue has also focused on the terms of reference utilized by Elbaum—"opening and closure"—and on the extent to which the new kabbalistic spirituality and indifference or antagonism to rational pursuits constituted an aberration from past traditions or a return to normalcy. In this chapter, we are concerned with cultural transformation only insofar as it reflects the decline of scientific interest among eastern and central European Jews. One major factor in the change of climate in Bohemia seems obvious but is hardly mentioned by recent interpreters: the battle of White Mountain of 1620, the ultimate victory of the Counter-Reformation, and the unleashing of the destructive forces of the ensuing Thirty Years War. A similar decline took place in Poland and Lithuania as well: the growing intolerance of the Catholic restoration, the increasing instability of the social order, Poland's declining international influence, and a general increase of obscurantism and anti-intellectualism. The Cossack pogroms of 1648 constituted a bitter culmination of this economic and political anarchy. While the Maharal and his students had planted the seeds of a new epistemological orientation regarding the sciences and Judaism, the cultural soil of Bohemia and Poland-Lithuania was inhospitable to the full flowering of this new vision, not so much because of Lurianic incursions as because of a general deterioration of cultural life. The seeds would have to germinate elsewhere.

One further dimension of Jewish scientific culture in this period deserves mention: the role of physicians and medicine. While physicians were at the center of Jewish scientific culture elsewhere in Europe (especially in Italy, as we shall see[138]), they were remarkably peripheral in central and eastern Europe. To be more precise, although physicians were politically and socially prominent, especially in eastern Europe, their intellectual impact was almost nonexistent.

135. This is basically the position of Elbaum, discussed above.

136. Baron's position, also mentioned earlier.

137. Cf. E. Reiner, "Itinerate Ashkenazic Preachers in the Early Modern Period," (forthcoming).

138. See chap. 3 below.

While the rabbinic leadership passionately embraced astronomy, it displayed a chilling indifference to medicine. Fishman has explored this question intelligently, taking into account the work of earlier scholars, so I will only summarize his findings in rounding out our discussion.[139]

The first Jewish doctors in Bohemia and Poland were émigrés from Spain and Italy. They were attracted to lucrative positions in serving the Polish king or nobility. Socially and intellectually, they were alien to the rabbinic establishment. They lived outside the Jewish community and their lifestyles made them suspect in the eyes of the religiously orthodox. By the seventeenth century, native Polish Jews were admitted to the medical faculties of Italian universities, especially Padua.[140] The cost of such an education excluded all but the most affluent Jewish merchant families. Upon their return to eastern Europe, they easily gained employment in the upper echelons of Christian society. As with their medieval counterparts, their medical contacts enhanced their economic and political power. Some became natural candidates for *shtadlanut,* political mediation between the Jewish and Christian communities and, in Fishman's words, "an important fixture on the social landscape of Polish Jewry."[141] Under exceptional circumstances, physicians like Emanuel de Jonah and Isaac Fortis even served as *parnasim* for the Council of Four Lands.[142] Others served as local *par-*

139. Fishman, "R. Moses Isserles," pp. 3–5. In addition to the works of Lewin, Gelber, Schipper, and Ringelblum that he cites, see M. Balaban, *Historja Zydow w Krakowie i na Kazim-ierzu,* 2 vols. (Cracow, 1931–36), L. Lewin, "Die jüdischen Studenten an der Universität Frankfurt a.d. Oder," *Jahrbuch der Jüdisch-literarischen Gesellschaft* 14 (1921): 217–38; 15 (1923): 59–96; 16 (1924): 43–86; G. Kisch, *Die Prager Universität und die Juden, 1348–1848* (Maehrisch-Ostrau, 1935); J. Litman, *The Economic Role of Jews in Medieval Poland: The Contribution of Yitzhak Schipper* (Lanham, 1984), pp. 176–77; R. Mahler, *Toledot ha-Yehudim be-Folin* (Merhaviah, Palestine, 1946), pp. 133–34; J. Warshal, "Żidzi polscy na Uniwersytecie padewskim," *Kwartalnik poświęçony badaniu przeszłości Żidów w Polsce* (Warsaw, 1913), I, sec. 3, pp. 37–72; S. Dubnow, "Jewish Students at the University of Padua in the Seventeenth and Eighteenth Centuries" (in Hebrew), *Sefer ha-Shana le-Yehudei Amerika,* ed. M. Ribolow and Z. Scharfstein (New York, 1931), pp. 216–19; and A. Gutterman, "Sephardic Jews on Polish Soil" (in Hebrew), *Pe'amim* 18 (1984): 53–79.

140. The Paduan experience is discussed in chap. 3 below.

141. Fishman, "R. Moses Isserles," p. 4.

142. See also the recent treatment of Dr. Mojzes Fortis in M. J. Rosman, *The Lords' Jews: Jews and Magnates in Old Poland* (Cambridge, Mass., 1990), chap. 6.

nasim, such as Jacob Winkler in Posen, David Marupk in Cracow, and Aaron Gordon in Vilna. In the seventeenth century, the Jewish doctor became the target of Polish anti-Semitic propaganda in a manner similar to what was occurring elsewhere in western Europe, especially in Germany. At the same time, more Jews were entering the medical profession as Jewish students were admitted to the medical schools of the universities of Frankfurt, Prague, and other cities. The impact of medicine on Jewish cultural and social life prior to the Enlightenment was insignificant. As Fishman points out, most doctors were perceived as social and religious deviants. The cultural role model of the rabbi-physician, which dominated Italian Jewry for centuries, generally did not exist in eastern Europe.

Fishman concludes by observing that although scientific study and activity were not alien to Jewish life in this region, "one is justified in viewing science as a secondary feature of Polish Jewish culture, rather than a primary one." He adds that it remained an elite phenomenon and never became a recognized social ideal. Furthermore, it was short-lived, limited to the period of Isserles' and his students' lifetimes, and eventually died out in the stifling antirational atmosphere of the mid-seventeenth century. The only vestige of this activity was what he calls a narrow "halakhic astronomy."[143] His assessment is widely shared by other scholars.

As I have tried to demonstrate, this evaluation is correct as far as it goes, but it does not go far enough. Jewish writing on purely scientific matters supports Fishman's conclusion. But from a broader perspective, one can observe the restructuring of Jewish religious thought in this era: the reassessment of the practical value of rational pursuits, the severing of physics from metaphysics, and the recognition of the study of nature as a separate and legitimate sphere of knowledge coexisting with the divine sapience of rabbinic and kabbalistic traditions. The major intellectual force in initiating this process was not Isserles but the Maharal. His theoretical contribution, although never fully implemented in eastern Europe, left an imprint elsewhere in early modern Europe.

It should now be evident why I insisted on describing the first of two historio-

143. Fishman, "R. Moses Isserles," pp. 21–23.

graphical debates before addressing the issue of science directly in this chapter. In the heated exchange about rationalism, not enough emphasis has been placed on the shifting context of the discussions about the relation between reason and faith before and during the era of the Maharal and his colleagues. Their writings expressed a new Jewish attitude toward nature and scientific activity.

Now it is time to turn to the debate between Katz and Ben Sasson over the supposed indifference of the Maharal and his circle to Christian culture, and to propose why it too is relevant to our topic. Ben Sasson and Kulka have suggested that the Maharal's critical formulation of the relationship of nature-study to faith owes much to its immediate Christian surrounding. Living in Prague, where religious and national ideologies dynamically interacted, so sophisticated a thinker as the Maharal could hardly have disengaged himself from this remarkable discourse. His views on the proper relation of science to Jewish faith were probably shaped by this environment, as were his views on national identity and education.

We have no hard evidence to substantiate the hypothesis developed by Ben Sasson and Kulka, but this need not restrain me from offering a plausible, albeit tentative, reconstruction of the genesis of the Maharal's thinking. In the light of Maharal's own reticence in disclosing the sources of his thought, especially if he had actually been aware of their Christian derivation, he would probably never have allowed such evidence to exist in the first place. Nevertheless, pointing to possible contacts, or at the very least, parallels between Jewish and Christian thinking on this issue still appears both justifiable and worthwhile. In the words of one historian searching for the roots of Copernicus' speculations: "As intangibles and unknown connections become involved, the historian's craft becomes more like that of the novelist who allows imagination to supply pieces that time has ravaged."[144] In the same spirit, I offer the following speculations about the roots of the Maharal's thinking on the place of nature in Jewish thought.

No doubt the Maharal's general voluntarist theology, his dismissal of Aristotelian metaphysics, and his legitimization of naturalistic pursuits within Judaism had precedents in earlier Jewish thought. We have mentioned above the clear parallels with the thought of Judah Ha-Levi and Naḥmanides. But Tamar Ross

144. Knoll, "Arts Faculty of the University of Cracow," p. 157.

has also pointed out the originality of the Maharal's position. Furthermore, in view of the special emphasis these themes receive throughout his diverse writings, the supposition that these medieval thinkers, remote both in time and place, constituted the Maharal's sole source of inspiration seems unconvincing. A more probable source of influence might have been the discussions on the nature of scientific knowledge and its relation to faith within the Protestant world. Both Calvinists and Lutherans, along with the aforementioned Czech brethren, inhabited the cultural space of Prague in close proximity to the Jewish community. On the issue at hand, the reflections of all three were not dissimilar. If the writings of any of these faith communities might have fallen into the hands of the Maharal, those of the Lutherans, a German speaking community, might have been the most accessible. Like David Gans, the Maharal could most easily have consulted sources written in German. But the Lutherans constituted only one possible avenue for these ideas; the latter were sufficiently diffuse to have reached this learned rabbi through multiple channels.

In recent years, several scholars have underscored the impact of nominalist ideas on both the birth of modern science and Reformation theology.[145] Critical to the thinking of the nominalists was the distinction between the absolute and ordained powers of God (*potentia absoluta* and *potentia ordinata*). The distinction

145. The literature is massive. I cite only a sampling which I consulted: H. Oberman, *Luther: Man between God and the Devil* (New Haven and London, 1989), pp. 114–23; idem, "Reformation and Revolution: Copernicus's Discovery in an Era of Change," in J. E. Murdoch and E. D. Sylla, *The Cultural Context of Medieval Learning* (Dordrecht and Boston, 1975), pp. 397–435; idem, "The Shape of Late Medieval Thought: The Birthpangs of the Modern Era," in C. Trinkaus and H. Oberman, eds., *The Pursuit of Holiness in Late Medieval and Renaissance Religion* (Leiden, 1974), pp. 3–25; idem, "Headwaters of the Reformation: Initia Lutheri–Initia Reformationis," in H. Oberman, ed., *Luther and the Dawn of the Modern Era* (Leiden, 1974), pp. 40–88; W. J. Courtnenay, "Nominalism and Late Medieval Religion," in *Pursuit of Holiness,* pp. 26–59; S. Ozment, "Mysticism, Nominalism, and Dissent," in *Pursuit of Holiness,* pp. 67–92; idem, *The Age of Reform, 1250–1550: An Intellectual History of Late Medieval and Reformation Europe* (New Haven and London, 1980), pp. 15–19, 38–60, 223–39; A. McGrath, *The Intellectual Origins of the European Reformation* (Oxford, 1987); D. Trapp, "Augustinian Theology of the Fourteenth Century: Notes on Editions, Marginalia, Opinions, and Booklore," *Augustiniana* 6 (1956): 146–274; H. Blumenberg, *The Genesis of the Copernican World,* trans. R. M. Wallace (Cambridge, Mass., 1987), pp. 135–67.

meant in theory that God has the ability to do many things that He does not will to do, has never done, nor ever will do. With the dialectic of two powers—one actual and one hypothetical—the notion of divine omnipotence was acknowledged without undermining the operation and predictability of the natural order. By the systematic application of this distinction between possibility and reality, speculative theology became pointless and irrelevant, and in the words of Heiko Oberman, man was set free "from the smothering embrace of metaphysics."[146] The world was now conceived as contingent upon the divine will, no longer an ontological necessity but the result of God's covenantal obligation. And with this new conception, intuition and immediate experience were given primacy in acquiring knowledge.

Despite his condemnation of some of the positions of the nominalists, Martin Luther was directly influenced by their understanding of the divine and secular realms through the impact of the *via moderna* and *via Augustinia moderna* during his early formative years. He openly objected to Aristotelian metaphysics; he sought God's reliable and certain word in Scriptures rather than in speculative theology. God's word was the sole foundation of ultimate truth and human experience the focus of perceiving the immediate world. Through this new demarcation, astronomy no longer competed with theology, nor was it impious for the believer in the divine word to fathom the heavens. Scripture was no longer read as a supernaturally revealed book of nature; it could only be grasped *extra rationem, sola fides. Theologia* no longer was to be understood as *scientia* but a higher *sapientia* solely constituting the ability to grasp the true sense of the sacred scripture. By concentrating on his experience and not on logical assumptions postulated beforehand, or on divine mysteries, and by recasting his understanding of the universe in terms of efficient rather than final causality, the scientist now faced the subject of nature openly; his imagination could soar freely so that mental experiments of all kinds were possible. A revolution in research methodology was taking place.[147] A new relation between the sacred and secular emerged whereby separation with coordination became an alternative to competition or subordination.

146. Oberman, "Reformation and Revolution," p. 408.
147. The language of Oberman, ibid., p. 410.

One additional element of the Lutheran position might also be mentioned. As Steven Ozment speculates, the young Luther may have represented a genuine synthesis of diverse traditions: a devotee of medieval spirituality trained simultaneously in the Ockhamist tradition. His theology might actually be characterized as a merger of nominalism and mysticism.[148] The Maharal's kabbalistic proclivities should be recalled in this regard.[149]

Is the intriguing parallel between the positions of Luther (and Calvin, or even the Czech Brethren) and the Maharal a mere coincidence? To my knowledge, there is no trace of a specific discussion of the dialectic of God's two powers in the Maharal's or, for that matter, in any other Jewish thinker's writing of the period. Yet the end result of the Maharal's sharp division between rabbinic truth and speculation about the natural world, his open break with Aristotelian metaphysics, his emphasis on divine will, the possibility of miracles, and the contingency of creation all suggest, at the very least, a remarkable consensus with his Protestant (and ultimately Catholic) neighbors. Both Jews and Christians had shifted to a "nominalist" mood in Prague and elsewhere. At the University of Cracow, for example, the nominalists Oresme and Buridan were studied assiduously.[150] Could Isserles too have absorbed something of this new orientation?

Our effort to locate the soil from which Jewish ideas spring is hazardous and ultimately inconclusive. And in the case of the Maharal and his co-religionists, as we have said, definite proof is probably unattainable anyway. Nevertheless, this comparative exercise should not be dismissed out of hand. In the light of what we now know about the Maharal and his cultural world, it seems safe to argue for the plausibility of this reconstruction. Having likely absorbed something of the nationalistic and educational theories of his environment, the Maharal might also have attuned himself to Protestant arguments about the relation of science and religion derived from late medieval nominalism. He then creatively adapted

148. Ozment, "Mysticism, Nominalism, and Dissent," p. 80.

149. On the Maharal's kabbalistic proclivities, see Elbaum, *Petiḥut ve-Histagrut*, p. 220; G. Scholem, *Major Trends in Jewish Mysticism* (New York, 1961), p. 339; Sherwin, *Mystical Theology;* B. Safran, "Maharal and Early Hasidism," in Safran, ed., *Hasidism: Continuity or Innovation?* (Cambridge, Mass., 1988), pp. 47–144

150. See the references to Wroblewski and Knoll in n. 61 above.

them to fit his own polemical and ideological needs and the circumstances of his own Jewish constituency. Whether or not the impetus for his position actually came from the outside, it profoundly influenced other Jewish thinkers for centuries to come. It offered Jewish enthusiasts of science a blueprint for establishing a cooperative partnership between scientific endeavor and religion in Judaism. More generally, it posited a new and constructive relation between the secular and sacred. With this new epistemological formula, Askhenazic Jewry of the early modern period had made a unique and enduring contribution.

3

Padua and the Formation of a Jewish Medical Community in Italy

Notwithstanding the openness of the Maharal and his students to the cultural ambiances of Prague and Cracow, neither city came close to offering the same intellectual stimulation that was available to Jews fortunate enough to be living in or to make their way to the old university towns of the Italian peninsula. For a Jewish student in search of a university education who found the means and fortitude to make the journey southward, crossing the Alps to the Veneto, with Padua as his final destination, the contrast was surely remarkable. By way of introducing the novelty of that experience, I offer the following Jewish "snapshots" of Padua in the seventeenth and eighteenth centuries.

In 1624, Joseph ben Judah Ḥamiẓ successfully completed his doctorate in philosophy and medicine at the University of Padua.[1] The event hardly seemed significant either for Padua or for its Jewish community. In the beginning of the seventeenth century, a constant trickle of Jews were among the hundreds of students who graduated each year from Padua's renowned medical school.[2] Nevertheless, Ḥamiẓ's graduation appears to have elicited an unusually favorable, even elated response from some of the most important luminaries of Italian Jewish culture in

1. A. Modena and E. Morpurgo, *Medici e chirurghi ebrei dottorati e licen-ziati nell'Università di Padova dal 1617 al 1816*, ed. A. Luzzato, L. Münster, and V. Colorni (Bologna, 1967), p. 8.
2. On Padua's medical school in the sixteenth and seventeenth centuries, see G. Whitteridge, *Willam Harvey and the Circulation of the Blood* (New York

this era. Undoubtedly, their reaction was encouraged by Ḥamiẓ's illustrious mentor, Leone Modena, who apparently undertook the responsibility of publishing an entire pamphlet of poems and approbations to honor his favorite prodigy.[3] Yet the participants' enthusiasm appears to far exceed the conventional

---

and London, 1917); C. B. Schmitt, "Science in the Italian Universities of the Sixteenth and Early Seventeenth Centuries," in M. Crosland, ed., *The Emergence of Science in Western Europe* (New York, 1976), pp. 35–56; idem, "Philosophy and Science in Sixteenth-Century Universities: Some Preliminary Comments," in J. E. Murdoch and E. D. Sylla, *The Cultural Context of Medieval Learning* (Dordrecht, 1974), pp. 485–537; J. Bylebyl, "The School of Padua: Humanistic Medicine in the Sixteenth Century," in C. Webster, ed., *Health, Medicine and Mortality in the Sixteenth Century* (Cambridge, 1979), pp. 335–70; N. Siraisi, *Avicenna in Renaissance Italy: The Canon and Medical Teaching in Italian Universities after 1500* (Princeton, 1987); C. Fichtner, "Padova e Tubingen: La Formazione medica nei secoli XVI e XVII," *Acta medicae historia patavina* 19 (1971–72): 43–62. See also the essays of F. D. Derroussiles, G. Ongaro, and C. Maccagni in N. Pozza, ed., *Storia della cultura veneta: Dal primo Quattrocento al concilio di Trento* (Vicenza, 1980), vol. 3, sections 2 and 3. References to the earlier standard works on Padua's university are found in these articles. See also the numerous essays in the *Quaderni per la storia dell'Università di Padova* (1968–).

On Jewish students at Padua, see Modena and Morpurgo, *Medici*; E. Veronese Ceseracciu, "Ebrei laureati a Padova nel Cinquecento," *Quaderni per la storia dell'Università di Padova* 13 (1980): 151–68; D. Carpi, "Jews Holding the Degree of Doctor of Medicine from the University of Padua in the Sixteenth and Beginning of the Seventeenth Centuries" (in Hebrew), in *Scritti in memoria di Nathan Cassuto* (Jerusalem, 1986), pp. 62–91 (repr. in D. Carpi, *Be-Tarbut ha-Renesans u-ven Ḥomot ha-Getto* (Tel Aviv, 1989); and in abbreviated form as "Note su alcuni ebrei laureati a Padova nel Cinquecento e all'inizio del Seicento," *Quaderni per la storia dell'Università di Padova* 19 (1986): 145–56; C. Roth, *Venice* (Philadelphia, 1930), pp. 285–93; V. Colorni, "Sull'ammissibilità degli ebrei alla laurea anteriormente al secolo IX," in *Scritti in onore di Riccardo Bachi, Rassegna mensile di Israel* 16 (1950): 202–16 (repr. in V. Colorni, *Judaica minora* (Milan, 1983); G. Kisch, "Cervo Conegliano: A Jewish Graduate of Padua in 1743," *Journal of the History of Medicine* 4 (1949): 450–59; J. Shatzky, "On Jewish Medical Students of Padua," *Journal of the History of Medicine* 5 (1950): 444–47; H. Friedenwald, *The Jews and Medicine,* 2 vols. (Baltimore, 1944), 1:221–40, 253–58; A. Ciscato, *Gli Ebrei in Padova (1300–1800)* (Padua, 1901); M. Soave, "Medici ebrei laureati nell'Università di Padova nel 1600 e 1700," *Il Vessillo israelitico* 24 (1876): 189–92.

3. The collection is entitled *Belil Ḥamiẓ* and was printed in Venice in 1624. It is reprinted in N. S. Leibowitz, *Seridim Mikitve ha-Pilosof ha-Rofe ve-ha-Mekubbal R. Yosef Ḥamiẓ* (Jerusalem, 1937), pp. 33–69.

response required by this literary exercise in public flattery. No less impressive is the wide spectrum of contributors to the pamphlet, ranging from Ḥamiẓ's classmate Benjamin Mussafia[4] to the "wise man of secrets," Azariah Figo, rabbi of Pisa.[5] For all these distinguished panegyrists, Ḥamiẓ's rite of passage into the hallowed corridors of licensed medical practice was deservedly cause for celebration and commendation to both Ḥamiẓ and his coreligionists.

Almost a hundred years later, the German orientalist Johann Jacob Schudt noted the phenomenon of Jewish graduation from Padua's medical school. In contrast to the accolades lavished upon Ḥamiẓ by his fellow Jews, Schudt found nothing praiseworthy about Padua's indiscriminate admission of "every igno- ramus and even the despised Jews," especially those from his own country. According to Schudt, such practice was unbecoming to so famous a university, whose only motivation in welcoming such unworthy degree candidates must have been its love of lucre, following the proverb: "We take the money and send the ass back to Germany."[6]

Two notices of Jewish medical graduates from Padua almost a century apart—the first adulatory, the second deprecatory—share, at least partially, a common insight. Padua's regularized and unprecedented admission and subse- quent graduation of hundreds of Jews was a matter of no small consequence to the university, to its Jewish graduates, and to the communities they eventually served. Indeed, neither Ḥamiẓ's associates nor Schudt were ever fully capable of appreciating the momentous significance of Padua's admission policy, spanning well over two centuries, for the development of Jewish culture and society in Padua, Venice, Italy, and the rest of Europe.

Both Jewish and medical historians have long acknowledged the presence of many Jews in Padua's medical school.[7] I have already alluded to the large per-

---

4. Benjamin Mussafia graduated from Padua a year later, in 1625 (see Modena and Mor- purgo, *Medici,* p. 10). On Mussafia as a doctor, see D. Margalit, *Ḥokhme Yisra'el Ke-Rofim* (Jerusalem, 1962), pp. 142–51.

5. On Figo, see chap. 6 below.

6. J. Schudt, *Jüdische Merkwürdigkeiten* (Frankfurt, 1714–18), 2:404; described in Frieden- wald, *Jews and Medicine,* 1:227–28.

7. See n. 2 above.

centages of students from central and eastern Europe who returned to serve as physicians in their respective communities.[8] Yet beyond mention of their sheer number, assorted biographical data about some famous graduates, and bibliographical references to their writings, the larger story of their encounter with one of the major centers of European culture in the early modern era remains generally untold. Padua, although not the only Italian university to welcome Jews,[9] was the foremost center for training Jewish physicians from the sixteenth century until well into the eighteenth, when it was superseded by more prominent medical schools in the north, such as the University of Leiden.[10] The Paduan experience is not distinctive merely because large numbers of Jews demonstrated a conspicuous interest in and capacity for medical practice. Medical practice, as we have already seen, was a well-established profession among Jews in both Moslem and Christian societies long before the sixteenth century. Nor does the mere admission of Jews to a European university define the novelty of Padua's Jewish encounter. Jews had long been affiliated with medical schools; many had been licensed by governmental authority; and many had fostered

8. See Warchal, "Żydzi polscy na Uniwersytecie padewskim," *Kwartalnik poświecony bandaniu przeszłości Żidów w Polsce* (Warsaw, 1913), I, 3, pp. 37–72, summarized by S. Dubnov, "Jewish Students at the University of Padua in the Seventeenth and Eighteenth Centuries" (in Hebrew), *Sefer ha-Shana le-Yehudei Amerika,* ed. M. Ribolow and Z. Scharfstein (New York, 1931), pp. 216–191; N. M. Gelber, "On the History of Jewish Doctors in Poland in the Eighteenth Century" (in Hebrew), *Shai le-Yishayahu* (Tel Aviv, 1956), pp. 347–71; and G. Kisch, *Die Prager Universität und die Juden, 1348–1848* (Mährisc-Ostrau, 1935); and references cited in chap. 2 above.

9. See, for example, Colorni, "Sull'ammissibilità"; L. Münster, "Laurea in medicina conferita ad un ebreo spagnolo a Napoli nel 1488," *XVᵉ Congreso Internacional de Historia de la Medicina* (Madrid, 1956), pp. 291–97; idem, "Laurea in medicina conferita dallo Studio Ferrarese ad un ebreo nel 1426," *Ferrara Viva* 3 (1961): 63–72; A. Franceschini, "Privilegi dottorali concessi ad ebrei a Ferrara nel sec. xvi," *Atti e memorie della Deputatione Ferrarese di Storia Patria* 19 (1975): 163–86; O. Scavalcanti, "Lauree in medicina di studenti israeliti a Perugia nel secolo xvi," *Annali della Facoltà di Giurisprudenza dell'Università di Perugia* 8 (1910): 91–129.

10. On Jewish medical students at Leiden, see J. Kaplan, "Jewish Students from Amsterdam at the University of Leiden in the Seventeenth Century" (in Hebrew), in *Meḥkarim al Toledot Yahadut Holland* (Jerusalem, 1979), pp. 65–75; H. S. Hes, *Jewish Physicians in the Netherlands (1600–1940)* (Assen, 1980). See also chap. 10 below.

substantial social and cultural liaisons with the upper echelons of Moslem and Christian society because of their medical practice.[11]

The Paduan experience is unique, however, because for the first time a relatively large number of Jews graduated from a major medical school and went on to practice medicine throughout Europe. Padua also was unique because it afforded the opportunity for intense socialization among Jews from remarkably variegated backgrounds—former conversos from Spain and Portugal, together with Italian, Ottoman, German, Polish, and other eastern European Jews. Graduates of the university maintained social and intellectual ties with each other and constituted a significant cultural force within their widely scattered communities. Moreover, Padua's university allowed its Jewish students constant social and cultural contact, both casual and formal, with non-Jewish students and faculty from diverse communities and ethnic backgrounds.[12] Above all, Padua offered hundreds of talented Jewish students a prolonged exposure to the study of the liberal arts, to Latin studies, to classical scientific texts, as well as to the latest scientific advances in botany, anatomy, chemistry, and clinical medicine.

From the perspective of Jewish cultural history, Padua's medical facility was thus more than a center for training Jewish physicians. It was also a major vehicle for the diffusion of secular culture, especially scientific culture, within the pre-emancipatory Jewish communities of Europe.[13] It provided one of the richest opportunities for Jews to familiarize themselves with the best of European civili-

11. See chap. 1 above. For an important example of a Jewish physician conferring degrees on his students outside the framework of a university medical school at the end of the fifteenth century, see D. Carpi, "R. Judah Messer Leon and His Activity as a Doctor," *Michael* 1 (1973): 277–301; repr. in *Koroth* 6 (1974): 395–415; in *Be-Tarbut ha-Renesans u-ven Homot ha-Getto* (Tel Aviv, 1989), pp. 57–84; and in abbreviated form in English as "Notes on the Life of Rabbi Judah Messer Leon," in *Studi sull'ebraismo italiano in memoria di Cecil Roth* (Rome, 1974), pp. 37–62.

12. Compare Shatzky, "On Jewish Medical Students," p. 446. On socialization between Jews and non-Jews, see below.

13. Shatzky, "On Jewish Medical Students," p. 444; Gelber, "On the History of Jewish Doctors," p. 351; N. Shapiro, "The Natural Sciences and Mathematics as Pathfinders for the Haskalah Movement" (in Hebrew), *Koroth* 2 (1958): 319–44.

zation, an encounter that was unavailable to the overwhelming majority of their coreligionists. Ultimately, so formative an experience was bound to have a profound effect on the cultural priorities, values, and even self-image of such Jews. It would also pave the way for similar opportunities for Jews at other university medical schools and other cultural centers throughout Europe well into the modern era.

Between 1617 and 1816 at least 320 Jews received medical diplomas from Padua, and assuredly many more attended classes without matriculating.[14] This is a dramatic rise from the 29 graduates who are recorded between 1520 and 1605.[15] Many of this number are well known for their contributions to Jewish culture and society: Joseph Delmedigo, Joseph Ḥamiẓ, Tobias Cohen, David Nieto, Solomon and Israel Conegliano, Isaac Lampronti, and Isaac Cantarini.[16] Others are hardly familiar at all. Only an exhaustive scrutiny of their lives and literary legacies will yield a full appreciation of their encounter with Padua. Such a task is clearly beyond the limitations of this book. What I have attempted to do in several chapters that follow is to provide more focused studies of the lives and thinking of some of the most illustrious members of this group, both graduates and other prominent members of their circles. My hope is that such studies will substantiate my observations about Padua's importance, as well as stimulating further study of Jewish medical graduates at Padua and at other Italian and northern European medical schools. As I have already suggested, this sizable body of university-trained physicians, together with the large number of converso graduates of Spanish, Portuguese, and Dutch universities, exerted a decisive intellectual and political impact on Jewish society. By way of introducing these studies, further elaboration of Padua's ambiance is required.

At the beginning of the sixteenth century, European students had good reasons for choosing the University of Padua. Its medical school was generally regarded as the best in Europe. Although the university was nominally Catholic,

14. Most names are listed in Modena and Morpurgo, *Medici e chirurghi;* additions are supplied by the more recent essays of Ceseracciu and Carpi mentioned in n. 2 above.

15. See Carpi, "Padua," pp. 64–65.

16. Delmedigo, Cohen, Nieto, and Lampronti are fully treated in succeeding chapters of this book. Ḥamiẓ, the Coneglianos, and Cantarini are also mentioned.

Protestant and subsequently Jewish students were not prevented from study-ing there. The high level of medical training Padua offered was consistent with the significant place a university-educated doctor held in Italian society. Unlike much of the rest of Europe, Italy had large numbers of university graduates who served a wide spectrum of social classes in both large cities and small towns.[17] Since the early fifteenth century Padua had been under Venetian control, and by virtue of its proximity to Venice the university became an official state insti-tution of the Veneto and the primary center for training its lawyers and doctors. The Venetian government's interest in and consistent support of the university reinforced the social standing of its medical graduates.[18]

Padua's success in attracting large numbers of foreign students—Germans, Flemings, Belgians, Dutch, Silesians, Poles, Russians, Hungarians, Spanish, French, Swiss, and English—was attributable to other reasons as well. Its prox-imity to Venice undoubtedly was a great asset. The excitement of so great a commercial and intellectual center surely was contagious to medical students interested in familiarizing themselves with different places, climates, diseases, and drugs. The ideal of enlarging one's cultural horizons, together with the mythology associated with the *peregrinatio medica,* undoubtedly resonated in the hearts and minds of Padua's students. And with humanities courses integrated into the scientific curriculum, Padua certainly was not stuffily parochial. The romantic ambiance of Renaissance architecture, art, theater, and music was no doubt augmented by excursions to exotic cultural treasures throughout Italy and beyond. Theoretically, at least, after class a Jewish medical student could enjoy both a hearty kosher lunch in the adjacent ghetto and an edifying excursion to view Giotto's paintings in a nearby church.[19]

17. See C. M. Cipolla, *Public Health and the Medical Profession in the Renaissance* (Cambridge, 1976), pp. 67–116; Bylebyl, "School of Padua," p. 336.

18. Bylebyl, "School of Padua," pp. 342–43; O. Logan, *Culture and Society in Venice, 1470–1790* (London, 1972), pp. 20–21, 46–47. On Paduan students who elected to take their degree from the Venetian College of Physicians, see R. Palmer, *The Studio of Venice and Its Graduates in the Sixteenth Century* (Padua, 1983).

19. I refer to the short walk from the Jewish ghetto to the Chiesa degli Eremitani. See Fichtner, "Padova e Tubingen," which discusses Thomas Bartholin's *De peregrinatione medica* (Hafnaie, 1674).

Padua's medical curriculum was based on a two-tier system of courses covering five years.[20] During the first two, students acquired a basic familiarity with logic and natural philosophy, primarily from the texts of Aristotle. During the last three years, students specialized in both theoretical and practical subjects, utilizing the basic texts of Hippocrates, Galen, Avicenna, and Rhazes.[21] The instructor of theory would treat the general principles of health and disease, while his colleague in medical practice would cover the same ground from a more pragmatic perspective. In addition, a student would enjoy an ample exposure to the rest of the liberal arts curriculum. At the beginning of the sixteenth century, for example, students were expected to master Aristotle's *Rhetorica* and *Poetica,* Cicero's *Topica, Tusculanarum quaestionum, Commentarii* and *Somnium Scipionis,* Sophocles' *Oedipus tyrannus,* some writings of Demosthenes, Horace's first book of *Odes,* Livy's *History,* and so on. All of this learning was anything but passive. Each doctor reading in arts and medicine was required to hold public disputations at least twice a year; seven students took part in each disputation. Every evening, informal disputations took place in the presence of instructors whose attendance was required at least one hour each day to solve any student problem. A typical graduate of the medical school accordingly received a doctorate of both philosophy and medicine.

Padua's curriculum underwent major changes throughout the sixteenth and into the seventeenth century. By the late 1700s, through the collaboration of the Hospital of St. Francis of Padua, daily hospital rounds became a standard fea-

20. My description of Padua's curriculum and social setting is based on the works of Bylebyl, Whitteridge, and Schmitt listed in n. 2 above. See also J. P. Tomasini, *Gymnasium patavinum* (Udina, 1645); J. Facciolati, *Fasti gymnasii patavini* (Padua, 1757); A. Favaro, *Atti della nazione germanica artista nello Studio di Padova,* 2 vols. (Venice, 1911–12); S. de Renzi, *Storia della medicina in Italia,* 5 vols. (Naples, 1845–48); H. F. Rashdall, *The Universities of Europe in the Middle Ages,* 3 vols., 2d ed., ed. M. Powicke and A. B. Emden (Oxford, 1936); P. O. Kristeller, "Philosophy and Medicine in Medieval and Renaissance Italy," in S. F. Spicker, ed., *Organism, Medicine, and Metaphysics* (Dordrecht, 1978), pp. 29–40; A. Favaro, *Saggio di bibliografia dello Studio di Padova* (Venice, 1922); D. Nardo, "Scienza e filologia nel primo Settecento padovano: Gli Studi classici di G. B. Morgagni, G. Poleni, G. Pontedera, L. Targa," *Quaderni per la storia dell'Università di Padova* 14 (1981): 1–40.

21. Further details are in Siraisi, *Avicenna,* particularly on how new information was introduced by instructors in teaching the classic texts. See also chap. 8 below.

ture of Padua's clinical training.[22] Such bedside teaching still was unparalleled outside of Italy even by the end of the sixteenth century. In the same period, botany emerged as an autonomous subject in the Paduan medical curriculum, and botanical gardens were established at the university.[23] Professors of botany often taught about the animal and mineral worlds as well. Herbaria often were supplemented by natural history museums. Observation and research in the natural sciences also led to experiments in alchemy and iatrochemistry.

The period also witnessed major developments in the teaching of anatomy and surgery. In 1594, the first permanent anatomical theater elevated the status of surgery at Padua considerably, while elsewhere in Europe its status was on the decline.[24] Finally, although inferior in the overall educational scheme, optics, mechanics, cosmography (astronomy and geography), and other mathematical subjects were integrated into the curriculum as important adjuncts to medicine.[25] By the end of the seventeenth century, the scientific education that Paduan medical students received was radically different from that of their medieval ancestors, who had focused primarily on the mastery of the classical medical texts.

The intellectual feast offered by Padua's curriculum provided one primary dimension of the learning experience; the social circumstances in which this learning took place provided another. Within the University of Arts and Medicine, all students were organized according to their "nations." Each nation elected a councilor to serve the rector. Most of the non-Italian Jewish students belonged either to the German or Polish nations and were assigned licensed lodgings in the city. Almost like religious confraternities or merchant guilds, the student nations constituted the primary social group for all students, providing them

22. L. Münster, "Die Anfange eines klinischen Unterrichts an der Universität Padua in 16. Jahrhundert," *Medizinische Montatsschrift* 32 (1969): 171–74; F. Pellegrini, *La Clinica medica padovano attraverso i secoli* (Verona, 1939).

23. M . A. Visentini, *L'Orto botanico di Padova e il giardino del Rinascimento* (Milan, 1984)

24. E. H. Underwood, "The Early Teaching of Anatomy at Padua, with Special Reference to a Model of the Padua Anatomical Theatre," *Annals of Science* 19 (1963): 1–26.

25. A. Favaro, "I Lettori di matematiche nell'Università di Padova dal principio del secolo XIV alla fine del XVI," *Memorie e documenti per la storia dell'Università di Padova* 1 (1922): 1–70.

mutual aid and comfort and free medical care.[26] Jewish students at Padua had no official "national" identity. They apparently were denied admission to the Polish nation,[27] but it remains uncertain whether the university's other nations may have admitted Jews. Most Jewish students probably sought living space and nurturing support within the local Jewish community.[28] Nevertheless, their intense exposure to the university afforded them ample opportunities for social and intellectual interaction with non-Jews.

Whether admitted to a nation or not, each Jewish student, whatever his origin, discovered at the university an environment quite different from any he had previously experienced. More often than not, he was unprepared linguistically, culturally, or socially for such an intense experience. With the exception of former conversos, no group of Jews had ever worked and studied so intimately among such an international population. Few Jews arrived in Padua with the educational prerequisites to assume the rigorous course load of an entering medical student. The social and cultural shock of entering the university world, from even the most enlightened of family backgrounds, was no less formidable. No doubt the extraordinary challenges posed to Jewish religious sensibilities and ritual practice were similarly compelling. Problems of dietary and Sabbath

26. See P. Kibre, *The Nations in the Medieval Universities* (Cambridge, Ma., 1948), especially pp. 43, 116–205; Favaro, *Atti della nazione germanica;* Cipolla, *Public Health,* pp. 6–7; *Omaggio dell'Accademia polacca all'Università di Padova* (Cracow, 1922).

27. See Warshal, "Żydzi polscy," p. 58.

28. My thanks to Prof. Daniel Carpi for helping me to clarify this point. Professor Carpi shared with me the following evidence from the *Minute Books of the Council of the Jewish Community of Padua,* 4, folio 40, 16b, dated 7 Nissan, 5418 (=1698). The document describes the request of an "important and honorable man," a certain Ḥayyim Polacco, for housing and financial support, including a loan, in order to allow him to receive "the crown of philosophy and medicine," since he is poor and has no other financial means. He promises to repay the loan on his return to his city and the loan is approved. While several graduates of Padua have the same family name in the lists compiled by Modena and Morpurgo, *Medici e chirurghi,* Ḥayyim Polacco's name does not appear, possibly indicating that despite the support he received, he did not matriculate. How typical this requested arrangement was for the vast majority of Jewish students at the university is yet to be determined. Yet it seems plausible that the Paduan Jewish community's material and spiritual support was critical to many of them.

observance were not the only obstacles in the path of the Jewish student. The emphasis on surgery and autopsies, many of which were performed on bodies obtained illegally, even from Jewish cemeteries, also was burdensome.[29]

Despite Padua's relatively tolerant policy toward non-Catholics, Jews still encountered special obligations and disabilities. Prior to 1615, the few Jewish students who succeeded in completing their academic requirements at the medical school generally gained the title of *magister*. Only in exceptional cases were they awarded the more prestigious degree of *doctoratus in artibus et medicine* through the personal intervention of the pope's representatives, the Comites Palatini, and only "outside the walls of the university" conducted in a private ceremony. Due to the transfer of authority in awarding degrees from these papal officials to the more secular Collegium Venetum by 1616, the number of Protestant and Jewish students naturally increased under the more flexible supervision of this governing body.[30] Nevertheless, the road to matriculation was far from easy, especially for Jews. They paid higher tuition than others; upon graduation they were burdened with an additional tax of 170 pounds of sweet meat to be delivered to Christian students.[31] No doubt such formal liabilities were only a small part of the abuses Jews encountered on a day-to-day basis in trying to compete with non-Jewish students. Thus Tobias Cohen, a graduate of Padua writing at the beginning of the eighteenth century, refers openly to the hardships he and other Jews experienced as medical students: "Why should a doctor spend his time, increase his expenses, inflict his body and endanger himself in his study at the academies of the Gentiles who had Jewish students?"[32]

Above all, the Jewish student had to resist the temptations of weakening or even losing his faith. No doubt Joseph Delmedigo's experience as a student at Padua at the beginning of the seventeenth century is reflected in the following advice: "This is a warning directed to those parents who cause their sons to

29. See Ciscato, *Gli Ebrei in Padova*, p. 209. Moses Vital Cantarini composed a treatise on the problem of using Jewish corpses for dissections. See *Hebraische Bibliographie* 16 (1874): 37.

30. See Carpi, "Jews Holding the Degree of Doctor," pp. 65–66.

31. See Kisch, "Cervo Conegliano," pp. 457–59; Ciscato, *Gli Ebrei in Padova*, p. 213; Friedenwald, *The Jews and Medicine*, 1:226–27.

32. Tobias Cohen, *Ma'aseh Tuviyyah* (Cracow, 1908; repr. New York, 1974), p. 82b; and see chap. 8 below.

sin by sending them to Padua 'to philosophize' before the light of the Torah has shined upon them so that the nature of faith would haven been implanted previously in their souls in order that they not turn away from it."[33] Elsewhere he alludes to the problem of medical studies involving more than the limited mastery of medical texts: "How good it would be that you would request medicine from medical texts and faith from the source of Israel and not from the 'children of strangers and aliens,' as the secular disciplines [are called]; therefore be faithful to the Lord your God."[34] No doubt the physician David Provençal, writing in the middle of the sixteenth century, had the same problem in mind when he proposed the establishment of a Jewish institution for higher learning to train doctors immune from the corrosive influences of general university life like that of Padua.[35] In similar fashion the Paduan graduate Solomon Marini wrote, at the beginning of the seventeenth century, of those he had seen who desired "to learn and understand philosophy without prior learning of our holy Torah."[36] And certainly at the beginning of the eighteenth century, the same issue remained critical for Tobias Cohen when he warned: "No one [Jew] in all the lands of Italy, Poland, Germany, and France should consider studying medicine without first filling his belly with the written and oral Torah and other subjects."[37]

Tobias resolved his problem, as did many other Jewish medical students at Padua, by taking advantage of an extraordinary Jewish network of educational and social services that prepared foreign students like himself and his classmate Gabriel Felix to enter the university. Thus he continued: "As I testify also regarding the numerous students of my wise teacher . . . Solomon Conegliano, some of whom become rabbis and some of whom become physicians to kings

33. Joseph Delmedigo, *Sefer Elim* (Odessa, 1864–67), p. 63. Compare the remark with a similar traditional concern discussed in M. Idel, "On the History of the Interdiction against the Study of the Kabbalah before the Age of Forty" (in Hebrew) *Association for Jewish Studies Review* 5 (1980): 15–20. Delmedigo is discussed in chap. 4.

34. Delmedigo, *Sefer Elim*, p. 92.

35. Provençal's proposal is found in S. Assaf, *Toledot ha-Ḥinukh be-Yisra'el*, 4 vols. (Jerusalem, 1939–43), 2:115–20. An English translation is in J. Marcus, ed., *The Jew in the Medieval World* (New York, 1965), pp. 381–88.

36. Leibowitz, *Seridim*, pp. 44–45.

37. *Ma'aseh Tuviyyah*, p. 82b.

and important princes; for I am the least notable among them all."[38] The Jewish doctor Solomon Conegliano's preparatory school for Jewish students desirous of entering the university surely arose as a necessary solution to a set of extraordinary challenges each was expected to overcome. Under the able direction of an illustrious graduate of Padua, Jewish students could master Latin, Italian, and other propaedeutic disciplines in order to prepare themselves sufficiently for university entrance. Moreover, Solomon's home obviously offered them an appropriate social and cultural setting, a kind of half-way house between their homes and the university. Most important, it provided the necessary spiritual reinforcement—"a filled belly of Torah"—to ward off all "heretical" inclinations fostered by Padua's cosmopolitan setting. Conegliano trained students not only for medical careers but also to become rabbis. Torah and medicine had always been the most complementary of disciplines. Together they provided the necessary training for Jews to assume leadership roles either in the Jewish community or among "kings and important princes."[39]

The absence of concrete documentation does not allow us to conclude that institutions like the Conegliano boarding school were a staple of Jewish life at Padua in earlier periods. What seems clear, however, is that Jewish students could not have flourished, indeed, survived, without such supportive institutions. Moreover, the fact that Jewish graduates of Padua maintained lively social and intellectual liaisons with each other long after their departure from the university leads one to believe that such tangible support for future graduates was always forthcoming. The remarkable camaraderie among Jewish doctors and rabbis demonstrated by the celebration surrounding the Ḥamiẓ graduation is only one example of many. Equally telling is the special fellowship between Abraham ha-Cohen of Zante, Shabbatai Marini, and Solomon Lustro at the end of the seventeenth century.[40] Tobias Cohen's medical encyclopedia con-

38. Ibid.

39. On Conegliano and his school, see the introduction to *Ma'aseh Tuyiyyah* as well as the preface written by Solomon Conegliano himself. D. Kaufmann, *Dr. Israel Conegliano und seine Verdienste um die Republik Venedig bis nach dem Frieden von Carolwitz* (Budapest, 1895); idem, "Trois Docteurs de Padove," *Revue des études juives* 18 (1889): 293–98.

40. See M. Benayahu, "R. Abraham ha-Cohen of Zante and the Group of Doctor-Poets in Padua" (in Hebrew), *Ha-Sifrut* 26 (1978): 108–40

tains introductory approbations by colleagues and friends that also illustrate the social context of Jewish medical activity.[41] The life and social involvements of Isaac ha-Cohen Cantarini in the seventeenth and early eighteenth centuries offer an equally impressive example of support and liaison with other Jewish medical students and doctors similar to those of Solomon Conegliano.[42]

The impression of social fellowship and mutual support among Jewish medical students before, during, and after graduation is strengthened by the disproportionate numbers of Jewish graduates from the same family. Names like Delmedigo,[43] Wallich,[44] De Castro,[45] Pardo,[46] Cantarini,[47] Cardoso,[48] Morpurgo,[49]

41. *Ma'aseh Tuviyyah,* introductions.

42. See M. Osimo, *Narrazione della strage compiuta nel 1547 contro gli ebrei d'Asolo e cenni biografici della famiglia Koen-Cantarini* (Casale Monferrato, 1875), pp. 67–93; H. A. Savitz, "Dr. Isaac Ḥayyim ha-Cohen Cantarini," *The Jewish Forum* 43 (1960): 80–82, 99–101, 107–8. His correspondence with the Christian Hebraist Theophil Unger was published by S. D. Luzzatto in *Ozar Neḥmad* 3 (1860): 128–50.

43. Abba di Elia Delmedigo (graduated 1625, and brother of Joseph); David Vita di Donato Delmedigo (1655); Joseph Isaiah di Jacob Delmedigo de Dattolis (1677); Abramo Delmedigo (1683); Emmanuel di Jacob Delmedigo de Dattolis (1686). On Joseph, see chap. 4 below.

44. Lazzaro Wallich (1626); Abram Wallich (1655); Isaac Wallich (1683); Leone di Abram Wallich (1692); Hirsch di Abram Wallich (1692); Jacob Wallich (1722).

45. Daniel di Rodrigo De Castro (1633); Ezekiel alias Pietro di Isacco alias Ludovico De Castro (1645); David di Abram De Castro (1700). See also Friedenwald, *Jews and Medicine,* 2:452–53. On the family in Hamburg, see chap. 10 below.

46. Daniel di Abram Pardo (1624); Abram di Daniel Pardo (1646). See also L. Della Torre, "La Famiglia Pardo," in *Scritti sparsi* (Padua, 1908), 2:251–56.

47. Clemente di Simone Cantarini (1623); Leon di Simone Cantarini (1623); Simon Cantarini (1654); Isaac Vita di Jacob Isacco Cantarini (1664); Vidal Moise di Angelo Cantarini (1686); Angelo di Vidal Moise Cantarini (1697); Grassin di Samuel Vita Cantarini (1703); Angelo di Grassin Cantarini (1705); Joseph di Simon Cantarini (1718); Angelo di Simon Cantarini (1722); Simon di Grassin Cantarini (1730); Vidal Cantarini (1748). See also n. 42 above.

48. Jacob Cardoso, son of the physician Isaac Cardoso and nephew of Abraham Cardoso, graduated from Padua in 1658. On Isaac, see Y. Yerushalmi, *From Spanish Court to Italian Ghetto* (New York, 1971).

49. David di Shemaria Morpurgo (1623); Aron Morpurgo (1671); Marco Morpurgo (1694); Samson di Salvador Moise Morpurgo (1700); Mario Morpurgo (1747); Moise Raffael di Jacob Morpurgo (1768); Joseph Morpurgo (1805). See also E. Morpurgo, *La Famiglia Morpurgo di Gradisca sull'Isonzo (1585–1885)* (Padua, 1909).

Winkler,[50] Maurogonato,[51] Loria,[52] Felix,[53] and Conegliano[54] often appear among the graduates of Padua throughout the sixteenth, seventeenth, and eighteenth centuries. In the cases of these individuals, educational, financial, and social support was available from older family members who had undergone the same experience some years earlier. When this intricate web of social relationships is examined beyond the confines of Padua and even beyond Italy, one discovers similar bonds among Jewish graduates of Padua as colleagues, as teachers and students, as correspondents, and as cultural and intellectual allies in Prague, Bingen, Frankfurt, Hamburg, Cracow, Salonika, and other cities.[55]

50. Leo di Isaaco Winkler (1629); Jacob di Leo Winkler (1669); Isacco di Leo Winkler (1699); Wolff di Jacob Winkler (1701). See D. Kaufmann, "Hundert Jahre aus einer Familie Jüdischer Aerzte—Dr. Leo, dr. Jakob, dr. Isak, dr. Wolf Winkler," *Allegemeine Zeitung des Judentums* 52 (1890): 468–71 (repr. in Kaufmann, *Gesammelte Schriften* (Frankfurt, 1915), 3:286–89).

51. Eleazoro di Sabbato Maurogonato (1620); Elia di Sabbato Maurogonato (1620); Jacob di Sabbato Maurogonato (1629); Geremia Maurogonato (1633); Sabbato Maurogonato (1678); Geremia di Sabbato Maurogonato (1708); Samuel di Sabbato Maurogonato (1708).

52. David Loria (1623); Isacco di David Loria (1663); David Vita di Isacco Loria (1696); Constanino di Josue Loria (1740). See I. Levi, "La famiglia Loria," *Il Vessillo israelitico* 52 (1904): 156–58. Carpi, "Jews Holding the Degree," pp. 82–83, adds Solomon Loria graduating in 1589.

53. Vitale di Moise Felix (1658); Gabriel di Moise Felix (1683). On the latter's relationship to Tobias Cohen, see Kaufmann, "Trois Docteurs" and chap. 8 below; on his relationship to Yair Bachrach, see D. Kaufmann, *R. Jair Chajim Bachrach (1637–1702) und seine Ahnen in Worms* (Treviri, 1894).

54. Salomon di Giuseppe Conegliano (1660); Israel di Giuseppe Conegliano (1673); Abramo Joel di Israel Conegliano (1686); Joseph di Leon Conegliano (1688); Joseph di Israel Conegliano (1703); Aron Conegliano (1707); Issachar di Israel Conegliano (1710); Zevulum di Israel Conegliano (1716); Naftali di Giuseppe Conegliano (1743); Beniamino di Moise Conegliano (1766); Giuseppe Conegliano (1774); Salomon di Naftali Conegliano (1775); Amadeo Conegliano (1783). See also n. 39 above.

55. In the absence of a comprehensive statistical study of all the graduates, my general impression cannot be proved conclusively at present. But even a simple study of the origins and points of return of graduates listed by Modena and Morpurgo, *Medici e chirurghi,* when available, offers numerous cross-references to each of these places, among others. It stands to reason, even lacking concrete evidence, that university-trained physicians in the same area maintained professional and other contacts with each other. For additional examples,

The graduation of hundreds of Jews from Padua's medical school in the early modern period led to the evolution of a definable social and cultural group of Jewish intellectuals—almost all of them physicians, many of them rabbis as well—who shared a common university background, a common cultural heritage, and common interests and values. They were linguistically and culturally assimilated but maintained close contact among themselves, with non-Jewish colleagues, and with the upper echelons of western and eastern European society. Many of them were cosmopolitan and often restless in spirit and maintained an unstable itinerant lifestyle. Indeed, the term *scientific society,* which has a particular connotation for seventeenth-century European culture, might also describe the emerging fraternity of Jewish medical graduates from Padua and other graduates of Spanish and northern European universities.[56]

---

compare Kaufmann's several essays on doctor-families emanating from Padua, including the Conegliano and Winkler in nn. 39 and 50, and his "Ein Jahrhundert einer frankfurter Aerzte-familie," *Monatsschrift für Geschichte und Wissenschaft des Judentums* 41 (1897): 128–33 (repr. in *Gesammelte Schriften,* 3:296–301); Gelber "On the History of Jewish Doctors in Poland;" and J. Leibowitz, "On the History of Jewish Doctors in Salonika" (in Hebrew), *Sefer Yavan* 1 (=*Sefunot* 11) (1971–77): 341–51; J. Nehama, "Les Médecins juifs à Salonique," *Revue d'histoire de la médecine hébraïque* 8 (1951): 27–50; Kisch, *Die Prager Universität,* all strongly suggesting contacts between Jewish physicians in Italy, the Ottoman Empire, and eastern Europe. To this, one might add several specific examples of obvious Jewish medical circles in Italy, such as the poet-doctors mentioned above and contacts between Lampronti, Cantarini, and Morpurgo (discussed in chap. 9 below); Delmedigo's correspondence with the Polish physician Broscius, a fellow graduate of Padua (see chap. 4); Tobias Cohen's contacts with doctors Felix and Conegliano, and more. One could also point to interactions between Paduan graduates and like-minded converso physicians: Isaac Cardoso's sending his son to Padua; Delmedigo's contacts with Menasseh ben Israel and his circle; De Castro's contacts with Padua; Mussafia's contact with Ḥamiẓ, and more.

56. Cf. M. Ornstein, *The Role of Scientific Societies in the Seventeenth Century* (Chicago, 1938). Some recent studies of specific societies include M. B. Hall, *Promoting Experimental Learning: Experiment and the Royal Society, 1660–1727* (Cambridge and New York, 1991); D. Lux, *Patronage and Royal Science in Seventeenth-Century France: The Académie de Physique* (Ithaca, 1989); A. Stroup, *A Company of Scientists: Botany, Patronage and Community at the Seventeenth-Century Parisian Royal Academy of Sciences* (Berkeley, 1990); W. Middleton, *The Experimenters: A Study of the Accademia del Cimento* (Baltimore and London, 1971). Additional references are cited in

The Jewish network's membership ties were less formal than those of actual scientific societies, perhaps to the point of being "invisible" at times,[57] but they existed nevertheless. They were nurtured by an enthusiasm and commitment to science and enlightenment, along with a growing impatience for obscurantism and parochialism; they were reinforced also by a swelling resentment and antagonism among non-Jews throughout Europe toward the "ubiquitous" Jewish doctor.[58] For such disparaging recognition could easily be taken by Jews as an ethnic badge of honor. Had not Jews always been associated with a tradition of scientific and medical achievement? The impressive accomplishments of Jewish physicians in recent times undoubtedly were a further acknowledgment of Jewish national honor. In the words of a Jewish doctor who will be more fully introduced in a later chapter: "Though scattered all over the world, they [the Jewish physicians] manage to maintain the unity and purity of their nationality. . . . Since the time when the world was created, no other nation has thus preserved its strength and integrity."[59]

Not one of the encomiasts who participated in Joseph Ḥamiẓ's celebrated college graduation could have fully anticipated the rich symbolism of so seemingly modest an occasion. For Padua offered Jews like Ḥamiẓ more than the limited opportunity of acquiring technical knowledge. It afforded them a radically novel learning experience, a new basis for sociability with non-Jews, and a unique environment for cultivating different, often conflicting, values. It pro-

---

the epilogue below. Note there my final point that these informal Jewish "societies" did not compensate for the fact that Jews, in the main, were excluded from real scientific societies.

57. An allusion to D. Crane's *Invisible Colleges: Diffusion of Knowledge in Scientific Communities* (Chicago and London, 1972). The emphasis here is less on actual scientific collaboration than on a professional group of medical practioners with shared values and natural intellectual ties within specific communities and beyond them. On the more "visible" links among converso physicians as a critical dimension of their Jewish identifies, see chap. 10 below.

58. See Friedenwald, *Jews and Medicine,* 1:31–68; S. Muntner, *Alilot al Rofim Yehudi'im be-Aspaklariyah shel Toledot ha-Refu'ah* (Jerusalem, 1953). On converso doctors and the Inquisition, see chap. 10 below.

59. Cited by Friedenwald, *Jews and Medicine,* 1:65, from Benedict de Castro, *Flagellum calumniantium seu Apologia* (Hamburg, 1631). For a more extensive treatment of this work, see chap. 10 below.

vided them a stage, a forum for wrestling with the inevitable tensions of living a Jewish life in a dramatically changing social and intellectual universe. They had entered merely to study medicine; they came out thoroughly transformed human beings.[60]

Meir Benayahu reminds us to examine the portraits of the Jewish doctors he has studied—Abraham Cohen of Zante, Shabbatai Marini, and Solomon Lustro.[61] They, like their illustrious contemporaries Joseph Delmedigo and Tobias Cohen, flattered themselves by having their own pictures printed on the opening leaf of their published writings. How stately, how solemn, how pretentious, and how "non-Jewish" they appear in their formal medical attire! Who would doubt that beneath the composed exteriors of these gentlemen lies an inner world of variegated and challenging life experiences, of intellectual ferment, of cultural strains and agitations, and perhaps even of psychological turmoil—a world not unlike that of subsequent generations of Jews striving to enter modern European society? The following chapters probe more deeply the life experiences and cultural attitudes of several of these individuals who left for posterity both their written thoughts and their visual images.

60. Compare also the general remarks of R. Bonfil, "Academie rabbiniche e presenza ebraica nelle università," in G. P. Brizzi and J. Verger, eds., *Le Università dell'Europa dal Rinascimento alle riforme religiose* (Milan, 1991), pp. 133–51.

61. Benayahu, "R. Abraham ha-Cohen of Zante," p. 119.

4

Can a Scholar of the Natural Sciences
Take the Kabbalah Seriously?

THE DIVERGENT POSITIONS OF LEONE MODENA AND

JOSEPH DELMEDIGO

Leone Modena's public display of satisfaction with the graduation of Joseph Ḥamiẓ from the medical school of Padua in 1624
was genuine and deeply felt.[1] Equally authentic was his angry
and pained response some fifteen years later to the shocking
news of Ḥamiẓ's infatuation with the kabbalah, eventually leading to an enthusiastic endorsement of the messiahship of the
notorious Shabbatai Ẓevi. Having encouraged his illustrious student to pursue rational and naturalistic inquiries, Modena must
have seen Ḥamiẓ's turn to mystical fantasies as a repudiation of
his prodigious studies and a betrayal of his mentor.[2] Modena's

---

1. See chap. 3 above.

2. On Ḥamiẓ, see N. Leibowitz, *Seridim mi-Kitve ha-Pilosof ha-Rofe ve-ha-
Mekubbal R. Yosef Ḥamiẓ* (Jerusalem, 1938); I. Tishby, "Documents on Nathan
of Gaza in the Writings of R. Joseph Ḥamiẓ" (in Hebrew), in *Netive Emunah ve-Minut* (Ramat Gan, 1964), pp. 30–51; E. Kupfer, "R. Joseph Ḥamiẓ
in Zante and His Work on the Education of Youth" (in Hebrew), *Sefunot*
[=*Sefer Yavan*] 2 (1971–78): 199–216; M. Idel, "Differing Conceptions of
Kabbalah in the Early Seventeenth Century," in *Jewish Thought in the Seventeenth Century,* ed. I. Twersky and B. Septimus (Cambridge, Mass., 1987),
pp. 154–97. Both Benjamin Richler and Moshe Idel have informed me of
another manuscript recently identified by Richler as being composed by
Ḥamiẓ. MS Parma De' Rossi 1285 deals with astronomical matters, with
kabbalistic references interspersed throughout. My thanks to both scholars
for this reference.

Ari Nohem, his well-known critique of the kabbalah completed in 1639, was to a large extent personally directed to his seemingly disloyal pupil.[3] My concern with Modena in this chapter is not with his general criticism of the place of kabbalah in Judaism, but more specifically with his pointed remarks about the study of nature, rationality, and the pursuit of the sciences that emerge obliquely from his polemic. He is also important to our subject because of his close intellectual and social relations with two of the major champions of the sciences within Jewish culture of his day: Joseph Delmedigo and Simone Luzzatto.[4] None of Modena's writings are devoted to the sciences per se. Nevertheless, his position becomes quite clear from several passages in *Ari Nohem,* especially when viewed in conjunction with his earlier enthusiasm for both Ḥamiẓ's medical career and the publication of Joseph Delmedigo's scientific text, the *Sefer Elim,* in Amsterdam in 1629.

Before examining Modena's position more closely, it might be useful to propose a general typology of conceptual schemes within the intellectual circles of Italian Jewry in Modena's lifetime and after. Such a proposal should be construed merely as a rough map of the complex intellectual terrain over which Modena, Ḥamiẓ, Delmedigo, Luzzatto, and some of the figures discussed in subsequent chapters trod.

In a first category I would place the intellectual fully committed to integrating rabbinic culture with the secular world and to explaining it, as well as possible, in terms comprehensible to human reason and experience. He is a true heir of Maimonides. Although he no longer shares Maimonides' confidence in the Aristotelian system, he identifies with the process of translating Judaism into a rational language of discourse and confronts, indeed invites, the dialogue between Jewish faith and universal reason. Surely Modena belongs in this cate-

---

3. *Ari Nohem* (Jerusalem, 1971), pp. 1–2. Modena also mentions the debates he held with his son-in-law, Jacob of the Levites, on the authenticity of the kabbalah. On Modena, see the introductory essays of the English translation of his autobiography, M. Cohen, ed. and trans., *The Autobiography of a Seventeenth-Century Venetian Rabbi* (Princeton, 1988), and H. Adelman, "Success and Failure in the Seventeenth-Century Ghetto of Venice: The Life and Thought of Leon Modena," Ph.D. diss., Brandeis University, 1985. As we shall see shortly, *Ari Nohem* was also directed to Joseph Delmedigo, as Adelman correctly notes (pp. 796–801).

4. Delmedigo is discussed in this chapter; Luzzatto is the subject of the next.

gory, as do his more rational colleagues Azariah de' Rossi and Simone Luzzatto, the Frances brothers, and Samson Morpurgo.[5] No doubt many of this group had been fortified in their positions by their exposure to the scientific ambiance of medical schools like Padua's. Although their intellectual positions were increasingly challenged by contemporaries, they held an influential position among Jewish and Christian intellectuals, as exemplified by Modena and Luzzatto.

Those who objected strongly to their rationalistic tendencies came from two camps, neither of which was so distinct as to either exclude or overlap with the other. In the first were the "pure" or "mythical" kabbalists, those like Moses Ḥayyim Luzzatto, Moses Zacuto, and their ancestors Menaḥem Azariah da Fano, Ezra Fano, and Aaron Berakhia of Modena. All expressed unequivocal intellectual and spiritual satisfaction with the vineyards of the kabbalah and gave relatively little weight to the pursuit of other forms of learning. Of course, not even this group had fully isolated themselves from the larger cultural concerns of their contemporaries. Luzzatto and Zacuto had integrated their kabbalistic concerns with baroque drama.[6] Luzzatto's messianic circle were hardly oblivious or firmly opposed to the naturalistic pursuits promoted especially in his native Padua.[7] And the two Fanos, while primarily interested in kabbalistic matters, were quite open to naturalistic pursuits, if the latter could be utilized to illumine their esoteric preoccupations.[8] In reality, no "pure kabbalist" or, for that matter, "pure rationalist" was visible in Italian Jewish culture.

5. On De' Rossi's relevance to science, see esp. chaps. 2 and 9. On Morpurgo and the Frances brothers, see chap. 7.

6. See, for example, P. Lachover, *Al Gevul ha-Yashan ve-ha-Ḥadash* (Jerusalem, 1951), pp. 29–58; J. Schirmann, "The Hebrew Drama in the Seventeenth Century" (in Hebrew), *Moznayim* 4 (1938): 624–35 (repr. in his *Studies in the History of Hebrew Poetry and Drama,* 2 vols. (Jerusalem, 1977), 1:25–38; and Y. Melkman, "Moshe Zacuto's Play *Yesod Olam*" (in Hebrew), *Sefunot* 10 (1966): 299–333.

7. See, for example, the interesting statement of Luzzatto's disciple Yekutiel Gordon on the near completion of his medical studies, in M. Benayahu, *Kitve ha-Kabbala shel Ramḥal* (Jerusalem, 1979), p. 76. See also S. Ginzberg, *The Life and Works of Moses Ḥayyim Luzzatto* (Philadelphia, 1931), pp. 112–13, 115–17, 136–37.

8. See D. B. Ruderman, *Kabbalah, Magic, and Science: The Cultural Universe of a Sixteenth-Century Jewish Physician* (Cambridge, Mass., and London, 1988), pp. 21–22, and the additional works cited in the notes.

A second group of thinkers demands our primary attention in this and subsequent chapters because, to my mind, they constitute the most important of
the three intellectual circles. Many of them were kabbalists—more open to the
sciences than the first group, yet firmly opposed to philosophy and especially
Aristotelian metaphysics. The same Joseph Ḥamiẓ, in the introduction to his *Or
Nogah*, delineates these three groupings and places himself squarely in the third:
"From the beginning, I always tried [compare Proverbs 8:23] to find a path to
follow the Torah and [rational investigation] so that one would not contradict
the other, and so that both—that which is based on reason and that which lies
beyond reason—could be upheld. . . . This was for me the straight path by which
a person might recognize that God placed intelligence within him not only to
distance him from what is beyond him but to draw him closer to what is before him. . . . [Accordingly,] one must understand nature in order to know what
is beyond nature."[9] Despite his teacher's misgivings, Ḥamiẓ pursued his kabbalistic interests without denying his background in medicine and naturalistic
studies. He integrated the two in the writings he later composed in Zante.[10] And
Ḥamiẓ was hardly alone in merging the physical sciences with Jewish esoteric
pursuits. Among the prominent Italian Jews with similar integrative proclivities
we might include Abraham Portaleone, Abraham Yagel, Isaac Cardoso and even
his brother Abraham, Azariah Figo, Solomon Basilea, Isaac Lampronti, David
Nieto, and many others.[11]

In the midst of Modena's frontal attack on the veracity of kabbalistic claims
to knowledge, he makes the following categorical statement in *Ari Nohem:* "All

9. Leibowitz, *Seridim*, pp. 15–17

10. See the references in n. 2 above, esp. the essays of Tishby and Kupfer.

11. Yagel is discussed in Ruderman, *Kabbalah, Magic, and Science*. Figo, Basilea, Lampronti,
and Nieto all receive extensive treatments below. On Isaac Cardoso, see Y. Yerushalmi, *From
Spanish Court to Italian Ghetto* (New York, 1971). On the academic background of his brother
Abraham and its place in the latter's messianic thinking, see N. Yosha, "The Philosophi-
cal Background of Sabbatian Theology—Guidelines toward an Understanding of Abraham
Michael Cardoso's Theory of the Divine" (in Hebrew), *Galut Aḥar Golah: Meḥḳarim be-Toledot
Am Yisra'el Mugashim le-Professor Ḥaim Beinart,* ed. Y. Kaplan, A. Mirsky, A. Grossman (Jeru-
salem, 1988), pp. 541–72. Portaleone's scientific interests have not yet been studied seriously.
See N. Shapira, "R. Abraham Portaleone, the Doctor, Encyclopedist, and His Book *Shilte
Gibburim* (1542–1612)" (in Hebrew), *Ha-Rofe Ha-Ivri* 33 (1960):111–12.

knowledge that you are able to know as a person living on this earth can only be a posteriori, especially with respect to the reality of God and His unity and the other divine matters. There is no knowledge that can be a priori except that of a prophet . . . and [quoting a rabbinic statement] a scholar is preferred to a prophet."[12] Elsewhere he declares: "Every science has a definition, either with respect to its subject, or purpose, as natural philosophy is the science of knowing the natures of created things, and astronomy that of knowing the position and movement of the stars."[13] "But what then is the kabbalah?" Modena asks. A rational, scientific mode of inquiry has come to judge "the science" of the kabbalah and finds it lacking. True science for Modena is to be located elsewhere in the investigation of the natural world: "For when God came to chastise Job, who expressed doubt in His providence and dominion over the world, He reminded him that he had not investigated *Ma'aseh Bereshit* [the biblical account of creation, identified by Maimonides as physics], from which he would recognize His greatness and ability, and His judgment in all the land, of the elements, plants, animals, and those that came into existence in the air, by the laws of heaven and the stars. For these are the investigations that enable man to know his creator. . . . Anything else than this is not known in such a manner . . . cannot be called science in any way."[14]

As if to clinch his argument, Modena later adduces the testimony of a most reliable source, Elijah Montalto, the prominent converso physician and scientific writer. Modena had apparently made his acquaintance during his sojourn in Venice and obviously viewed his career and vast scientific learning as a model which Ḥamiẓ might have emulated. The story he relates illustrates dramatically the confrontation between scientific rationality and kabbalistic sapience. Speaking directly to Ḥamiẓ, Modena writes:

> It is impossible not to tell you what happened more than twenty-five years ago . . . when you were still a small boy. R. Yedidiah Galenti arrived here, the emissary from the land of Israel, and about the same time as his coming,

12. B.T. Babba Batra 12 and elsewhere. See *Ari Nohem,* p. 16.
13. Ibid., p. 14.
14. Ibid., pp. 18–19. On the challenge of defining kabbalah as a science, compare Ruderman, *Kabbalah, Magic, and Science,* pp. 150–54.

the wonderful scholarly doctor R. Elijah Montalto was sick on his deathbed. Many of the learned Torah scholars went to visit him since he was modest and related well to other people despite his vast erudition. While we were there, Galenti began to tell of the miracles and wonders of the Ari [the Safed kabbalist Isaac Luria], of blessed memory, from the aforementioned [kabbalist] writings and also from the unwritten testimony of Joseph Delmedigo. When he had finished most of his discourse, the physician [Montalto], of blessed memory, gathered his strength, sat up in bed, and began to scream in a loud voice. We did not know what had happened to him and thought that he had been seized by pains due to his illness. And in his shouting, he uttered the following in Spanish: "I can no longer be silent and endure this any longer. Let the truth live! All this is a lie and a falsehood. No signs can we observe, for there is no longer any prophet or anyone among us who knows for how long [compare Psalm 74:9]. Either he is a sorcerer or all these are lies, and do not tell me any more of this."[15]

Montalto's deathbed rage undoubtedly encapsulated Modena's immediate frustration in losing the loyalty of his supposedly enlightened student to the blandishments of kabbalistic "lies and falsehoods." But even taking into account the tinge of personal bitterness accompanying his strongly worded polemic with Ḥamiẓ, Modena's position in *Ari Nohem* on what constitutes true knowledge appears to reflect his long-held view quite accurately. In his statement— solicited together with those of three other Venetian rabbis, including Luzzatto—introducing the publication of Delmedigo's scientific tome, he took a remarkably similar position. After mentioning his pleasurable personal encounters with Delmedigo in Venice, he calls him a true scholar whose wisdom "is like divine knowledge glorifying him by lighting the candle of the splendor of our nation in natural and divine sciences necessary for divine worship, as the author of the *Guide [of the Perplexed,* Maimonides], the crown of intelligence, indicated, demonstrating to the nations of the world that God did not also speak

15. Ibid., p. 80. The most recent work on Montalto is B. Cooperman, "Eliahu Montalto's 'Suitable and Incontrovertible Propositions': A Seventeenth-Century Anti-Christian Polemic," in *Jewish Thought in the Seventeenth Century,* pp. 469–97. Cooperman translates part of the above passage on p. 490.

to them but [only] to us.[16] But [this knowledge] disappeared among the many 'self-proclaimed holy ones and purified' sages of our people, who would close their eyes from seeing the leather cover of [such] a book among them, hiding their limited intelligence and ignorance in a holy covering and relating to such [works] with strangeness and alienation."[17] Modena mentions *Sha'agat Aryeh,* which he wrote to combat these scholars' falsehoods. The work he recalls repre-sented his short, incomplete response to the anonymous critique of rabbinic Judaism called the *Kol Sakhal.*[18] But one wonders whether he really had in mind his yet-to-be-completed *Ari Nohem,* his other "roaring lion" (the meaning of the titles of both works). His praise for a true scientific book that was obviously unappreciated by "self-proclaimed holy ones . . . who close their eyes" to its wisdom, hiding "their limited intelligence" in mystical fantasies, seems to relate more appropriately to this later work.

Be that as it may, the passages in *Ari Nohem* and in Modena's approbation of *Sefer Elim* are linked by a common perception of what constitutes true knowl-edge embodied by two of the most outstanding Jewish scientific luminaries of Modena's era: Elijah Montalto and Joseph Delmedigo. How ironic, therefore, to discover that the second target of Modena's barbed missiles in *Ari Nohem* was none other than Joseph Delmedigo himself! Was this the same author who had called himself a disciple of Galileo, related the new Copernican cosmology with unrestrained enthusiasm, and advocated the study of mathematics, mechanics, and astronomy in contemporary Jewish society? Had this remarkable student of the sciences also lost his mind and the right path by joining the disreputable camp of kabbalistic frenzy and superstition? How was it possible for two Jewish graduates of Padua to embrace the kabbalah after having undergone so intense an exposure to academic and scientific learning?

16. Apparently a reference to his well-known interpretation of Deut. 4:6, what Isadore Twersky calls Maimonides' "outer-directed awareness." Cf. *Guide of the Perplexed,* 2:11, 3:31; and I. Twersky, *Introduction to the Code of Maimonides (Mishneh Torah)* (New Haven, 1980), pp. 385–87.

17. Joseph Delmedigo, *Sefer Elim* (Amsterdam, 1629; repr. Odessa, 1864–67), opening.

18. See Adelman, "Success and Failure," chap. 21, and T. Fishman, "*Kol Sachal*'s Critique of Rabbinic Tradition: A Solution to the Problem of Galut," Ph.D. diss., Harvard Univer-sity, 1986.

Modena was reacting to Delmedigo's second book, *Ta'alumot Ḥokhmah,* published two years after *Sefer Elim* under the supposed editorship of Delmedigo's disciple Samuel Ashkenazi.[19] In striking contrast to the first work, the second consists of two parts: an anthology of writings primarily by others and a sprawling discussion of various metaphysical issues called *Novlot Ḥokhmah,* heavily relying on the kabbalah and apparently written by Delmedigo himself.[20] Modena was especially irritated by the only composition in the first part that Delmedigo had written, *Maẓref la-Ḥokhmah.* It was allegedly a refutation of a book composed in 1491 by Joseph's ancestor Elijah Delmedigo called *Beḥinat ha-Dat,* which was also included as the first work in the anthology. What particularly interested Joseph about this philosophical treatise were Elijah's critical comments on the kabbalists, including the allegation that their classic *Sefer ha-Zohar* had been written in the Middle Ages and was not a work of ancient and sacred provenance.[21] Modena was not only familiar with Elijah's position; he identified with it, defended it, and expanded upon it in *Ari Nohem.* To behold such a pious defense of the kabbalah from the pen of so prominent a scientist and intellectual ally, along with the other eclectic writings in this strange volume, distressed him immensely.

Modena mentions *Maẓref la-Ḥokhmah* several times and responds directly to its specific arguments in defense of the authenticity and antiquity of the kabbalistic tradition. Joseph Delmedigo had claimed that although the kabbalah was of ancient origin, the rabbis of the Talmud and the *Gaonim,* the leaders of world Jewry under medieval Islam, did not refer to it since they were preoccupied with legal matters, not spiritualist ones. Delmedigo adduced a scientific parallel to make his point: "In all the medical texts one would not find any hint of the craft of seafaring or carpentry."[22] Modena understandably rejected this argument, defining the Talmud as encyclopedic. The rabbis were not specialists in

19. *Sefer Ta'alumot Ḥokhmah* (Basel, 1629–31)

20. For a full description of the work's contents, see I. Barzilay, *Yoseph Shlomo Delmedigo (Yashar of Candia): His Life, Works, and Times* (Leiden, 1974), pp. 103–21.

21. The most recent treatment of Elijah Delmedigo and the Kabbalah is K. P. Bland, "Elijah del Medigo's Averroist Response to the Kabbalahs of Fifteenth-Century Jewry and Pico della Mirandola," *Jewish Thought and Philosophy* 1 (1991): 23–53.

22. *Maẓref la-Ḥokhmah* (Warsaw, 1890), p. 81; Barzilay, *Yosef Shlomo Delmedigo,* p. 286.

one craft; they commanded knowledge in all areas and wrote profusely about everything.[23] Modena was particularly galled by Delmedigo's characterization of Saadia Gaon, the medieval philosopher, which he discusses at length. After citing a long passage from Saadia in which the philosopher seemingly distances himself from the kabbalah, he examines Delmedigo's forced explanation: "If the Gaon Rabbi Saadia . . . did not speak of this kabbalah, along with others like him, it wasn't because they didn't know about it or because he didn't believe in it, but only because he was speaking in a philosophic manner at that time."[24] Modena clearly could fathom neither the possibility of a person writing as a philosopher while simultaneously believing in mysticism, nor the opposite— writing in favor of mysticism while upholding a scientific, rational point of view, as in the case of Joseph Delmedigo. Saadia had no affection for the kabbalah, according to Modena, and despite Delmedigo's masquerade as a kabbalist, it was inconceivable to him that such an author could countenance so ludicrous a position.[25]

Modena realized, however, that Delmedigo's plea for the coexistence of philosophy and the kabbalah had been articulated by others. He referred specifically to the notion of Israel Sarug, the reputed emissary of Lurianic kabbalah in Italy, who had taught the kabbalah in a philosophic manner.[26] He also noted that Ḥamiẓ had entertained similar correlations between the Platonic ideas and the kabbalistic *sephirot* or the Pythagorian notion of transmigration with that of the kabbalah. In this context, he cites two passages from Delmedigo's writing, the first strongly aligning Plato with the kabbalah,[27] the second attempting to explain the kabbalistic notion of "points" as corresponding to the atomism of the ancients.[28] Modena objects to the claim that the ancient philosophers derived

23. *Ari Nohem,* pp. 35–36.

24. *Maẓref la-Ḥokhmah,* p. 80.

25. *Ari Nohem,* pp. 37–38.

26. On Sarug, the classic work is G. Scholem, "Israel Sarug, the Ari's Disciple?" (in Hebrew), *Zion* 5 (1940): 214–41; the most recent work is M. Idel, "Beween the Kabbalah of Jerusalem and the Kabbalah of Israel Sarug" (in Hebrew), *Shalem* 6 (1992): 165–73.

27. *Maẓref la-Ḥokhmah,* p. 107.

28. *Sefer Ko'aḥ ha-Shem* in *Ta'alumot Ḥokhmah,* pp. 198a–203b; Barzilay, *Yosef Shlomo Delmedigo,* pp. 294–96; Idel, "Differing Conceptions," pp. 185–90.

their notions from the kabbalah. On the contrary, such parallels demonstrate the recent origin of Jewish mystical teachings and its ultimate derivation from Gentile pagan sources.[29]

Such misguided eclecticism was surely unbecoming to so exalted a scientist as Delmedigo. The only explanation for his bizarre stance, Modena finally claims, is that Delmedigo was dissimulating: he adopted his incongruous defense of the kabbalah in order to please a political patron. Modena refers to the following passage of Delmedigo, one immediately following his discussion of Saadia, that appears to reveal his utter insincerity:

> Here I am writing against the philosophers and on behalf of the kabbalists, since I was asked to do so by one of the dignitaries of the Jewish community whose heart is attracted at the moment to the kabbalah. Being attached to him by ties of love, I turned away from my own studies to satisfy his request. Should he be in a different mood by tomorrow and, entertaining a predilection for philosophy, ask me to praise and extol it, I shall eagerly undertake such a vigorous defense of it. I submit to you a major principle: you must not think to fathom the mind of authors on the basis of the views they express in their books. God alone knows the mysteries of the human heart. . . . There is neither a teacher nor a father who reveals to his disciple or son whatever is in his heart with regard to such matters.[30]

For Modena, this statement transparently indicates that Delmedigo "presented himself as a defender of the wisdom of the kabbalah while praising it when his real intention was to diminish and degrade it with all his strength. And truly he is a cunning scholar and a master of all the sciences." To clinch this assessment, he finally points out how Delmedigo extolled the magical wonders of the kabbalist Isaac Luria while in the same breath publicizing the trickery of a Polish father who shamelessly presented his infant as a prodigy. In the final analysis, claimed Modena, Delmedigo's views of such stories were identical with those of Montalto cited above.[31] Modena would not allow Ḥamiẓ to view

29. *Ari Nohem*, p. 53.

30. *Maẓref la-Ḥokhmah*, pp. 80–81. I generally follow Barzilay's translation in *Yosef Shlomo Delmedigo*, pp. 242–43.

31. *Ari Nohem*, pp. 78–79.

Delmedigo as a role model for his distressing turn from science to mysticism. Underneath Delmedigo's guileful and insidious exterior was a man committed only to his reason and scientific methodology, cut in the image of Modena himself.

Modena's seemingly thorough detective work regarding Joseph Delmedigo's apparent deceit was surely welcomed by those nineteenth-century scholars of Jewish thought who, like Modena, sought to reclaim his image for the rationalistic camp of Judaism. To Abraham Geiger,[32] Heinrich Graetz,[33] and Israel Zinberg,[34] among others, Delmedigo was a figure of heroic proportions, carrying a solitary torch of enlightenment and science through a Jewish desert of legalism, parochialism, and spiritualist and messianic superstition. He was a true seventeenth-century precursor of their valiant efforts to rehabilitate Jewish life and culture, and although he seemingly lacked the courage to stand publicly by his private convictions, there remained no doubt about what those convictions were. His parading of kabbalistic pieties was surely meant to protect himself from the wrath of his orthodox coreligionists. His authentic ideas about science, Judaism, educational reform, and rabbinic and kabbalistic thought could not be expressed in public, and therefore he adopted camouflage and subterfuge in his writing.[35]

Modena's intuition was seemingly confirmed in 1840 with the dramatic publication by Abraham Geiger of a private letter Delmedigo supposedly wrote to one of his Karaite disciples. An earlier version of this epistle, usually called "the Aḥuz letter" after its opening word, had been published as the beginning of *Sefer Ma'ayan Ganim*.[36] In its original form, it mildly criticized rabbinic culture, spoke of the kabbalah in a positive though puzzled manner, and strongly advocated the study of the sciences among Jews. Geiger claimed to have come upon a dif-

32. Abraham Geiger, *Melo Chofnajim* (Berlin, 1940).

33. H. Graetz, *Divre Yeme Yisrael,* ed. S. Rabinowitz (Warsaw, 1917), 8:186–93.

34. I. Zinberg, *A History of Jewish Literature,* trans. B. Martin (Cincinnati and New York, 1974), 5:155–74.

35. The subtitle of Zinberg's depiction reads: "Delmedigo's True Face and Strange Mask" (p. 163).

36. *Sefer Ma'ayan Ganin,* in *Sefer Elim,* pp. 126–35.

ferent and fuller version of the letter. Still preserved in manuscript, uncensored and unrestrained, it apparently exposed Delmedigo's true feelings, which were hidden in the printed version. Most notable of these was an utter disdain for all kabbalistic ideas and writings and a concomitant appreciation for Karaite exegesis and literature.[37] We shall consider this letter again later in the chapter. Suffice it to say at this point that the evidence Geiger presented, together with his learned analysis of Delmedigo's life and thought, left its mark on all subsequent scholarship. His parallel findings on Modena—who, according to Geiger, had also camouflaged his heretical views on rabbinic law and culture[38]—meant that Geiger and his reform-minded contemporaries had located two seventeenth-century "reformers" of Judaism. In both studies, Geiger's scholarship brilliantly served his ideology of Judaism.

The most important contribution of the study of Delmedigo since Geiger's was the ambitious and comprehensive study of Isaac Barzilay.[39] While fully aware of the tendentious excesses of nineteenth-century scholars, Barzilay shared their unabashed enthusiasm for Delmedigo as a scientific rationalist. His portrait was consistent with his earlier and later studies of the Berlin Enlightenment. In his well-known essay "The Italian and Berlin Haskalah," Barzilay had followed his teacher Salo W. Baron in suggesting an organic connection between the two.[40] While noting differences between the two cultural epochs, Barzilay still viewed the Italian "enlightenment" as an adumbration of the German one. In his study of "antirationalism" in Italian Jewish thought, he essentially described the Jewish cultural milieu of Italy as polarized between rational and antirational camps, where ultimately a commitment to one camp precluded a sympathetic involvement with the other.[41]

In presenting Delmedigo as a champion of rational interests, Barzilay acknowledged the extraordinary challenge of establishing the real "intellectual and

37. Geiger, *Melo Chofnajim,* Hebrew section, pp. 1–28.

38. Geiger, *Leon da Modena, Rabbiner ʒu Venedig (1571–1648) und seine Stellung ʒur Kabbalah, ʒum Talmud und ʒum Christenhume* (Breslau, 1856).

39. Barzilay, *Yoseph Shlomo Delmedigo.*

40. Barzilay, "The Italian and Berlin Haskalah," *Proceedings of the American Academy for Jewish Research* 29 (1961–62): 15–54.

41. Barzilay, *Between Reason and Faith: Anti-Rationalism in Italian Jewish Thought (1250–1650)* (The Hague, 1967).

psychological identity of the man."[42] Having painfully digested and outlined every page of Delmedigo's massive writings, Barzilay could not fully concur with Geiger in "dismissing the pietist element [of Delmedigo's thought] as mere camouflage, as a stratagem for concealing his heretical views."[43] In struggling for a more balanced assessment, Barzilay accepted Geiger's view only with respect to *Mazref la-Ḥokhmah,* Delmedigo's purported defense of the kabbalah, but not with respect to the kabbalah in general. He acknowledged that the spiritual elements of the kabbalah in his writing were too extensive and too profuse to be dismissed out of hand. They had to be considered integral to his thought, part of the process of Delmedigo's "quest and search," raising questions and doubts and undermining the dogma of all systems.[44]

Nevertheless, Barzilay appeared increasingly impatient with the massive dosages of kabbalistic thought in Delmedigo's work, especially the *Ta'alumot Ḥokhmah.* In contrast to his appreciative portrait of Delmedigo's involvements in astronomy, mathematics, mechanics, and applied technology, Barzilay visibly wrestled with the irritating fluctuations between rationalism and mysticism in the *Novlot Ḥokhmah* and *Orah* and their long discussions of emanation, light, divine contraction, and creation. He ultimately elected to understand these discussions regressively—that is, evolving from philosophy to mysticism to spiritualism and crude superstition.[45] The first part of *Ta'alumot Ḥokhmah,* with its eclectic anthology of philosophical and kabbalistic writings, is meant to suggest for Barzilay the obvious superiority of the former over the latter.[46] By printing the Lurianic texts, Barzilay maintained, Delmedigo meant to refute them and to show how absurd they really are.[47] Barzilay noted Delmedigo's seemingly tortured attempts to philosophize the kabbalah. He held up the example of his correlations between kabbalistic points, atoms, and the technology of printing. But Barzilay was convinced that this search for solutions to the great problems of creation and existence, no matter how sincerely motivated, was doomed to

42. Barzilay, *Delmedigo,* p. 25.
43. Ibid., p. 169; see also p. 241.
44. Ibid.
45. See esp. ibid., pp. 196–98, 249.
46. Ibid., pp. 107–8.
47. Ibid., p. 266.

failure. In the final analysis, Lurianic kabbalah was "nothing but a myth leading to superstition and witchcraft. . . . When rationalized, it was only a new garb for the ancient views of the atomists, on the one hand, and for the logos of the Neo-Platonists, on the other."[48]

In other words, despite Barzilay's earnest attempt to appreciate the totality of Delmedigo's writing, to search for a common thread binding its disparate and apparently contradictory elements, there was a marked tendency to privilege the refreshing consistency and rational analysis of the image of Delmedigo presented in *Sefer Elim* over that encountered in *Ta'alumot Ḥokhmah*.[49] In the end, the boundaries in the struggle between the forces of reason and superstition of the seventeenth century were still clearly drawn. Barzilay's Delmedigo, despite the mixed signals in his complex writings, opted for the rational camp. He was a true critic of rabbinic Judaism, especially the predominance of kabbalah in his day.[50] He associated with Karaites in order to vent his own spirit of rebellion against rabbinic Judaism.[51] He severely criticized Jewish education and displayed the first inferiority complex among modern Jews, and, as his rootless life demonstrates, Delmedigo remained "a stranger to his own age and to his own contemporaries."[52]

In the almost twenty years since the publication of Barzilay's pioneering study, the directions of historical research with respect to the history of both science and Jewish thought have radically shifted. Barzilay was not acquainted with Frances Yates's provocative reading of Giordano Bruno's scientific thought, published some ten years before his own, or with her controversial essay on the Hermetic origins of modern science.[53] Since the 1960s, the contentious and

48. Ibid., pp. 292–96; the citation is from p. 296.

49. Note ibid., p. 218: "Yashar is modern in *Elim,* totally emancipated from the medieval Weltanschauung. Contrariwise, he is wholly medieval in *Novloth,* both with regard to his views and to his use of the method of formal dialectics."

50. Ibid., pp. 305–10.

51. Ibid., pp. 311–14.

52. Ibid., pp. 315–22; the citation is from p. 322.

53. F. A. Yates, *Giordano Bruno and the Hermetic Tradition* (London, 1964) and "The Hermetic Tradition in Renaissance Science," in *Art, Science, and History in the Renaissance,* ed. C. S. Singleton (Baltimore, 1967), pp. 255–74.

stimulating discussion of her thesis on the relations between occult and scientific mentalities has greatly enriched our understanding of the cultural climate of Copernicus, Kepler, Galileo, Newton, and many others, as well as the capacity of scientific thinkers and experimenters to absorb and to live comfortably with spiritualist, occult, and prophetic elements in their understanding and appreciation of the natural world. Despite the extremity of some of Dame Yates's formulations, a general consensus among historians of science has emerged about the cultural complexity of the age in which modern science was born, about the coexistence of mystical and rational elements among scientific thinkers, and about the need to view scientific thought in its broader intellectual, religious, and social contexts.[54]

The last twenty years have also witnessed a significant remapping of Jewish cultural and intellectual development in the era of Delmedigo. I refer to the reevaluation of Scholem's grandiose reconstruction of kabbalistic thought in the early modern period by Moshe Idel, Yehudah Liebes,[55] and others,[56] and specifically to the study of Jewish thought in Italy.[57] Idel's studies, in particular, of Yohanan Alemanno,[58] of Italian kabbalistic thought,[59] of Leone Ebreo,[60] of

54. On "the Yates thesis," see B. Vickers, ed., *Occult and Scientific Mentalities in the Renaissance* (Cambridge, 1984) and P. Curry, "Revisions of Science and Magic," *History of Science* 23 (1985): 291–325, both of whom list earlier references.

55. See, for example, M. Idel, *Kabbalah: New Perspectives* (New Haven and London, 1988), and Y. Liebes, *Studies in Jewish Myth and Jewish Messianism* (Albany, 1993).

56. See Introduction above.

57. Idel, "Particularism and Universalism in Kabbalah, 1480–1650," in D. B. Ruderman, ed., *Essential Papers on Jewish Culture in Renaissance and Baroque Italy* (New York and London, 1992), pp. 324–44; idem, "Major Currents in Italian Kabbalah between 1560 and 1660," *Italia Judaica*, vol. 2: *Gli Ebrei in Italia tra Rinascimento et età barocca* (Rome, 1986), pp. 243–62 (repr. in *Essential Papers*, pp. 345–68).

58. Idel, "The Magical and Neoplatonic Interpretations of the Kabbalah in the Renaissance," in B. Cooperman, ed., *Jewish Thought in the Sixteenth Century* (Cambridge, Mass., 1983), pp. 186–242 (repr. in *Essential Papers*, pp. 107–69).

59. Idel, "Major Currents."

60. Idel, "Kabbalah and Ancient Theology in R. Isaac and Judah Abravanel" (in Hebrew), in *The Philosophy of Love of Leone Ebreo*, ed. M. Dorman and Z. Levy (Haifa, 1985), pp. 73–112.

Leone Modena,[61] and of Menasseh ben Israel[62] have underscored the syncretistic nature of Jewish cultural development in Italy and beyond, the powerful hold of Renaissance quests to correlate disparate cultural experiences, and the consistent tendency of kabbalistic thinkers in Italy from the late fifteenth to the seventeenth centuries to integrate kabbalah with Neoplatonism and magic. My own writing on Abraham Yagel, Delmedigo's older contemporary, has suggested how magical, kabbalistic, and scientific elements could coexist in the thinking of a Jewish intellectual equally enamored of the new scientific discoveries.[63] Alexander Altmann's[64] and especially Nissim Yosha's recent study of Abraham Herrera,[65] Delmedigo's contemporary in Amsterdam, have demonstrated the still powerful influence of Renaissance understandings of ancient theology and Neoplatonism on Jewish thought and the need to explain Lurianic myth in the language of philosophy in precisely the cultural milieu in which Delmedigo flourished. In short, the cultural space Christians and Jews shared in the seventeenth century has come to be understood in a more nuanced and complete way and more in its own cultural terms than as a mere prelude to Enlightenment and nineteenth-century developments. Contextualizing Delmedigo's thought in the light of this new scholarship makes him appear a less isolated figure than Barzilay portrayed him to be, less a precursor of another age and more a product of his own. Most important, his proclivity to integrate kabbalah, Neoplatonism, magic, and science appears less ludicrous and considerably more serious than Barzilay and Geiger initially assumed.

A young researcher, Joseph Levi, has recently undertaken the task of re-

61. Idel, "Differing Conceptions of Kabbalah in the Early Seventeenth Century".

62. Idel "Kabbalah, Platonism and Prisca Theologia: The Case of R. Menasseh ben Israel," in *Menasseh Ben Israel and His World*, ed. Y. Kaplan, H. Méchoulan, R. Popkin (Leiden, 1989), pp. 207–19.

63. Ruderman, *Kabbalah, Magic and Science* (Cambridge, Mass., 1988) and *A Valley of Vision: The Heavenly Journey of Abraham ben Hananiyah Yagel* (Philadelphia, 1990).

64. Altmann, "Lurianic Kabbalah in a Platonic Key: Abraham Cohen Herrera's Puerta del Cielo," *Hebrew Union College Annual* 53 (1982): 317–52; repr. in Twersky and Septimus, *Jewish Thought in the Seventeenth Century*, pp. 1–38, and in Altmann, *Vor der Mittelalterlichen zur moderen Aufklarung* (Tübingen, 1987), pp. 172–205.

65. Yosha, "Abraham Cohen Herrera's Philosophical Interpretation of Lurianic Kabbalah" (in Hebrew), Ph.D. diss., Hebrew University, 1991.

conceptualizing Delmedigo's work. Although his study is still incomplete, I cannot pass over his emerging position in silence in this discussion of Delmedigo's image in recent scholarship.[66] Levi expresses dissatisfaction with previous scholarship on Delmedigo on precisely the grounds that I have suggested: its inability to root him in the cultural matrix of his times and its reluctance to reveal the immanent connections between his kabbalistic and scientific works. Levi emphasizes the common literary elements in his two major works, *Sefer Elim* and *Ta'alumot Ḥokhmah.* In both anthologies, Delmedigo creates a "triadic dialogue" between teacher, student, and advanced student, who mediates between the other two in a manner not dissimilar to the Galilean dialogues. Although Delmedigo's works remain unfinished and preliminary, they propose a new direction, a questioning of authority, an enthusiastic confidence in the new sciences, and an evolving religious philosophy based on pre-Aristotelian philosophies and Galilean methodology. His positive evaluation of Plato emerged in no small part from a similar stance adopted by his mentor, Galileo. Both Galileo and his Jewish disciple sought to understand the natural world outside the framework of Aristotelian physics, notwithstanding their strong indebtedness to it in shaping their conceptual discourse. Delmedigo's increasing interest in the kabbalah, along with his attempt to correlate it with Neoplatonism and atomism, should be understood as part of his questioning of scholastic metaphysics and his openness to discovering alternative philosophical positions. Levi also emphasizes Delmedigo's community of interest, the support he received from Modena, Luzzatto, and other rabbis in Venice, Amsterdam, and Pesaro, despite the lack of appreciation about which he also complained. Despite his

66. Levi is presently concluding his doctoral dissertation on Delmedigo at the Hebrew University under the supervision of Moshe Idel. The unpublished papers Dr. Levi has generously shared with me are entitled "Science and Tradition in Jewish Thought: The Case of Delmedigo and His Contemporaries," a lecture presented at a conference on "Science and Religion in the Seventeenth Century," Johns Hopkins University, April 1985; and "Yosef Shelomo Delmedigo: His Jewish Disciples and Contemporaries in Northern and Southern Europe: Between Modern Philosophy and Science and the Medieval Tradition," a paper prepared for the conference "Venezia e gli Ebrei," sponsored by Fondazione Cini, Venice, June 1983. I also listened to his paper presented at the annual meeting of the Association for Jewish Studies in Boston, December 1988, entitled "Joseph Shelomo Delmedigo: A Jewish Follower of Galileo Galilei and Giordano Bruno."

ties to Karaites and non-Jews, and despite his criticisms of rabbinic Judaism, he was never a heretic and remained loyal to the Jewish tradition.

Levi also attempts to periodize Delmedigo's intellectual development, to better comprehend the process by which the seemingly disparate elements in his thinking came together or remained in tension with each other. From Padua Delmedigo adopted his critical stance toward Aristotle, his emphasis on the primacy of the senses, his praise of mathematics as a "mythical" tool, his interest in mechanics, Copernican cosmology, and the separation of science and faith. When he left Padua for other Mediterranean Jewish communities and eventually Poland, his Paduan assumptions confronted directly the stark realities of Jewish and non-Jewish life. In this later period, Levi argues, Delmedigo adopted kabbalistic, atomistic, and Neoplatonist positions and tried to integrate them all into his thought. While the new Lurianic kabbalah came through Jewish sources, the Karaites may have facilitated his interest in atomism. His conflict with Polish Jewry and its rabbis was not simply a clash along intellectual lines but also had social and economic dimensions, including the inevitable tension between Delmedigo's Sephardic mentality and the Ashkenazic one he encountered.

Levi acknowledges that the integration of these disparate elements was never complete. Delmedigo never fully resolved the tensions between his interest in mechanics and practical science and his metaphysics; between his attempt to demarcate religious and scientific truths and his presentation of mathematics and Copernican science in a religiously charged, mystical language; and between his disparagement of popular magic and superstition and his openness to alchemy, Hermes, demonology, and animistic views of nature. But all this reflects for Levi not a ruse, not the strategy of a heretic parading cynically in pious clothing. Rather, it indicates an authentic search for meaning in an intellectual world of scientific uncertainties and in a Jewish world steeped in kabbalistic theosophy.

There is need for a more systematic examination of the philosophical, scientific, and kabbalistic sources that informed Delmedigo's writing. He himself identifies many of his sources, both Jewish and non-Jewish, and offers a full inventory of authors of the mathematical and physical sciences that he consulted,[67]

---

67. In addition to the scientific authors cited frequently in *Sefer Elim,* see the list Delmedigo offered to the Polish astronomer Broscius, published by I. Halperin in "Exchanges between

but more work remains to be done in this area. That Delmedigo read Galileo, Bruno,[68] Kepler, or Brahe is self-evident from his citations, but one still misses the actual weight of their influence—and that of other unidentified sources— in evaluating his overall corpus. As Robert Bonfil pointed out years ago, Delmedigo's excursus on the active intellect—and, we might add, his discussions of light, emanation, and contraction—require more systematic treatment than the general descriptions offered by Barzilay.[69] Detailed analyses such as that of Idel's recent discussion of Delmedigo's correlations between atomism and Judaism,[70] dismissed by Barzilay as an intellectual failure,[71] allow us to appreciate how earnest and serious Delmedigo was in his endeavor to view Lurianic concepts as useful intellectual tools. Nissim Yosha's careful study of Herrera's similar attempt to reconcile Luria and Renaissance Neoplatonism provides another important context for Delmedigo's metaphysical speculations. Although Yosha finds no evidence of mutual influence between the two, he points out that Herrera served on the board of censors of the Amsterdam Jewish community that studied and eventually approved of Menasseh ben Israel's publication of *Sefer Elim*.[72] Even more significant is Yosha's comparison of Herrera's and Delmedigo's extended discussions of the Lurian notion of contraction (*zimzum*), revealing a basic disagreement in interpretation but vividly demonstrating how Delmedigo's fascination with the concept in resolving the philosophical problem of creatio ex nihilo did not evolve in a vacuum but was addressed with equal

---

Broscius and Delmedigo" (in Hebrew) in his *Yehudim ve-Yahadut be-Mizrah Eropa* (Jerusalem, 1968), p. 391 (originally published in B. D. Weinryb and S. Zeitlin, eds., *Studies and Essays in Honor of Abraham Neuman* [Philadelphia, 1962], pp. 640–49). Levi also suggests the influence of Guidobaldo del Monte and Giambattista della Porta on Delmedigo.

68. Bruno is not mentioned by name, but see Barzilay, *Yosef Shlomo Delmedigo*, p. 168. Many of Delmedigo's other sources are discussed throughout Barzilay's chapters on the various sciences.

69. See Bonfil's review of Barzilay's book in *La Rassegna mensile di Israel* 42 (1976): 107–09.

70. Idel, "Differing Conceptions of Kabbalah."

71. Barzilay, *Yosef Shlomo Delmedigo*, pp. 292–96.

72. Yosha's "Abraham Cohen Herrera's Philosophical Interpretation" refers to the essay by J. d'Ancona, "Delmedigo, Menasseh ben Israel, en Spinoza," in *Bijdragen en Mededeelingen van het Genootschap voor de Joodsche Wetenschap Nederland* 6 (1940): 105–52; and see Yosha, "Herrera," pp. 18–20.

seriousness by at least one other contemporary Jewish thinker.[73] Idel's brief discussion of Menasseh ben Israel's commitment to ancient theology and of his particular interest in Leone Ebreo's dialogical treatise on love reveals as well a shared perspective with the scientific author he promoted and published in Amsterdam.[74] All of the above underscore the significance of moving away from the nineteenth-century characterization of Delmedigo to a wider and deeper view of his place in seventeenth-century Jewish culture and of his creative merger of post-Aristotelian physics and kabbalistic metaphysics.

Such a task is clearly beyond the limits of this chapter. What I would like to offer instead are some initial suggestions as to how one might read Delmedigo's most controversial works: the aforementioned *Mazref la-Ḥokhmah*, his putative defense of the kabbalah, and his *Mikhtav Aḥuz*, particularly its second recension published by Abraham Geiger, his biting and uncompromising condemnation of kabbalistic thought and literature. More than any other works in the Delmedigan corpus, they offer two antithetical and seemingly irreconcilable positions. Although Delmedigo's writings contain many smaller inconsistencies, these two compositions present the greatest obstacle to viewing him as a consistent and balanced thinker. As we have seen, Geiger and Barzilay eliminated the contradiction between the two positions by assuming that Geiger's version of the Aḥuz letter was wholly authentic and that the *Mazref* was actually an exercise in dissimulation, passing itself off as a defense of kabbalah when in actuality it impudently made a mockery of it. I am not convinced that either interpretation is correct, and since these two works are so critical in understanding what Delmedigo actually believed, a tentative rereading may be order, if not to settle the question, at least to open it again.

Barzilay devotes considerable space in his book, including a special chapter, to disproving that *Mazref la-Ḥokhmah* is a credible defense of the kabbalah.[75] He admits that among Delmedigo's contemporaries, only Leone Modena detected "its true nature." Such sophisticated students of Jewish and non-Jewish litera-

73. Yosha, "Abraham Cohen Herrera's Philosophical Interpretation," part 2, chap. 5, esp. p. 159.

74. See n. 62 above.

75. Most of his discussion is found in chaps. 16–18, esp. chap. 18, entitled "*Mazref la-Ḥokhmah:* A Concealed Anti-Cabbalistic Work," pp. 280–91.

ture as Ḥayyim Ya'ir Bacharach and Moses Zacuto found fault neither with the book nor with the sincerity of its author.[76] It never seems to have crossed Barzilay's mind that Modena may have been a less than objective critic, since he had good reason to undermine the genuineness of Delmedigo's arguments. He was justifiably alarmed that two distinguished graduates of Padua, both of whom he had supported at critical moments in their scientific careers, had seemingly been seized by the "kabbalistic delirium." *Ari Nohem,* so he thought, was his last opportunity to persuade Ḥamiẓ to pursue the intellectual path to which Modena had previously steered him. That the author of *Sefer Elim* would dare to justify the kabbalah, and indirectly Ḥamiẓ's infatuation with it, was surely too much for him to bear. Modena had no choice but to challenge the book's authenticity for his own peace of mind and to save face with his student. The question we might ask is: Is Modena's reading of *Maẓref* in the heat of his bitter polemic the only way to understand the book, or can it be approached from a different perspective, one emerging from the legitimate assumption that many scientific minds in the seventeenth century were open to and fascinated by mythical and magical notions of reality?[77]

I begin with one of Barzilay's prime examples in challenging the author's sincerity: Delmedigo's discussion of the supernatural powers of the sages to make golems (artificial human beings). After faithfully summarizing the gist of

76. Barzilay, *Yosef Shlomo Delmedigo,* pp. 280–81.

77. I offer my reading despite the tempting possibility that the image of Delmedigo as a dissimulator would make him very much a child of his age. See P. Zagorin, *Ways of Lying: Dissimulation, Persecution, and Conformity in Early Modern Europe* (Cambridge, Mass., 1990). But note Zagorin's discussion (pp. 9–10) of Leo Strauss's famous thesis in *Persecution and the Art of Writing* (Glencow, 1952), where he cautions that the Straussian interpreter might torture and manipulate a text to produce a result guaranteed in advance. I wonder whether the Geiger-Barzilay reading of *Maẓref* might be an example of such overreading. One might also raise the more general question of why Delmedigo was obliged to dissimulate in the first place. Was Jewish society so intolerant that Delmedigo actually feared persecution? Certainly Azariah de' Rossi, Simone Luzzatto, and even Modena himself publicly expressed controversial views of rabbinic tradition or the kabbalah without being persecuted for them. The fate of Da Costa and Spinoza in Amsterdam was, of course, different. A comprehensive comparative study of the limits of tolerance within the Jewish and Christian communities of early modern Europe would be useful.

Delmedigo's argument extolling these wondrous abilities, Barzilay concludes: "It is, no doubt, with tongue in cheek that Yashar [Delmedigo] appears to be suggesting to his contemporaries to look up to the Talmudic sages and the medieval Jewish wonder workers as examples for scholarly emulation; it is they who followed the right path and method in the study of nature and things divine. It requires, indeed, very little insight to discern Yashar's sarcasm in displaying the miraculous deeds of the sages of Israel as patterns for emulation by the scientists and technologists of his own time, and presenting their legendary feats as the realization of the scientific method and ideal."[78]

If one is convinced as Barzilay is that equating Jewish golem-making with practical science is ludicrous, then one must assume that Delmedigo is being sarcastic here. But there is surely another way to read this passage. In the light of recent scholarship on the extensive discussions about creating life among both Jews and Christians in the Renaissance—among such thinkers as Agrippa, Lazzarelli, Reuchlin, Alemanno, Yagel, Cordovero, and others—we should be cautious about dismissing the possibility that Delmedigo was utterly serious about such matters.[79] Abraham Yagel's detailed discussion of the practical knowledge of the Jewish magus, whom he identifies as the most exalted natural philosopher since he alone is capable of making a golem, should not be read as a ruse,[80] and neither should Delmedigo's. The latter anchors his discussion in the words of a respectable authority, Abraham Bivago, who differentiated between the useless speculative knowledge of the ancients, by which he meant the followers of Aristotle, and the productive and useful knowledge of the Jews.[81] We have already seen this argument utilized by other Jewish thinkers, most notably Naḥmanides, as an argument for the uniqueness of Jewish scientific activity in contrast to the inferior science of the Aristotelians.[82] Similarly for Del-

---

78. Barzilay, *Yosef Shlomo Delmedigo*, p. 258, discussing *Maẓref la-Ḥokhmah*, pp. 47–48.

79. See esp. the new synthesis of M. Idel, *Golem: Jewish Magical and Mystical Traditions on the Artificial Anthropoid* (Albany, 1990), expanding on the pioneering work of G. Scholem, *On the Kabbalah and Its Symbolism* (New York, 1965), chap. 5. All the above thinkers are treated by Idel.

80. See Ruderman, *Kabbalah, Magic, and Science*, pp. 102–20.

81. *Maẓref la-Ḥokhmah*, pp. 47–48; and see Idel, *Golem*, pp. 165–67.

82. See chap. 1 above.

medigo, in contrast to the creators and inventors Rabbi Yoḥanan ben Zakkai and Elazar ben Arakh, Aristotle and his followers—Avicenna, ibn Roschd, Themistius, and Yoḥanan the Grammarian— were also useless thinkers and writers who couldn't even move a wing.[83] That the activity performed by the rabbis can be favorably compared with the work of alchemists, mineralogists, and the like follows logically from the above and is precisely Yagel's message as well. By offering as further evidence the reputed stories about Abraham ibn Ezra and Solomon ibn Gabirol, both enlightened philosophers respected for their rational pursuits, and then citing his trusted contemporary Judah Moscato, Delmedigo was hardly being sarcastic. That he matter-of-factly discounted the attribution of a commentary of *Sefer Yeẓirah* to Saadia might be taken to mean how serious he was about the entire matter, for in enlisting authoritative testimony he would not countenance an incorrect citation. Be that as it may, Delmedigo was not making a novel argument in seeing golem-making as a productive scientific activity worthy of emulation and admiration. Nor was it a false argument for him. Rather, it was his way of sanctioning scientific and technological activity in Judaism and of promoting its relevance to the scientific culture of his day.[84]

Given Barzilay's predilection to assume that Delmedigo exhibits contempt for the kabbalah on almost every page of *Maẓref,* his readings of the text often seem forced and less than accurate. When Delmedigo writes: "I do not know who gave the preachers the right to exact new meaning and divulge new mysteries," bringing "up from darkness its profound meanings," Barzilay is correct in seeing it as a condemnation of the preachers' misinterpreting of the Torah, "whose opinions originate in darkness."[85] But is this a blanket condemnation of the kabbalists in general as he suggests? By immediately quoting Judah Ḥayyat and Meir ibn Gabbai on the need to avoid divulging kabbalistic secrets in so reckless a manner, Delmedigo is clearly criticizing not the kabbalah but only the irresponsibility of popular preachers who divulge their secrets to the masses.[86]

83. *Maẓref la-Ḥokhmah,* p. 43, and Barzilay, *Yosef Shlomo Delmedigo,* pp. 258–59.
84. See *Maẓref la-Ḥokhmah,* pp. 48–50; compare Barzilay, *Yosef Shlomo Delmedigo,* pp. 255–59.
85. *Maẓref la-Ḥokhmah,* p. 57, and Barzilay, *Yosef Shlomo Delmedigo,* p. 251.
86. See *Maẓref la-Ḥokhmah,* p. 57.

Barzilay claims to expose Delmedigo's authentic feelings about cantillation marks and accents in the Bible that provide a rich resource for kabbalistic exegesis. By observing that the Jews of his native Crete make no distinction between long and short vowels and by citing the argument of Elijah Levita in favor of a late origin for the vowels and accents, Delmedigo must have been trying to undermine the credibility of their usage for fathoming the secrets of sacred scripture.[87] But this is not necessarily the point Delmedigo wants to impart. His comment on Crete could easily be taken in a disparaging way, as an indication of the boorishness of its citizenry and its lack of high culture. Delmedigo had sarcastically pointed out in the same passage how the Greek he had learned in his childhood had little relation to ancient Greek and thus he was obliged to learn the latter as if he were mastering a new language.[88] In other words, the Cretians were hardly reliable transmitters of ancient culture! More telling is the authority Delmedigo cites after mentioning Levita's arguments, conveniently left out in Barzilay's summary: Azariah de' Rossi and his long refutation of Levita in defense of the antiquity of the vowel points.[89] It is hard to imagine how Delmedigo could enlist so serious a contemporary scholar unless he actually believed in the antiquity of the cantillation notes in the first place.

Barzilay similarly misunderstands Delmedigo's derogatory comments on *gematria* and *notarikon* as revealing "the contempt in which he held these artificial techniques."[90] Delmedigo does not deny their value altogether, since they still function as "deserts after the meal" rather than "the body of Torah." He merely upbraids those who misuse them since "they are light things into which a complete scholar should not thrust himself." They are merely "an opening and beginning" to arrive at higher truths, a stratagem by which "one is awakened to understand one thing from another, to investigate more and to fathom the real meaning of the secret." When misused by preachers so that they are conceived

87. See Barzilay, *Yosef Shlomo Delmedigo,* pp. 253–55.

88. *Maẓref la-Ḥokhmah,* p. 51 and Barzilay, *Yosef Shlomo Delmedigo,* pp. 31–32.

89. *Maẓref la-Ḥokhmah,* pp. 52–53, citing Azariah de' Rossi, *Me'or Einayim* (Vilna, 1866), Imre Binah, chapter 59 entitled: "On the Antiquity of the Cantellation Marks".

90. Barzilay, *Yosef Shlomo Delmedigo,* p. 255.

as ultimate secrets, they are dangerous—but not for the true kabbalist, who sees them as a means to a higher end.[91]

A close reading of Delmedigo's discussion of Maimonides and the mystical tradition does not sustain Barzilay's claim that Delmedigo attempted to show that the philosopher actually "belonged to the early mystics."[92] Delmedigo does provide a string of quotations about Maimonides' possible leanings but leaves the subtlest analysis for last—that of Moses Alashkar, who discusses quite clearly the limits of the rational quest and the possibilities the kabbalah opens up for penetrating the secrets of nature, "for providing the keys of wisdom and the explanation of that which is hidden from me." In other words, perhaps mirroring Delmedigo's own mind-set, Alashkar provides a plausible explanation of how a rationalist might be attracted to mystical reflection. Delmedigo concludes: "You can see how Maimonides and all the sages knew and wrote about the wisdom of the kabbalah," clearly a lesser claim than actually belonging to the mystic camp.[93]

Delmedigo's discussion of the witch of En Dor and his long inventory of classical, Christian, and Jewish sources on the existence of angels, spirits, and demons similarly betray for Barzilay Delmedigo's complete skepticism about such beings: "He must have felt that the texts were so obviously absurd that by just printing them, even without comment, they could safely be relied upon to refute the views contained in them."[94] He finds utterly incredible the following statement of Delmedigo: "With our eyes we see things daily that reason refuses to accept; yet they actually appear to be true, and perhaps our judgment is determined by our imagination rather than by our reason; moreover, it is further substantiated by wondrous activities [of nature], like the magnet that possesses many great and wonderful properties, as I wrote in a long composition on it . . . ."[95] This is followed by a citation from Abraham Shalom's

91. *Mazref la-Hokhmah,* pp. 59–60.
92. Barzilay, *Yosef Shlomo Delmedigo,* p. 284.
93. *Mazref la-Hokhmah,* pp. 68–69.
94. Barzilay, *Yosef Shlomo Delmedigo,* p. 266.
95. I have retranslated Barzilay's inexact and partial translation from *Yosef Shlomo Delmedigo,* p. 263 *(Mazref la-Hokhmah,* p. 69). Delmedigo's reference to his work on the magnet

Neve Shalom, a work of philosophical pedigree referring to the *Mineralogia,* a text on natural wonders ascribed to Aristotle, which Barzilay deems "ludicrous evidence in support of the irrational and the occult."[96]

There is no need to adduce "the towering edifice of authority," as Sidney Anglo once called it, in support of the existence of spirits and demons in Delmedigo's day from from the Bible, Talmud, and classical writers to Roger Bacon, Albertus Magnus, Marsilio Ficino, Henry Cornelius Agrippa, Jean Bodin, Robert Burton, and many more.[97] Delmedigo's *testimonia* for these beings are hardly ludicrous when judged by the sensibilities of seventeenth-century Jewish and Christian culture. Moreover, as I have discussed in the case of Abraham Yagel, demonology in this era was more than pseudo-science and superstition. At its best, it represented a rational attempt to explain the unknown and could often contribute to the scientific discourse of the sixteenth and seventeenth centuries.[98]

Delmedigo's statement about our eyes seeing what our reason cannot accept is especially significant when compared with the following statement of Yagel, reacting to Gersonides' denial of demonic existence and an incident of alleged demonic activity he recorded in Mantua: "Therefore, you see that the intention of this philosopher is to deny that demons have any reality . . . to all of which the senses testify the opposite [is the case]. . . . For the conclusions of Gersonides are philosophical; however, the senses testify to the contrary of his words. If he actually had seen with his own eyes the incident we described that happened in Mantua, how could he falsify [the impressions based on] his senses and upon his imagination?"[99] Delmedigo's sentiment is obviously identical to that of Yagel, both expressions of a larger epistemological debate in their era about

---

might refer to his discussions in *Ma'ayan Ḥatum* in *Elim,* pp. 407, 410, 428, 438, as cited by Barzilay, p. 149.

96. *Maẓref la-Ḥokhmah,* p. 69, and Barzilay, *Yosef Shlomo Delmedigo,* p. 264. See M. Steinschneider, *Die hebraischen Ueberseṭzungen des Mittelalters und die Juden als Dolmetscher,* 2 vols. (Berlin, 1893), 1:236, n. 916, who refers to the work as that of pseudo-Aristotle.

97. S. Anglo, "Melancholia and Witchcraft: The Debate between Wier, Bodin and Scot, in *Folie et déraison à la Renaissance* (Brussels, 1976), p. 210.

98. See Ruderman, *Kabbalah, Magic, and Science,* chap. 3 and the extensive bibliography cited there.

99. Quoted in Ruderman, *Kabbalah, Magic, and Science,* p. 46.

what was real or unreal, rational or irrational, and whether one should rely on inate knowledge or that based on the senses. Delmedigo's analogy between the possibility of demonic activity and the occult properties of magnets is also understandable in light of his quest and those of his scientific contemporaries to establish criteria of intelligibility in a natural order that had not revealed all of its manifold secrets.[100] Note finally his reference to Shalom's citation of Aristotle, an ironic touch indicating that the peripetic sage was capable of being led by his senses and imagination, even when they appeared to contradict his rational inclinations!

I come finally to the most daunting obstacle to accepting the sincerity of Delmedigo's kabbalistic defense: his portrait of Saadia, followed immediately by his statement that he writes this work for a patron he is pledged to satisfy regardless of what the latter requests.[101] Both of these passages, as we have seen, led Modena to accuse his colleague of dissimulation. I readily concur with Barzilay that these passages offer the most damaging assault on Delmedigo's credibility when read in isolation in the quotation cited above. But let us attempt, at the very least, to understand Delmedigo's words in a somewhat different manner. By linking the statement about his own writing to his portrayal of Saadia, Delmedigo saw himself in Saadia's image as an intellectual who could function on two simultaneous levels: that of a philosopher-scientist and that of a kabbalist. Just because a person might choose to write as a philosopher in one instance should not preclude the possibility of his writing as a kabbalist in another, and one should not automatically assume that such shifts are necessarily dishonest. When Delmedigo admitted that he was writing to please the man who commissioned him to write this work, was this unambiguous proof that he was dishonest and intensely disliked the kabbalah? And if his effort in subterfuge was to be fully realized, why would he tip his hand by revealing what a hypocrite he was, embarrassing himself to his readers and especially to his patron?

Rather than a simple confession of dishonesty, I would interpret Delmedigo's remarks on a more profound level. They point to the complexity of thought,

---

100. See esp. S. Clark, "The Scientific Status of Demonology," in Vickers, *Occult and Scientific Mentalities in the Renaissance,* pp. 351–74.

101. *Maẓref la-Ḥokhmah,* pp. 80–81 and Barzilay, *Yosef Shlomo Delmedigo,* pp. 242–43.

of human existence, of the diverse influences that affect the writer or teacher—intellectual, spiritual, political, and social. They also suggest that the reader should never view the world naively and arbitrarily in black-and-white terms. Delmedigo points out that Maimonides too never fully divulged his true intentions,[102] suggesting perhaps a rationale for the earlier allusion regarding the philosopher's openness to the kabbalah. Delmedigo's last line that "there is neither a teacher nor a father who reveals to his disciple or son whatever is in his heart" is surely not a prescription for dishonesty with respect to the most sacred and trusting relationships between sons and fathers, students and teachers. It is more a pedagogic strategy: a good teacher who wishes to communicate his values effectively cannot reveal everything he knows. Delmedigo is consciously ambiguous here, but he is neither cynical nor disrespectful to either his reader or his patron.

While the above passage is well known and often discussed, Delmedigo's final statement in *Mazref,* in which he again mentions his patron, is usually passed over in silence. It should, however, be considered in conjunction with the first:

I began to write this apologetic treatise in the city of Hamburg, but a plague ravaged my neighborhood and I was forced to flee. So I came to the city of Gluckstadt, that is, a city of good luck, although it holds neither luck nor blessing . . . and it is sufficient for me that my words will be pleasing to the master upon whose request I composed them. However, those beginning students of philosophy will surely mock me, claiming that Rabbi Yoseph of Candia deserted wisdom or forgot his teaching while a foolish spirit invaded him. They will continue to speak in a manner of adolescents who lack equilibrium and whose effervescent wine has not quieted down. But I was aware that their words would not please those elders who have acquired wisdom. Even if their charges against me increase, accusing me of still not arriving [at the level] of a shepherd of a flock, I shall declare to them that it is better to be called a fool all my days rather than to do evil before God even for an

102. *Mazref la-Ḥokhmah,* pp. 80–81.

hour, as R. Akiva ben Mahalal stated to his associates and as it is found in chapter five of [Mishnah] Eduyot.[103]

The mood of this last statement stands in dramatic contrast to that of the first. Should we assume that Delmedigo's last lines also belie his true thoughts? On the contrary, they convey to me an authentic sense of the author's genuine convictions. Ironically, Delmedigo sees himself taking an unpopular stand, in displaying his courage and moral conviction, by defending the kabbalah rather than criticizing it. Like Akiva ben Mahalal, he will not bend to the conventional wisdom of his intellectual peers, those sophomoric scholars who have only begun to philosophize and still have not acquired true wisdom. If we can accept this statement as an authenic reflection of Delmedigo's actual motivation in writing the *Maʒref,* then Modena, Geiger, and Barzilay have missed the mark completely. Delmedigo was not a secret heretic dressed in the pious clothes of a kabbalist. Rather, he quietly believed in the truths of the kabbalah while presenting himself as an enlightened natural philosopher. Only when pressed by his patron did he summon the courage to publicly declare his true convictions, notwithstanding the criticisms he expected to bear. Of course, I cannot state in all certainty that this final statement is more trustworthy than the first, although I suspect it might be. But, at the very least, it neutralizes the force of the first and leaves the question of Delmedigo's ultimate loyalty probably as he would have preferred to leave it, in a state of utter ambiguity and uncertainty. Be that as it may, I hope that my reading of *Maʒref la-Ḥokhmah* will raise doubts about the conventional view of this book in modern historiography.

As we have seen, modern scholars have given considerable weight to the "Aḥuz letter" as an important indicator of Delmedigo's views on rabbinic culture, Karaism, and especially the kabbalah. Barzilay succinctly summarizes how the document first came to light.[104] The original version of the letter, addressed to his Karaite disciple Zeraḥ ben Nathan, was published at the opening of four scientific studies called *Ma'ayan Ganim* in Menasseh ben Israel's edition of *Sefer Elim* in 1629. As Barzilay notes, despite some unflattering remarks about rab-

103. Ibid., p. 132, citing Mishnah Eduyot 5:6; also compare Akiva ben Mahalal's saying in Avot 3:1.

104. Barzilay, *Yosef Shlomo Delmedigo,* pp. 99–100.

binic culture in Poland and a strong endorsement for the study of the sciences within the Jewish community, there is nothing unusual or inconsistent about either the substance or tone of Delmedigo's remarks. However, by the second decade of the nineteenth century, a longer version of the letter came to light that included a scathing attack on the kabbalah and an elaborate inventory of Jewish writings approved by Delmedigo, including a generous sampling by Karaite authors. It was first published in part by Judah Leib Miesis in his *Sefer Kinat ha-Emet* in 1828. Six years later it appeared in its entirety in an anthology of Karaite writings called *Pinnat Yikrat* by Isaac ha-Ḥazan in 1834. Abraham Geiger republished the entire letter with a long introduction to Delmedigo in his *Melo Chofnajim* of 1840. He explains in the introduction that he had received the manuscript from the Karaite Ḥakham of Halicz and through the intervention of S. L. Goldenberg of Tarnopol. Geiger knew of the excerpt published by Miesis but was unaware of Isaac ha-Ḥazzan's complete edition appearing six years earlier.

Israel Zinberg, in his chapter on Delmedigo, quoted extensively from Geiger's version of the letter and added a few salient facts about its discovery. Zinberg claimed that in the same year that Geiger published the letter, Abraham Firkovich published it in Guslow under the title *Iggeret ha-Yashar*.[105] What Zinberg probably meant was the aforementioned 1834 publication of the letter by Isaac ha-Ḥazan, where the same title appears. Zinberg added that Ḥayyim Michael, a noted Hebrew bibliographer, suspected that the Karaites who had first "discovered" the text had indeed falsified it.[106] Heinrich Graetz had previously remarked that Leopold Zunz shared this view.[107] Zinberg discounted these suspicions and reported that he had inspected a manuscript in the Firkovich collection, copied in Troki sometime in the seventeenth century. It was highly probable, Zinberg claimed, that this was a copy made from the original text by a Rabbinite who identified Zeraḥ as a member "of the community of Karaites." From this description, it appears that Zinberg examined the same text published by Isaac ha-Ḥazan in 1834. Convinced that this text was authentic while *Maẓref la-Ḥokhmah* was inauthentic, Zinberg readily offered his own judgment of Del-

105. Zinberg, *History*, 4:164.
106. Ibid.
107. Graetz, *Divre Yeme Yisrael* 8:189, n. 3.

medigo: "He represents himself supposedly as a defender of the wisdom of the kabbalah but in fact he is its definite opponent."[108]

In addition to these scant publishing details, we might briefly consider some biographical information about these nineteenth-century scholars who first brought to light the new version of the Aḥuz letter. Judah Leib Miesis (1798–1831) was a radical member of the Galician Haskalah known for his outspoken criticism of traditional Judaism. In the volume where the excerpt containing Delmedigo's denunciation of the kabbalah appears, he bitterly attacks the superstitious views of rabbinic Judaism, especially those of the kabbalah. The complete title of the work sets the tone for the entire volume: "The Book of the Zeal for Truth . . . on the Origin of the Opinions and Customs of the Children of Israel. . . . From Most of the Sages of the Children of Our People on the Matter . . . of Demons, Magic, and Transmigration . . . ." This is hardly an exercise in dispassionate scholarship. Delmedigo's uncompromising assault on the kabbalist tradition was a perfect fit for Miesis's polemical anthology.[109] Less radical than Miesis was Samuel Leib Goldenberg (1807–46), the editor of the Hebrew periodical *Kerem Ḥemed,* who was also affiliated with the Haskalah in Galicia.[110] Abraham Geiger's pioneering role in the development of Reform Judaism is well known. Although blessed with great scholarly gifts, he was not adverse, as we have seen, to utilize them to support his own ideological positions. His tendentious scholarship on Delmedigo's contemporary Leone Modena has been pointed out before.[111]

Zinberg's claim that the new version of the Aḥuz letter originated in one of the manuscripts owned by Abraham Firkovich (1786–1874) is not an unimportant detail in reconstructing the trail of those men responsible for the new "discovery." Firkovich, the zealous advocate of Karaism's independence from rabbinism, was well known not only as a consummate collector of rare manu-

108. Zinberg, *History,* lists the manuscript as n. 523 in the Firkovich collection (p. 164). The quote is on p. 172.

109. On Miesis, see Zinberg, *History* 10: 34–43 and Klausner, *Toledot ha-Sifrut ha-Ivrit ha-Ḥadashah* (Jerusalem, 1960), 2:267–82.

110. On Goldenberg, see Klausner, *Toledot,* 2:37–38.

111. See E. Rivkin, "Leon Da Modena and the Kol Sakhal," *Jewish Quarterly Review* 40 (1949): 146–52; Adelman, "Success and Failure," 1:77–94.

scripts but as a brilliant forger who had few compunctions about "fortifying" original texts with his own emendations and interpolations. He was not only a champion of Karaite interests but a severe critic of Hasidism. Once in Berdichev he feuded with a Hasidic teacher who referred to the Karaites as heretics and atheists. His fierce antagonism to rabbinism in general and Hasidism in particular is plainly articulated in a memorandum he prepared for the Russian government on the Jewish question, in which he chillingly recommended the extermination of the Hasidim. Despite the efforts of several nineteenth-century scholars to demonstrate that the Firkovich materials were often unreliable, the full extent of his tampering with texts is still not known.[112] The two Firkovich collections presently housed in the Public Library of Leningrad have only recently been available to Western researchers. The Institute for Microfilmed Hebrew Manuscripts at the National and University Library in Jerusalem is in the process of microfilming the entire collection. As of this writing, the Firkovich manuscript of the Aḥuz letter is not yet available for study.[113]

Whether or not one might soon determine conclusively if the manuscript of the second version of Delmedigo's letter to Zeraḥ is authentic, it seems reasonable to be suspicious about the circumstances of the letter's sudden appearance in the 1820s in light of the evidence presented above and of its discoverers' ideological convictions. Despite Delmedigo's complex and often contradictory postures vis-à-vis the kabbalah and rabbinic Judaism, his brazen vilification of the kabbalah in this epistle is unlike that in any of his other writings. He pokes fun at the supernatural powers of the kabbalists, ridicules their beliefs in demons and metempsychosis into animals, and claims that all of their ideas are taken from Christianity.[114] His enthusiasm for Karaite science, Karaite literature, and

112. On Firkovich, see H. L. Strack, *Abraham Firkowitch und seine Entdeckungen* (Leipzig, 1876); A. Harkavy, *Altjüdische Denkmaler aus Krim* (St. Petersburg, 1876); J. Mann, *Texts and Studies in Jewish History and Literature* (New York, 1972), 2:695–97; and Z. Ankori, *Karaites in Byzantium* (New York, 1959), index.

113. My thanks to Dr. Tzvi Y Langermann of the institute for this information. He does report on the recent arrival of another manuscript of the Aḥuz letter listed as MS. Budapest Seminary 40 in the institute. This may have been copied by I. S. Reggio and is very similar to the version published by Geiger.

114. See esp. Geiger, *Melo Chofnajim,* pp. 6–10.

even Karaite liturgy appears somewhat overzealous.[115] How implausible would it be to assume that this letter was forged or at least doctored by Firkovich alone or with several collaborators? However the text was finally put together, its final delivery to Geiger and its dramatic publication would appear to represent a collusion of interests between Maskilim antagonistic to Talmudic and Hasidic Judaism and Karaites interested in publicizing their historic impact on rabbinic culture, who also held little affection for either rabbinic legalism or mysticism. I am in no position to determine whether the Geiger version of the Aḥuz letter was forged. I offer instead some brief questions and observations from a comparative reading of both versions of the letter that heightens my suspicions all the more.

It is obvious that Geiger's version of the letter is based in part on the version that appeared in *Sefer Elim*. Not only are the first five pages identical, as Geiger points out, but several subsequent lines of the first version appear to be inserted in the second.[116] What is more interesting is what the second version leaves out. Understandably, it removes the modest praise of the kabbalah Delmedigo offers in two places in the original letter, including a suggestive remark about the connection between mathematics and mysticism, as well as an expression of his openness to study the *Sefer Ha-Zohar* even though he confesses he does not understand its mysteries.[117] Less understandable is the removal of his complementary portrait of his colleague Simone Luzzatto, whom he calls the greatest rabbinic scholar of mathematics of his generation. In the original version Delmedigo singles out two scholars, besides Zeraḥ himself, among a tiny minority of contemporaries who are still committed to the study of the sciences: Luzzatto and the Karaite scholar Jacob Iskandrandi (the Alexandrian).[118] In the second version, only the latter portrait is preserved.[119] If Delmedigo had indeed composed the second version, why would he have consciously left out the only contemporary rabbinic student of the sciences worthy of mention, a rabbi to whom he was indebted for his enthusiastic endorsement of *Sefer Elim*

115. Ibid., pp. 12, 13, 14, 15, 20.
116. Compare *Sefer Elim*, pp. 130–31, with Geiger, *Melo Chofnajim*, pp. 11 and 13.
117. *Sefer Elim*, pp. 132, 134.
118. Ibid., p. 131.
119. Geiger, *Melo Chofnajim*, p. 13.

and a scholar with whom he had much in common? On the other hand, it would certainly have been in the interest of nineteenth-century Karaites to point out that Delmedigo could only share his scientific interests with their ancestors, and that despite the contributions of Jewish luminaries of the past, the rabbinic world of Delmedigo's era was conspicuously devoid of secular knowledge. Thus Delmedigo could not even mention one solitary rabbinic colleague who excelled in the sciences other than himself!

A reading of the remainder of the letter elicits the following questions, to which I have no clear answers: Why the presentation of an elaborate curriculum of enlightened Jewish studies in the second version, in contrast to the more restricted one in the first? Is the excessive praise of Maimonides and the emphatic plea for the study of the Hebrew language in the second version more characteristic of Maskilic concerns than of Delmedigo's?[120] Why the positive view of Isaac Abravanel, who is the subject of constant criticisms throughout the *Novlot Ḥokhmah?*[121] And why is Delmedigo sparing in his praise of Eliezer Ashkenazi, who is even criticized obliquely for his brief discussion of the existence of demons, while elsewhere Delmedigo lionizes him without reservation?[122] Was Delmedigo actually familiar with the unpublished historical writing of his countryman Elijah Capsali?[123] Was he actually referring to Abraham Yagel's *Gei Ḥizzayon* in his list of recommended books, and if so, how was he able to see this still unpublished work?[124] In this letter Delmedigo thanks his parents for giving him the opportunity from a tender age to read the Greek of the ancient philosophers.[125] However, in *Mazref* he complains that the Greek he learned as a child was useless in reading ancient Greek, which he was obliged to learn from the start.[126] How does one reconcile these two observations? Finally, how might one explain the differing versions of a bitter reference Delmedigo makes about

120. See ibid., pp. 16, 18.

121. See ibid., pp. 17–18, 21; compare, for example, *Novlot,* pp. 6b–7a, 25a–b, 86b, 99b–103a, *Mazref,* p. 73

122. See Geiger, *Melo Chofnajim,* p. 22; compare *Novlot,* pp. 40b, 46a, and Barzilay, *Yosef Shlomo Delmedigo,* p. 191.

123. See Geiger, *Melo Chofnajim,* p. 23.

124. Ibid., p. 23

125. See ibid., p. 24.

126. Cf. *Mazref la-Ḥokhmah,* p. 51, and Barzilay, *Yosef Shlomo Delmedigo,* pp. 31–32.

rabbinic ignorance of astronomy? In the first version, Delmedigo attributes this statement to Maimonides; in the second he states it directly, perhaps accentuating the sharpness of his critique.[127]

Other anomalies might be forthcoming from an even closer examination of the text, particularly its manuscript version. I hope that I have at least raised the question as a serious concern for future scholarship. In the absence of a final verdict about the second Ahuz letter, three possibilities thus present themselves: 1) Geiger's version is authentic and thus the rest of Delmedigo's kabbalistic writings are a hoax; he clearly composes them as a dissimulator. 2) Geiger's version, except for the parts lifted from the first versions, is a complete forgery. Thus the rest of his writings, especially his *Novlot Hokhmah* and *Mazref la-Hokhmah,* legitimately reveal his integrationist approach with respect to science and kabbalah. Despite occasional contradictions and inconsistencies, his work as a whole holds together quite well. 3) Geiger's version of the letter was actually composed by Delmedigo, but in the hands of Firkovich and his collaborators it has been subjected to emendations and elaborations, all meant to promote Karaite and Maskilic interests. When the original core of the letter is identified, the extremity of Delmedigo's position regarding rabbinism and kabbalah will disappear. The integrationist perspective of possibility 2 is then generally valid.

Assuming my tentative conclusions about the *Mazref la-Hokhmah* and the second version of *Mikhtav Ahuz* are correct, Barzilay's reconstruction of Delmedigo's subsequent thought requires considerable revision. In the three categories of thought mentioned at the beginning of this chapter, suggested by Joseph Hamiz, Delmedigo would find his place in the third group of thinkers, Hamiz's own group, who "tried to find a path to follow the Torah and [rational investigation] so that one would not contradict the other" and who understood "nature in order to know what is beyond nature."[128] In joining this camp, Joseph Delmedigo would become its most distinguished representative in both his mastery of the sciences and his eagerness to establish bridges between them and kabbalistic theosophy. Leone Modena would have had every right to feel abandoned.

---

127. See *Sefer Elim,* p. 131; compare Geiger, *Melo Chofnajim,* p. 13.
128. See n. 9 above.

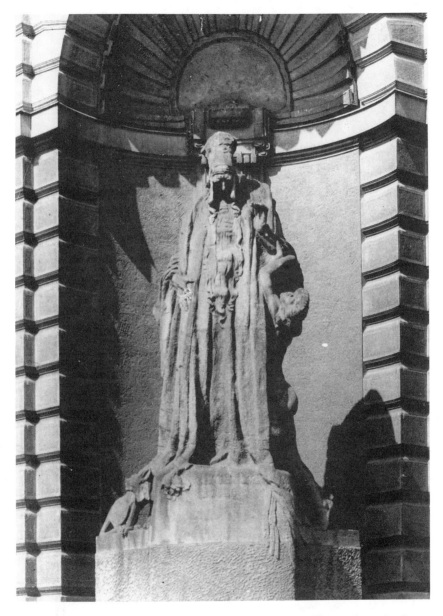

Fig. 1. Ladislas Saloun's hewn-stone monument of the Maharal of Prague, located at the entrance to the Prague Town Hall. (All illustrations in this section are courtesy of the Library of the Jewish Theological Seminary of America.)

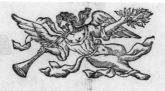

NELL' OCCASIONE DEL PRENDER
LA LAUREA DOTTORALE
IN FILOSOFIA, E MEDICINA
IL MOLTO ILLUSTRE, ED ECCELLENTE SIG.
SALOMON CONIGLIANO
Figliuolo del Celebre e rinomato Eccellente Signor
DOTTOR CERVO CONIGLIANO M. F.

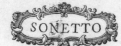
SONETTO

ביום שהוכתר בכתר. הרפואה והפילוסופיאה הכבוד. דגומר משכיל ונבון כמהדר
שלמה קוניליאנו
בן הקצין אביר ונשיא הרופאים הרופא המובהק כמהדר נפתלי קוניליאנו נר"ו · עליו יציץ נזרו · אכי"ר

L faper la virtù ti diede il Cielo
SALOMON, nel bel fior di fresca Etade;
Onde scoprir l'occulta veritade;
Di natura ai fecreti alzand' il velo;

חכמה ומדע מֵעַל נתְנו
אֵלֶיךָ שְׁלֹמֹה נַעַר עוֹדְךָ
הוֹצִיא תַּעֲלוּמוֹת לְאוֹר שְׁכְלָךָ
מִצְפוּנוֹת בְּרִיאָה לְךָ לֹא נִטְמֵנוּ

Succo vital de velenofo ftelo;
Sudafti a eftrar a prò di tue contrade;
Tanta a fanarci avrai TU poteftade;
Che la morte al tuo piè deporrà il telo;

הַיָקֹרֶת לַחוּצִיא מוֹלֵל לָנוּ
יַגַעַתָ וּמַצְאת כִּלְבָבֶךָ
הַמוֹר מַשְׂכֵּל תַּשְׂפִּיל יָדְךָ
כִּי רְפָאוֹת לְחַלְיֵינוּ בְּךָ מַצְאָנוּ

Di piante, ed erbe già facefti verbo;
Quanta virtù l'iopo, e 'l Cedro impingua;
Pirlarne com' il Re Savio ti piacque.

דִברְתָ עֲלֵי עֵץ עַל צִיץ וְשִׂיחַ
מֵאֲרֶו וְאֲחַזוֹב טוֹבוֹת יְבָאוּ
כִּשְׁלֹמֹה בְּחָכְמָה בְּמוֹ תַּשִׂיחַ

Non ti fu impofto un nome fi fuperbo
In van: ma forfi un di dirà ogni lingua;
La SALOMONE a TE fimil non nacque.

שֵׁם לֹא נָתְנוּ לְךָ לָרִיק וָתֹהוּ
בִּשְׁמוֹ · בֵּי כְּפִי בֹל וְשֶׁמַע שֵׁח
כִּי מֵנוּ בְּמוֹתֶךָ לֹא קָם כָּמוֹרֵנוּ

Tradotto da Meffimo Todefco Finzi.

משֶׁרֶת לְהַמְ"ל
שמחה קאלימאני

Fig. 2. A broadside consisting of a Hebrew poem by Simḥah Calimani with Italian translation by Todesco Finzi, in honor of Solomon Conegliano's graduation from the medical school of Padua in 1660. Jewish Theological Seminary mic. 9027, vol. 5, n. 24.

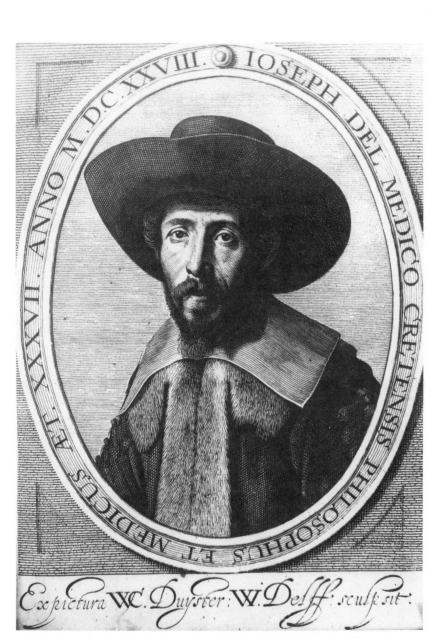

Fig. 3. Portrait of Joseph Delmedigo from *Sefer Elim* (Amsterdam, 1629).

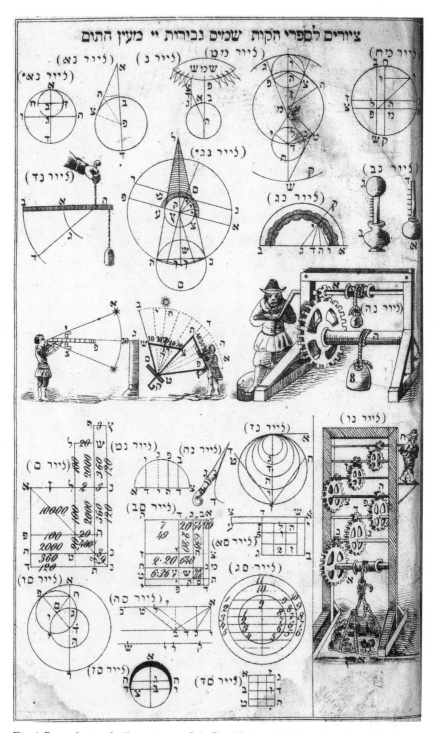

Fig. 4. Page of scientific illustrations in *Sefer Elim* (Odessa, 1864) based on those found in the first edition (Amsterdam, 1629).

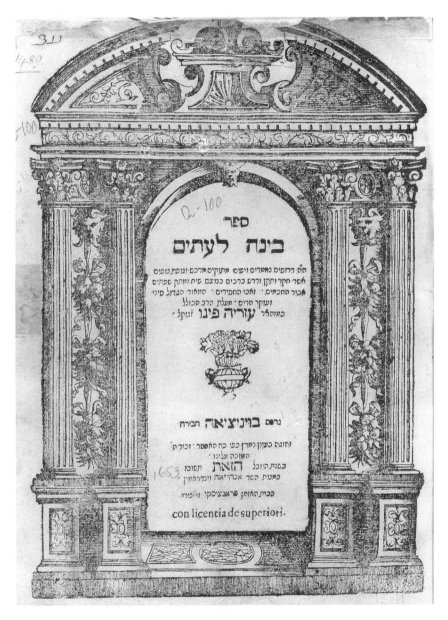

Fig. 5. Title page from Azariah Figo's sermon collection *Binah le-Ittim* (Venice, 1653).

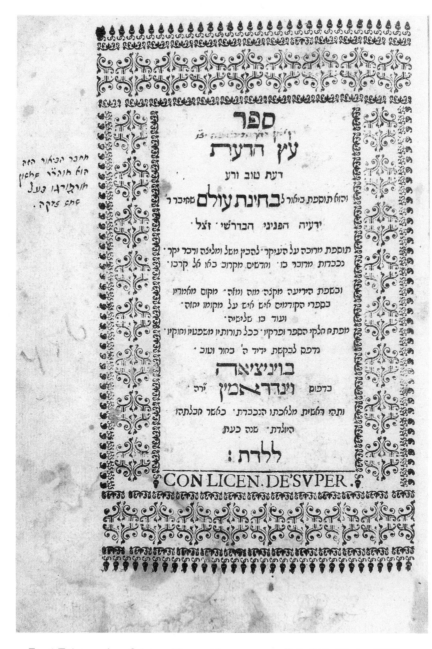

ספר
עץ הדעת
דעת טוב ורע
והוא תוספת וביאור לבחינת עולם שחיבר ר'
ידעיה הפניני הבדרשי · זצל'

תוספת מרובה על העיקר · להבין משל ומליצה ודבר יקר ·
נכבדות מדובר בו · וחדשים מקרוב באו אל קרבו ·

ובכספת היריעה מקנה מזה ומזה · מקום מאמריו
בספרי הקודמים איש איש על מקומו יהיה ·
ועוד כו שליטים ·
מפתח חלקי הספר ופרקיו · וככל תורותיו משפטיו וחוקיו ·
מדפס לבקשת ידיד ה' כמוך וטוב ·

בויניציאה
בדפוס וינדראמין יר"ה

ותהי ראשית מלאכתו הנכבדת · כאשר קבלתהו ·
היולדת · שנה כעת ·

ללדת ׃

CON LICEN. DE'SVPER .

Fig. 6. Title page from Solomon Morpurgo's commentary *Eẕ ha-Da'at* (Venice, 1704) on Jedaiah Bedersi's ethical work *Sefer Behinat Olam*. Morpurgo's name is omitted.

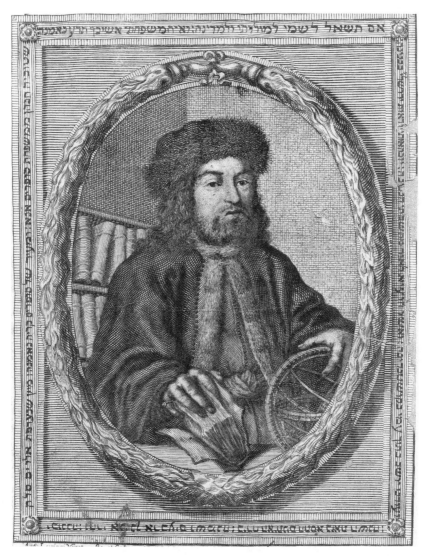

Fig. 7. Portrait of Tobias ha-Cohen from the first edition of his *Ma'aseh Tuviyyah* (Venice, 1707).

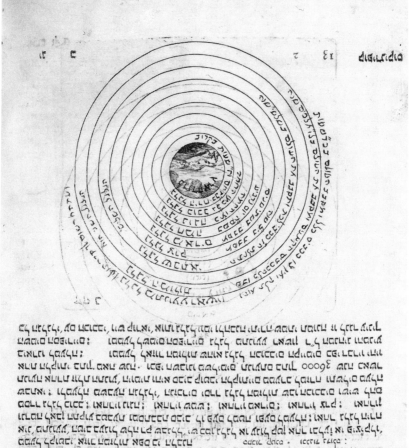

Fig. 8. Diagram with explanatory text of the geocentric universe according to Ptolemy in *Ma'aseh Tuviyyah* (Venice, 1707), p. 50a.

קופירניקום הנ״ל יסדר השמש במרכז העולם ורוצה שהוחר המסבב וגלגל
ככבי הנבוכים מתנועעים סביב השמש ועמהם טונה כדור הארצי
באחד מככבי הנבוכים ואומר שהארץ תשלים הקפתה בשנה אחת ממערב למזרה באופן
שתנועתה שנתירת לא תעכב את תנועתה היומירת מה שיש לה סביב מרכזה בתוך
כ״ד שעורת :
תנועת הכוכבים הנבוכים היא כל כך ישרה כאלו נעשית במחוגה ועל ידי עגול שקושב
הארץ נוטה ממנו כ״ב מעלות וחצי :

הנה כפי סברת קופירניקוס השמש במרכז העולם וסביב לו גלגל כרתב ואהריו
גלגל נוגה · ולהיותם קרובים לו הקפתם יותר קטנה והוא ממערב למזרח
קודם כלות השנה · ואח״כ מסדר כדור הארץ ואומר שיש לו שלש תנועות ר״ל
תנועה יומירת · תנועה שנתית · ותנועת המאזנים · ועל ידי תנועה זו כפי דברינו
יבואר השתנות האורך אשר נרגש מימי איפירקוש ועד הנה · וגם כן יבואר מפני
מה בזמנינו קוטבי הארץ אינם מכוונים ונמצאים בנקודה שהיו נמצאים בימי איפירקוש ·
לפי שהארץ כפי דבריו כל יום מתנועעת ממערב למזרח תנועה יומית וכושכת עמה
הלבנה התלויה במעגל שלה כאשר תראה ותבין בתמונרת זו חקוקה ומחוגה וכחונה לפניך
ואח״כ מארים · ואח״כ צדק · וכסדר הזה וכו' :

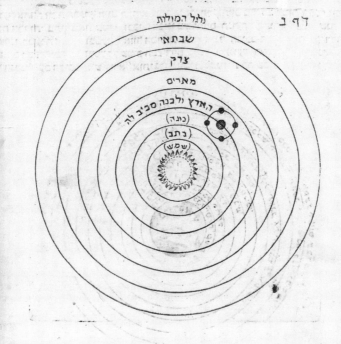

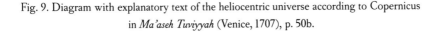

Fig. 9. Diagram with explanatory text of the heliocentric universe according to Copernicus
in *Ma'aseh Tuviyyah* (Venice, 1707), p. 50b.

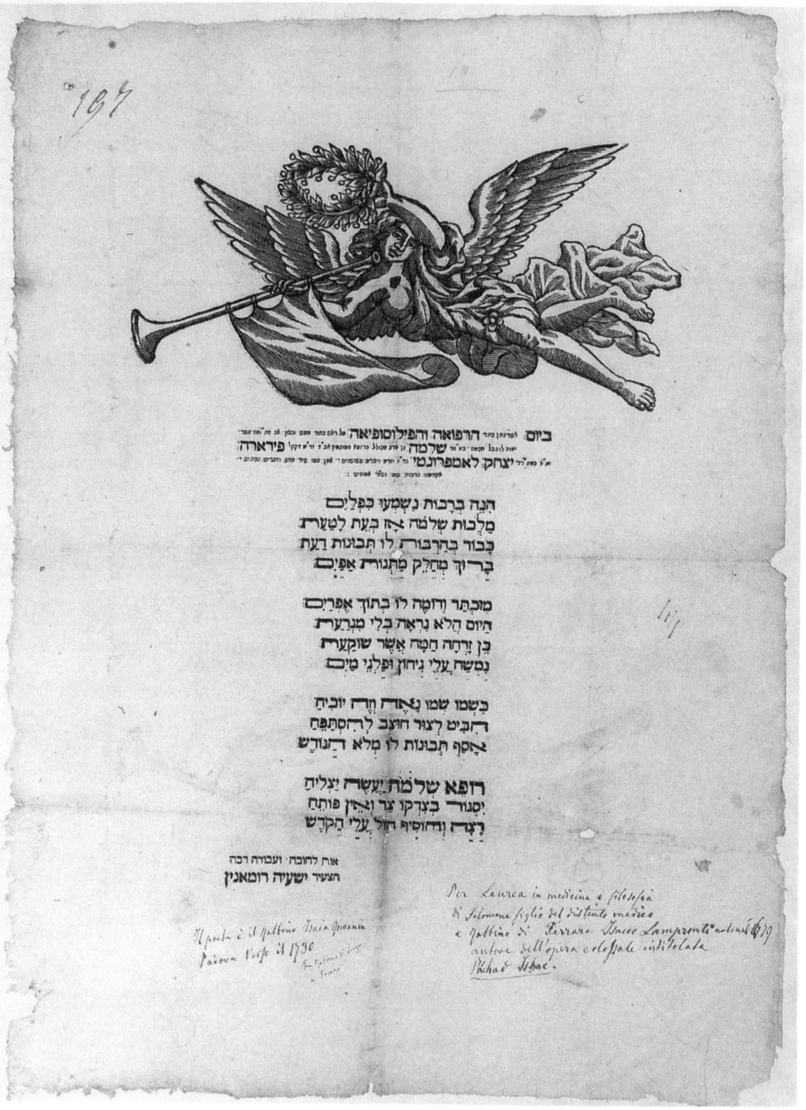

Fig. 10. Broadside of a Hebrew poem written by Isaiah Roman in honor of the graduation of Solomon, son of the celebrated Isaac Lampronti of Ferrara, from Padua's medical school in 1734.

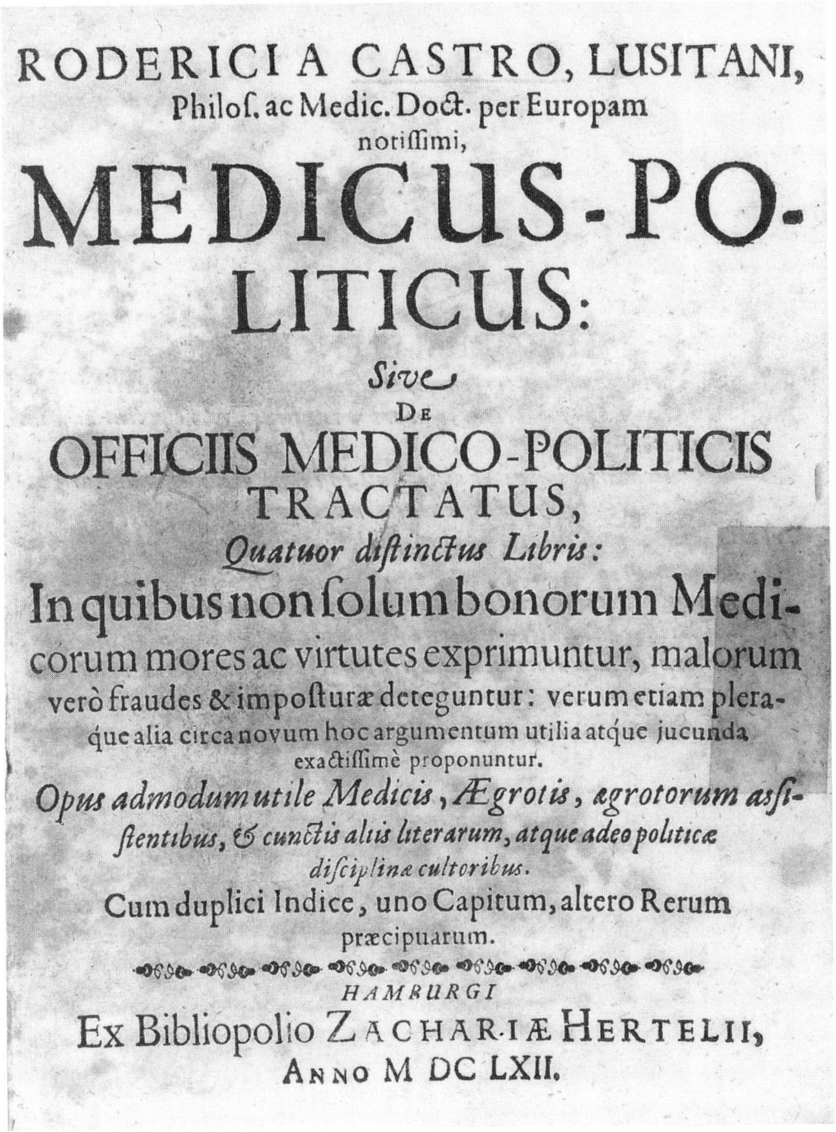

RODERICI A CASTRO, LUSITANI,
Philof. ac Medic. Doct. per Europam
notiffimi,

MEDICUS-PO-
LITICUS:

Sive

De

OFFICIIS MEDICO-POLITICIS
TRACTATUS,

Quatuor diftinctus Libris:

In quibus non folum bonorum Medi-
córum mores ac virtutes exprimuntur, malorum
verò fraudes & impofturæ deteguntur: verum etiam pleraque alia circa novum hoc argumentum utilia atque jucunda
exactiffimè proponuntur.

Opus admodum utile Medicis, Ægrotis, ægrotorum asfi-
ftentibus, & cunctis aliis literarum, atque adeo politicæ
difciplinæ cultoribus.

Cum duplici Indice, uno Capitum, altero Rerum
præcipuarum.

HAMBURGI

Ex Bibliopolio ZACHARIÆ HERTELII,
Anno M DC LXII.

Fig. 11. Title page of the converso physician Rodrigo de Castro's *Medicus politicus*
(Hamburg, 1614).

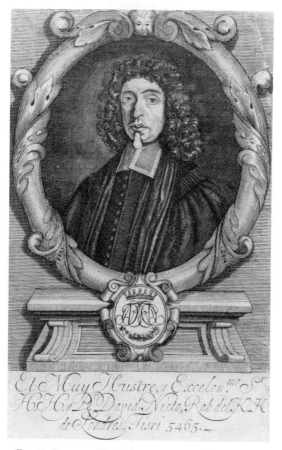

Fig. 12. Portrait of David Nieto, the *ḥakham* of the Spanish-
Portuguese congregation of London, dated Tishre
[September–October] 1704.

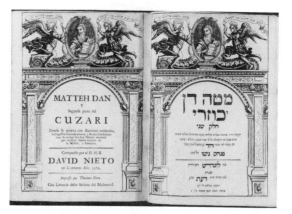

Fig. 13. Title page of part 2 of David Nieto's *Mateh Dan*,
also called *Ha-Kuzari ha-Sheni,* published in London
in 1714 in Hebrew and Spanish.

Science and Skepticism

If it were not for a brief remark by Joseph Delmedigo regarding Simone Luzzatto's extraordinary skills as a mathematician, no one might have associated this erudite but somewhat contentious Venetian scholar with the sciences in the first place. Recent interest in Luzzatto, who functioned as rabbi for almost sixty years until his death in 1663, has centered almost exclusively on his apologetic *Discorso circa il stato de gl'Hebrei et in particolar dimoranti nell'inclita Città di Venetia* (Venice, 1638), addressed to the Doge and Senate of Venice, eloquently defending the political and economic rights of Venetian Jewry.[1] Luzzatto's extant writing is sparse compared to that of his older contemporary Leone Modena. Most intriguing of all is the fact that his two major works, the *Discorso* and a philosophical work entitled *Socrate,* were both written in Italian and addressed to a non-Jewish readership. Although several responsa and letters of Luzzatto are extant in Hebrew, the most illustrious Venetian rabbi of the seventeenth century (other than Modena himself) left an anomalous legacy almost completely unrelated to rabbinics or

---

1. The two most important publications on this work are B. C. I. Ravid, *Economics and Toleration in Seventeenth-Century Venice: The Background and Context of the Discorso of Simone Luzzatto,* American Academy for Jewish Research Monograph Series, no. 2 (Jerusalem, 1978), and the Hebrew translation of the *Discorso (Ma'amar al Yehudei Venezia)* by D. Lattes, with introductions by R. Bachi and M. A. Shulvass (Jerusalem, 1950).

religious teachings of any kind.[2] Perhaps Heinrich Graetz was not as far off the mark as more recent scholars have suggested in viewing Luzzatto as a skeptic.[3] Certainly Bernard Septimus is correct in equating Luzzatto's portrait of Philo, the first-century philosopher who could have educated contemporary Jews but unhappily wrote for non-Jews, with Luzzatto himself.[4]

There are two problems with studying Luzzatto as a religious thinker and natural philosopher. In the first place, his intriguing *Socrate* has been virtually unstudied. No scholar has even described the work fully, let alone mentioned reading it in its entirety.[5] The sole discussion of its political ideas is partial, misleading, and ultimately flawed, as we shall see below.[6] In the second place, as Septimus points out,[7] it is difficult for the modern researcher to disentangle the public Luzzatto from the private one. In the absence of substantial writing in Hebrew, can one assume that his writings to Christian audiences reflect his own positions authentically? The *Discorso* is overtly apologetic; Jewish culture is presented in a manner consonant with Christian cultural and political values and tastes and in a language appropriate to Christian rhetorical style and modes of conceptualization. The circumstances surrounding the writing of *Socrate* are much more obscure. Besides the few hints Luzzatto offers in his preface, it remains unclear why he wrote the work, to whom it was directed, and who actually read it. Did he assume that by publishing a highly learned treatise in Italian, it would escape the attention of even his most learned coreligionists, and

2. Shulvass, in his introduction to *Ma'amar,* succinctly describes Luzzatto's extant Hebrew writings.

3. Graetz is cited in Ravid, *Economics and Toleration,* p. 94, n. 97.

4. B. Septimus, "Biblical Religion and Political Rationality in Simone Luzzatto, Maimonides and Spinoza," *Jewish Thought in the Seventeenth Century,* ed. I. Twersky and B. Septimus (Cambridge, Mass., 1987), p. 420.

5. Shulvass, in his study of Luzzatto's writings in *Ma'amar,* knew the work only from its title page, which we shall see is misleading.

6. I refer to A. Melamed, "Aḥotan ha-Ketanah shel ha-Ḥokhmot: Ha-Maḥshavah ha-Medinit she ha-Hogim ha-Yehudim ba-Renesance ha-Italki," Ph.D. diss., Tel Aviv University, 1976, pp. 393–417. Despite his generally useful discussion of Luzzatto, Melamed's partial reading of *Socrate* significantly misconstrues the essential position of the author, as I point out below.

7. Septimus, "Biblical Religion," p. 400.

that therefore he had the license to take positions he would never dare offer in Hebrew? On the other hand, since it was more common by the mid-seventeenth century for Italian Jews to read and write Italian, and Hebrew literacy was seemingly on the decline,[8] did he intend that his work would be read by Jews? Writing in dialogic form where a variety of opinions are expressed, and even Socrates' position remains somewhat veiled, Luzzatto was not making it easy either for the reader of his generation or for a modern one to fathom his real intention. And finally, might we conclude that the position Socrates seems to adopt at the end of his trial is identical with the position of its Jewish author? None of these fundamental issues lends itself to easy resolution. In the absence of any previous scholarly reading of *Socrate* and having only a partial synthesis of the *Discorso,* any characterizations of Luzzatto's thought must be tentative.

The analysis that follows is restricted to Luzzatto's understanding and appreciation of the natural world and the sciences. Other dimensions of his religious and political thought are beyond the scope of this chapter. Nevertheless, this more limited focus constitutes a central component of his thinking and might offer a most promising beginning to a more comprehensive treatment of the thinker, especially of *Socrate.* Unquestionably, it reveals a common universe of discourse with his older rabbinic colleague Leone Modena, but at the same time a much deeper and more sophisticated grasp of some of the current philosophical, scientific, and political theories of his day.

In the approbations in Delmedigo's *Sefer Elim,* Luzzatto's praise of the work is found immediately after that of Modena.[9] That all three scholars were intimately linked in their appreciation of naturalistic studies is the most telling impression the approbations convey. As we have seen, Modena testifies to his contacts with Delmedigo during his visits to Venice as a student of medicine at the neighboring University of Padua. He sings his praises and designates him a true scholar. No less stinting in his accolades is Luzzatto, who calls Delmedigo "a redeemer" of human sciences "knowledgeable in every secret regarding naturalistic, divine, and mathematical fields, ascending to the firmament, incomparable in all these

---

8. See the remarks of Judah del Bene in his *Kiss'ot le-vet David* (Verona, 1646), 2:9. I discuss del Bene in chap. 6.

9. *Sefer Elim,* beginning.

wisdoms." Like Delmedigo himself, Tobias Cohen, and many others,[10] he alludes to the low cultural level of the Jewish community, suggesting that the quality of Delmedigo's composition will somehow quiet "those who refer to us with arrogance and disdain, claiming that we are lacking in knowledge and that any sagacity has been removed from us. For today the scholars of Greece and Rome shall declare: 'They indeed possess a mind; they produced their witnesses and they testified altogether [compare Is. 43:9]. Would that such words be engraved in the Latin language, attributing to us glory and majesty!'"[11]

On another occasion, Delmedigo returns the compliment in kind in singling out Luzzatto as "a great leader of the Jews whose name is famous, the erudite rabbi Simḥah [Simone] Luzzatto, may God protect and preserve him, who knows every aspect of the mathematical sciences and has entered [all] of its chambers. . . . I did not know if he actually composed a work on geometry or astronomy."[12] Delmedigo's evaluation of Luzzatto's learning constitutes the most substantial evidence—other than Luzzatto's own writing—of his serious involvement in mathematics and astronomy and his proficiency in both.[13] His participation with Modena in promoting a Hebrew work on the sciences was thus neither perfunctory nor mere political flattery. In a community severely deficient in scientific knowledge in Delmedigo's eyes, his appreciation of Luzzatto's singular expertise should not be taken lightly. He might also have included Modena in his adulation, but Modena apparently was a mere champion of education in the sciences among Jews; Luzzatto was actually a serious student of the sciences in his own right.

Given the political focus of Luzzatto's *Discorso*, the natural world and its study would not appear to be central to the work's objectives. Nevertheless, the

10. On Tobias, see chap. 8 below.

11. Note how Luzzatto attributes gaining recognition to publishing in Latin. Perhaps this also helps to explain his interest in publishing in Italian.

12. *Sefer Elim* (Odessa, 1865), p. 131.

13. Other evidence of Luzzatto's reputation in the sciences has recently been noticed in the *Libro grande* of the Jewish community of Venice ("versati nelle scienze"), in a poem by Modena, and in a book by Giulio Morosini, the Venetian apostate ("grandemento acreditato per le scienze"). See D. Malkiel, *A Separate Republic: The Mechanics and Dynamics of Venetian Jewish Self-Government, 1607–1624* (Jerusalem, 1991), p. 203, n. 178, for references.

work is replete with references to nature and to the study of the natural world in the Jewish curriculum. One might argue that such references were merely meant to portray the Jewish community in the most favorable light before its Venetian sovereigns. No doubt Luzzatto consciously strove to underscore those qualities of Jewish cultural life that would make a positive impression on the Catholic government of Venice. When he states that "it is a known fact" that Jews are closer to the Catholics than to the Protestants, that Jews and Catholics share an understanding of the biblical text that requires the mediation of an interpretative tradition, and that both claim that repentance can ameliorate sin,[14] he is surely trying to win points with the city's religious majority. On the other hand, his characterization of Italian Jewry is more than empty flattery; it accurately reflects the comingling of Judaism and Catholicism in the age of the Italian ghettos.[15] Similarly, Luzzatto's remarks about nature might convey his own ideal of Jewish culture, if not its actual appearance.

Keen observations of nature abound throughout Luzzatto's treatise. No doubt his analogies to medicine and nature are a commonplace of contemporaneous political writing. But they resonate in a peculiar way to anyone familiar with *Socrate,* particularly the long speech Luzzatto assigns to Hippias. Furthermore, they are so numerous and so individualized that they should not be considered as mere rhetorical flourish. Take for example the analogies to 'the Jewish problem" that he adduces in the preface to the work. To demonstrate his point that the Jewish people as a whole should not be held responsible for the crimes of certain individuals, he points out that a farmer cultivates his soil by removing the weeds among his fine grasses, not by destroying the entire field; that good health is only noticeable in the context of illness; and that the movement of a swift current is only detected when someone confronts an obstacle that retards his motion.[16] In the introduction to the *Discorso,* he likens the Jews to the Stoic notion of a thin terrestrial vapor combined with the Atomist notion of indivisible and invisible particles. When both come together, they nourish and sustain

14. *Ma'amar al Yehudei Venezia,* p. 152.

15. Cf. D. B. Ruderman, ed., *Essential Papers on Jewish Culture in Renaissance and Baroque Italy* (New York, 1992), Introduction, pp. 24–32; see also my remarks on del Bene in chap. 6 below.

16. *Ma'amar,* p. 77; Ravid, *Economics and Toleration,* pp. 52–53. For other natural analogies, see *Ma'amar,* pp. 74–75, 106, and 107–8.

the public treasury of the state.[17] Such far-fetched analogies might be dismissed if they did not reveal an intimate understanding of ancient theories of nature, fully and dramatically confirmed by the lengthy discussions in *Socrate*.

The reference to a Stoic notion should be seen in conjunction with two others. Luzzatto writes: "Since God created the world with only one nature, He watched over it to unite all its parts and to nourish them in harmonious fashion. Thus He commanded that all humanity would relate to each other in brotherhood as one, since every person is obliged to see himself as a citizen of one universal republic."[18] The notion of a universal nature ruled in harmony by natural laws obliging each individual to see himself as a citizen of the world is Stoic through and through. When viewed together with the long discourse of Hippias in *Socrate* and with Luzzatto's later reference to the most significant Stoic philosopher of his own era, Justus Lipsius, the reference takes on added significance.[19]

Another Stoic notion of nature soon follows, this one appropriated to explain the peculiar psyche of the Jewish nation. Luzzatto refers to the concept of anti-peristasis—that a condition or quality hostile or contrary to an existent condition or quality often fortifies and enlivens it. Thus severe cold surrounding the heat of a newborn child enhances its inner heat, and the sense of danger aroused by an enemy enhances the courage of a besieged nation. In similar fashion, the Jewish people's alienation from the religion and customs of their neighbors reinforced their faith in God and their ancestral traditions.[20]

Luzzatto repeatedly underscores the significance of understanding the natural world in his response to the charges of Tacitus against Judaism. He ridicules Tacitus for not understanding the naturalistic benefits of leaving land uncultivated during the sabbatical year.[21] He mentions explicitly that the high priest prayed not only for his household and community but for the parts of nature:

17. *Ma'amar*, pp. 79–80; Ravid, *Economics and Toleration*, p. 53.

18. *Ma'amar*, p. 113.

19. Luzzatto's reference to Lipsius is found in the *Ma'amar*, p. 147. On Stoicism in *Socrate*, see my fuller discussion below.

20. *Ma'amar*, p. 121.

21. Ibid., p. 136.

"the land, the water, the wind and fire."[22] He points out that the miraculous can be appreciated only by an expert in the normal course of the world. A musician can identify dissonance only because of his expertise in harmony; a doctor discerns illness by grasping the standards of health. Similarly, one cannot "declare the wonders of God" without being a naturalist.[23] The inference that natural philosophy leads to greater piety is also suggested by Hippias in *Socrate*.[24]

Luzzatto's discussion of the types of scholars within the Jewish community further demonstrates his consistent preoccupation with the study of nature. He emphasizes that rabbinic sages cannot interpret Jewish law without a mastery of the natural sciences, particularly astronomy.[25] In this context he mentions the confusing theories of the cosmos from Ptolemy to Copernicus and his expectation that the rabbis must command some expertise in this bewildering discipline.[26] In his discussion of philosophers, he singles out Gersonides and his less-known astronomical writing, a work he claims to be far superior to the *Almagest* of Ptolemy.[27] His remarks suggest an intimate acquaintance with this highly technical Hebrew work, at least those parts Luzzatto was able to locate. Among the other philosophers, Ḥasdai Crescas is cited for his critique of Aristotle and specifically for his significant influence on the skeptical writing of Giovanni Francisco Pico Mirandola, a major source of Pyrrhonist skepticism in early sixteenth-century Italy.[28] We shall return to this reference in examining the skeptical foundations of *Socrate*.

It is clear from Luzzatto's depiction of the kabbalists that his view toward them is similar to that of Modena. He states categorically that Jews are not required to accept their views. Their greatest following is in eastern Europe, he contends, implying that more sophisticated Italian Jews would not take them so seriously.[29] His manner of presenting their ideas is to correlate them with

22. Ibid., p. 128.
23. Ibid., p. 134.
24. See below.
25. *Ma'amar,* pp. 139–40.
26. Ibid., p. 140.
27. Ibid., pp. 142–43.
28. Ibid., p. 143.
29. Ibid.

ancient philosophies—Pythagoreans, Stoics, skeptics, Neoplatonists, gnostics, and nominalists, as if to attenuate both the uniqueness and the antiquity of kabbalistic notions.[30] Luzzatto's presentation was certainly written with an eye to his Christian audience, seeking to translate esoteric concepts into a language comprehensible to non-Jews. At the same time, there is no reason to doubt that Luzzatto's loyalties lay elsewhere. Kabbalah for Luzzatto was merely another form of occult philosophy comparable to other philosophical schools of the ancient world. Through such a comparison, its sanctity and authority were reduced in size and stature; its claims on truth were no more or less credible than those of other schools.

Luzzatto fittingly concludes his discussion by emphasizing Jewish education in the sciences: "They [the Jews] consider it a commandment from the Torah to reflect on natural things in order to gain thusly a closer knowledge to ascertain the greatness of the Creator; and above everything, they consider it an obligation to study the science of the stars because of its importance in fixing the calendar and because this science functions as a gate and an opening to the knowledge of God's greatness and majesty, as written in the Psalms [89:3]: 'In the heavens, You establish Your faithfulness,' that is, through the heavens God prepares and orders the hearts of men to have faith as one looks at the expanse of the heavenly bodies and their speed of movement, the stability of their seasons, and the permanence of their periods." He adds finally that even in a time when Jews are enslaved in their exile and cannot immerse their minds fully in the sciences, they are still obliged to do so since their faith depends on it. Moreover, those few intellectuals in every generation who do pursue the sciences ultimately sustain and protect their communities. For in times of persecution and endangerment, only the activity of the mind on the part of these individuals allows them to win the confidence of the governments under which they live.[31] As the rabbi of the Jewish community of Venice, Luzzatto thus perceived his training in the sciences as having political consequences both for himself and for his community. His intellectual activity directly contributed to the positive public image of his constituency. Conversely, one might argue, he assumed that

30. Ibid., pp. 144–46.
31. Ibid., p. 148.

the untutored kabbalists sullied that image and undermined the credibility of Jews in the eyes of the Christian leadership.[32]

The full title of Luzzatto's *Socrate,* published in Venice in 1651, ostensibly suggests the major message of the work: *Socrate overe dell'humano sapere esercitio seriogiocoso di Simone Luzzatto Hebreo Venetiano opera nella quale si dimostra quanto sia imbecile l'humano intendimento, mentre no è diretto dalla divina rivelatione,* that is, the utter futility of human knowledge without the guiding hand of divine revelation. Such a pious affirmation surely seems fitting to the spirit of Counter-Reformation Italy, for Christians and Jews alike, and would appear to have easily gained the assent of both communities. That the book is not all it appears to be is suggested by two curious features. In the first place, the author is a "Venetian Hebrew" who had just assumed the chief rabbinical office of the city. Why he would devote such energy to explicating the trial of Socrates to a seventeenth-century Italian readership is hardly self-evident. In the case of the *Discorso,* Luzzatto had good reason to defend boldly and eloquently the rights of Jews. *Socrate,* however, is a different matter altogether. There is hardly anything particularly Jewish about the book. Although Luzzatto openly acknowledges his religious identity, he appears to address only issues of universal import. He does not claim to speak as a Jew to Christians, only as a Venetian to fellow Venetians. That Luzzatto would elect to write for an audience beyond his immediate coreligionists is not unprecedented in Jewish cultural history; the examples of Leone Ebreo and Moses Mendelssohn immediately come to mind.[33] But surely the act was unusual, daring, and puzzling, as in the case of Leone.

In the second place, the reader of this substantial work comes away with the distinct impression that the title is considerably misleading. While Luzzatto allows his various speakers to speak occasionally about God and divine providence, there is little if anything about divine revelation in the work. In fact, the

32. For a similar idea, see the debate between Morpurgo and Basilea discussed in chap. 7 below.

33. For a summary of some recent work on Leone Ebreo, see D. B. Ruderman, "The Italian Renaissance and Jewish Thought," *Renaissance Humanism: Foundations, Forms, and Legacy,* ed. A. Rabil, Jr. (Philadelphia, 1981), 1:407–12. On Mendelssohn's *Phaedon,* see A. Altmann, *Moses Mendelssohn: A Biographical Study* (University, Alabama, 1973), pp. 140–58.

religious message, when identifiable, is most faint and indirect. The major issue is not the certainty of divine guidance but human insecurity and uncertainty. The title promises a stronger spiritual orientation than the book delivers. One might assume that Luzzatto was simply conveying the convictions of the pagan Socrates and not his own, that a Christian or Jewish teaching would be an unwelcome anachronism. But *Socrate* was not intended merely to reproduce the historical record. It represents an intellectual critique and a social and political commentary on Luzzatto's own time. He is never reluctant to allow his ancient characters to refer to contemporary discoveries and ideas from Galileo's telescope, to Copernican astronomy, to Paracelsian chemistry, to contemporary discussions of geometry, optics, and navigation.[34] But on contemporary theology he is remarkably silent.

Luzzatto's dedication and preface only faintly convey his motivation for writing the book. To its dedicatees, Doge Francesco Molino and the Collegio of Venice, the author offers the sage Socrates, the oracle of human prudence, whose wisdom is comforting in any time but especially during "the present combustions of a most serious war against a most formidable enemy." Seven years of violence of immense forces have finally given way to a "constant and mature prudence."[35] Luzzatto prays in the name of his ancestors for a satisfactory outcome for the Venetians. He obviously refers to the war of Crete fought against the Turks, in which Molino had held major responsibility as head of Venice's navy.[36] As a gesture of his support as a good citizen of Venice, Luzzatto offers his erudite tome. Like his contemporary, Judah del Bene, who excoriated the Turks and fully supported the Catholic side,[37] Luzzatto fully identified himself as a Venetian. Having argued on behalf of Jewish loyalty to Venice in the *Discorso,* he was demonstrating it in the dedication of *Socrate.*

34. These are all mentioned below.

35. *Socrate,* dedicatory page: "Serenissimo prencipe et eccellentissimo collegio . . . in ogni tempo, & massime nelle presenti combustioni di gravissima guerra contro potentissimo nemico . . . onde per il corso d'anni sette fu esprimentato che la violenza benche munita d'immense forze, languisce & soccombe alla opposizione di constante & matura prudenza."

36. On Molino and the war of Crete, see A. da Mosta, *I Dogi di Venezia* (Milan, 1966), pp. 464–66; W. Carew Hazlitt, *The Venetian Republic: Its Rise, Its Growth, and Its Fall,* A.D. *409–1797* (London, 1915), 2:224–37

37. On del Bene, see chap. 6 below.

The only notices of his Jewish identity other than that on the title page are five citations of biblical verses throughout the book: two from Ecclesiastes, one from Leviticus, one from Job, and one from Proverbs. The first three appear in the opening pages of the volume; the last two, including the most significant of all, appear toward the end. Luzzatto first quotes Ecclesiastes 9:18 ("Wisdom is more valuable than weapons of war") by way of offering his words of wisdom in a time of war.[38] That he symmetrically closes the argument of the book with another quotation from the same text may be more than coincidence. Nor may it be fortuitous that Solomon, not a contemporary theorist of *ragione di stato* but the quintessential Jewish sage, opens by offering the Venetian leadership the most sensible strategy to extricate themselves from their costly conflict. In a gesture of humility, Luzzatto then offers his second biblical reference to the meal offering (Leviticus 2 and elsewhere): "In the Mosaic law it is noted that the Divine Majesty is satisfied with a little flour," comparing it with his own humble offering to the Doge.[39] And in the reader's preface, he offers the third, this time from Solomon's Proverbs (30:18): "Three things are beyond me; four I cannot fathom: . . . How a snake makes its way over a rock."[40] The last citation captures the essential theme of the entire book: the enigmatic quality of the natural world. Although humans attempt to comprehend the faint footprints embedded in nature, they can never fully grasp its essence; they can only approach understanding with modesty and discretion, liberating their souls from the presumptuous opinions of arrogant scholars and their despotic authority. Socrates pronounces "the subversion of human knowledge," adopting a mode of reflection that is "tentative, skeptical, and doubting" rather than "dogmatic and assertive."[41] Luzzatto returns to the same message in the closing of his work, where his final Solomonic reflection is uttered. With the gentle and discreet hand of a polished writer, he artistically situates the lengthy and convoluted

38. At the beginning of the dedication.

39. "che ramemorandosi che nella Legge Mosaica si trova registrato, che la Divina Maestà appagavasi di poca farina, che in segno di divotione povere meschino l'appresentava, si compiaciano parimente aggradire questo ben che minimo saggio di dottrina."

40. Preface to reader: "& Salamone nelli proverbij frà li quattro che nel camino non producono di loro segnale, fù annoverato il serpente, che sopra duro fasso si striscia."

41. ". . . che tutto ciò che pronontiò Socrate nelle everssione dell'humano sapere, fù più tosto per modo tentativo, septico, & dubbitativo, che dogmatico & assertivo."

reflections of the Greek sages of his dialogue between the two unadorned poles of Hebraic sagacity spoken by the biblical king.

Following the dedication and preface, Luzzatto offers a synopsis of the book's basic argument.[42] Utilizing his summary but expanding upon it, I present my own epitome of the book, emphasizing his extended discussions about the natural world. Since the book is not well known and, to my knowledge, has never before been fully described, such an effort seems appropriate prior to any analysis of my own.

In ancient Athens, the members of the Delphic Academy congregate to liberate Reason, who had been imprisoned and oppressed by human authority. They install a special receptacle where people can place secret denunciations regarding the abuses of reason and its diffusion of improper doctrines. Socrates is subsequently accused of subverting human science and is brought to trial. He defends himself by arguing that the uncertainty of human knowledge stems from the unresolvable controversies among the ancient scholars over the principles of natural things. He claims to have abandoned the unattainable quest for certain knowledge and in its place seeks only the "glimmer of the probable" (il barlume del probabile).[43] A full account of ancient hypotheses on the origin of the universe follows, including those with contemporaneous overtones such as the views of Aristotle, Plato, the atomists, and even the chemical philosophers (gli chimici).[44] As we shall see, one of the most characteristic features of such discussions is Luzzatto's inclusion of recent theories and discoveries about the natural world to bolster and reinforce ancient skeptical arguments.

From this preliminary exposition of theories, Socrates offers his initial impression about the futility of human beings ever knowing the truth, about the unstable, arbitrary, and capricious nature of human knowledge, the unreliability of sense perception, and the incapacity of the human intellect to conceptualize any object.[45] To illustrate his position, he takes advantage of information only available to one living in the seventeenth century. Emphasizing the severe limitations of the unaided eye to observe the heavens, he offers a detailed and

42. *Socrate,* pp. 3–4.
43. Ibid., p. 16.
44. Ibid., pp. 16–33.
45. Ibid., pp. 33–92.

accurate summary of Galileo's telescope and the observations of the moon, planets, and heliocentric universe.[46] Although these observations might appear to strengthen the position that human beings are indeed capable of observing and knowing quite a lot about their universe, Socrates is careful to balance these new achievements with the weight of human liabilities. Demonstrating a remarkable mastery of optics, he subsequently discusses various theories about the process by which the eyes receive rays of light in order to see. This allows him to diminish the significance of the recent advances by emphasizing once again the distortions and errors endemic to all human observation.[47]

Following detailed excurses on the nature of color,[48] the internal senses,[49] the imagination,[50] memory,[51] and the intellect,[52] Socrates considers the larger question of the purpose of knowledge and reflects on the dizzying multifariousness of the natural world. With the discerning eye of the naturalist, he offers a splen-

46. Ibid., pp. 94–95: "& massime doppo che fù sufragato dall'egregio adminicolo del cannachialo che dimonstrò l'errori & falacie, che l'antichità normata dall'humano discorso giudicava vere & sincere dottrine, stimò questa che la via lattea fosse sublunare, e terestre esalatione, ma l'occhio aiutato da tal criterio & instrumento, hora ci insegna che sia una congerie di minutissime stelle fisse, nelle più sublime parti del cielo esistenti: crese quella che la luna fosse corpo terso & polito c'instruisce questo che de molto cavità & prominentie sia ingombrata; ci persuase facilmente quella che solamente alla luna avenga diversità di apparenza, ci dimonstrò questo che venere parimente apparisce, intiera, dimezzata & falcatta; stimò quella che l'istessa Venere & Mercurio attorniassero la terra come fanno li altri pianeti, ci avisò questo che non la terra, ma il Sole come loro centro questi circondano & intorno ad esso si ravolgono; guidicò quella che sette fossero li erranti pianeti, ci accertò questo che all'intorno di Giove con loro periodi particolati si rivolgessero quattro altri globi, benche da esso circa il Zodiaco siano traportati & rivolti, & anco ci insegnò che Saturno non solamente uno pianeta sia; ma certo consortio di tre corpi, che in anni trenta con moto conforme la terra circuiscono. approbò quella che il Sole autore del mondano calore ne fosse egli privo. ci informò questo che il globo solare fosse occupato da molti mongibelli & vesuvji, che vomitando fuochi, & oscure esalationi . . . ."
47. *Socrate,* pp. 96–98
48. Ibid., pp. 101–5
49. Ibid., pp. 105–13.
50. Ibid., pp. 114–22.
51. Ibid., pp. 123–31.
52. Ibid., pp. 132–33.

diferous portrait of the earth's topography and the movement of the seas, the course of rivers and the appearance of mountain ranges, the variety of plants and animals and even human cultures and customs. By including the new data about the human species derived from dissections and from the discovery of the natives of Africa, he ponders whether such overwhelming diversity bespeaks a kind, beneficent, and purposeful universe or a frightening, monstrous, and calamitous one. In the light of such discoveries, one might conclude that ignorance is blissful, while knowledge torments.[53]

Having deflated the presumption of nature's bountiful and harmonious purpose, Socrates steers his interlocutors to the subject of how one knows. He again listens to a wide diversity of hypotheses, none of which is conclusive or reassuring.[54] When one of the participants, Archelao, offers his opinion that knowledge constitutes the understanding of the causes of things, Socrates again introduces recent data to confound the position that nature benefits human beings. He begins by inquiring about the disproportion of natural resources among differing localities: why some regions are blessed with natural irrigation and others arid, why the sea is tempestuous in certain areas and gentle in others, why the Mediterranean terminates arbitrarily in Syria, depriving the other peoples of Asia of an active commerce, and why the narrow land separating Africa from Asia impedes trade vessels from traveling between the Mediterranean and the "rich Indes."[55] From the natural impediments of the sea and land, he turns to dispel

---

53. Ibid., pp. 166–71, esp. p. 167 on the human species : "ma che il contrario pare che osservasse nella humana spetie, che di tal equalità punto non si curò, ritrovandosi cadauno homo, tanto diferente di virtù, conditione, costumi, & opinioni dal altro, che rassembra che cadauno d'essi constituisca affato diversa spetie; onde se l'anatomia interna dell'animo si potesse praticare, come la disecatione del corpo, s'osservarebbero la più portentose monstruosità che gia mai la imaginatione formalizare si potesse, ne l'Africa di hereirocliti parti fecondissima madre, ne la licentiosa libertà di poeti & pittori, tale ne formarebbero & fingerebbero, da che presero origine quelli tre celebri pronontiati che appo il volgo passano per adagij, homo homini Deus, homo homini lupus, homo homini homo, che forse questo ultimo meglio espresse la fierezza dell'humane genere."

54. *Socrate,* pp. 175–206.

55. Ibid., p. 212: "onde seguendolo li altri sapienti, chi mai di essi investigò & rinveni il fine per cui alcuni regioni della terra sono à satietà irrigate da prolifico humore, & altre affatto di esso destitute; & altre dalle illuvioni di fiumi sormerse? che ricercò perche alcuni paesi

the common assumptions that animals are created for human usage, singling out the poisonous vipers of Africa.[56] Even an element of uncertainty and incongruity afflicts mathematical demonstrations.[57] All of these examples suggest that comprehending the causes of things is not the ultimate goal of human knowledge; if it were, human beings would prove woefully inept.

Pausing to present and then criticize the deductive syllogism of Aristotle[58] and the inductive methods of "false alchemy,"[59] Socrates considers the final position of Cratilo, which in the end approximates his own. According to this view, certain questions concerning time, motion, and space can never be resolved with certainty. The unfathomable dimensions of the sun, of atoms, and of geometry make a mockery of human reason. In the end, speculations on such matters inevitably end in disagreement "and tension between sensory perception and the mind."[60] Cratilo acknowledges that human beings can only function in the realm of the probable, reserving "secure truth" to God. He adds that while a full understanding of the external universe alludes us, human beings require only a mediocre level of cognition for ordering human affairs, which he

sono piani & commodi alli usi humani & altri alpestri & sterili? chi indagò per quall'oggetto il mare in alcuni lochi della terra con furioso flusso l'assalta, & immediate la rilascia come accade nel mare occidentale Settentrionale, & in altri lochi con mediocri aggressi, regressi con essa scherza, & in altre positure come nella lunghezza del mare mediteraneo solamente con reciproco & alternante corso non crescendo ne diminuendo la lambisce? per qual scopo l'istesso mare nel lido della Soria termina, & non più oltre si estende, privandoci di ageuole comercio con li popoli più interni della vastissima Asia? qual mira hebbe l'opefice universale nell'impedire la navigatione alla Grecia, Italia, & altre Provincie mediteranee con l'infraporre quel stretto istimo & poco di terra fra l'Asia & Africa, in modo che ci rimane impedito lo transitare con vascelli alle ricche indie?"

56. Ibid., p. 213.

57. Ibid., pp. 213–14: "che ne anco le scientie matematiche che tengono fra le altre di certezza il principato nè di causa efficiente nè finale nelle lore ferme demostrationi punto si servono."

58. Ibid., pp. 215–20.

59. Ibid., pp. 223.

60. Ibid., pp. 230–35, concluding: "che il discorso nell'osservarle, che implicano in se stesse repugnanze & contrarietà affatto intolerabili & inadmissibili. riducendosi alla fine qualunque speculatione à termine di litigio & tenzone fra il senso & la mente."

terms *prudenza*.[61] Having narrowed the expectations of human understanding to the social and political order, he moves on to a rigorous consideration of nine definitions of *prudenza*.[62]

The lengthiest speech on the subject, and the one of most relevance to the subject of this chapter, is that of Hippias.[63] As if oblivious to all that has previously been said about the inscrutability of the natural world, Hippias confidently argues that the surest model of our social and political relations on earth is provided by the "midwife" of nature.[64] He eloquently argues that although human beings lack the capacity to understand everything outside themselves, nevertheless they can grasp distinctly the regular pattern of existence by which nature instructs men to act. In several carefully constructed chapters, Hippias's argument unfolds from a macrocosmic to a microcosmic perspective. First he demonstrates how speculation on the celestial movements enhances one's understanding of the administration of human government.[65] Just as the planets simultaneously revolve around the sun as they revolve on their own axes, the citizens and leaders of the state concern themselves with both the general good and their private interests. From four hypothetical models of planetary motions, he derives four kinds of governments, ranging from best to worst.[66] Similarly, the variegated relations between the sun, moon, and earth suggest for Hippias analogues with respect to the interactions of princes, courtiers, and their subjects.[67]

Civil *prudenza* can also be learned from the actions of nature in the sublunar world, according to Hippias. Employing the Aristotelian notion of the earth

61. Ibid., pp. 236–37.

62. Ibid., pp. 238–56.

63. Ibid., pp. 256–77. This is well summarized in Hebrew by Melamed, "Aḥotan ha-Ketanah," who incorrectly identifies it with the position of Luzzatto. See below.

64. Ibid., p. 257.

65. Ibid., p. 260: "Profitti per la prudenza morale & civile che si tragono della speculatione de cieli in universale . . . dalla speculatione de motti celesti apprese l'humana prudenza l'ottima administratione della Republica."

66. Ibid., p. 261: "ci amaestrano parimente li cieli e instruiscono che quattro modi di governi sono. il prime ottimo, il secondo buono, il terzo cativo, il quattro pessimo."

67. Ibid., p. 262.

suspended in the center of the universe, either remaining in a stable position or being pulled by various celestial movements, Hippias concludes that a nation is more stable when surrounded by stronger states than when it is surrounded by weaker ones. He similarly demonstrates the qualities of the four elements and their analogues in the social order; animals and plants offer other social and political lessons.[68] Finally, he compares the processes of the human body with those of the body politic. So, for example, the liver delivers blood like a leader who passes out food to the needy; the heart is like the treasury of the state, while the brain is equivalent to its political advisers.[69]

For Hippias, nature offers humanity the only solution to overcome the wretchedness and precariousness of its existence. The splendor and majesty of the "grand machine" of nature is there to emulate. It not only offers advice on rendering life worthwhile; it constitutes man's ultimate master and teacher. When we follow its signals and walk in its footsteps, "it is impossible to fail and to deviate from the right path."[70] Furthermore, it reveals the universality of the human experience. When man abides by the the laws of nature, he not only learns to serve his nation but becomes a loyal citizen of the universe. And the universal norms that function in the physical and social realms ultimately suggest a supreme cause admired and revered by all. In fact, for Hippias true human science and philosophy fortify faith in God and his providence and protect human beings from impiety and superstition, "preparing the human soul for a sentiment of true religion." Knowledge of "the grand theater of the universe" is to be contrasted to the useless and debilitating mental exercises of the scholastics. The former is accessible to all; it is satisfying and ennobling.[71]

68. Ibid., pp. 263–67.

69. Ibid., pp. 267–68.

70. Ibid., p. 272: "onde essendoci la natura ottima maestria, e direttrice, e che giamai non falisce nelle sue operationi se non per superfluità ò deficientia over contumacia della materia, che incontra, & che alle mani li perviene, mentre che noi seguiamo li suoi vestigi & constantemente insistiamo nelle sue orme, ci riesce impossibile il falire, & dal retto deviare."

71. Ibid., pp. 273–75: "ci sugerì l'intendimento che teniamo di una suprema cagione, il cui sapere admiramo, potenza riverimo & bontà amamo . . . . [Science and philosophy remove impiety] [274]: "preparando l'animo humano al sentimento della vera religione, ma di più s'impiegò a rintuzzare la pazza superstitione . . . essendo l'empij privi di alcun sentimento

Socrates refrains from approving Hippias's speech. Instead, he suspends his judgment until listening to the rebuttal of Timon.[72] Timon reverses most emphatically the direction of Hippias's remarks in favor of a full-fledged skepticism. Exploring the movements of the stars is an effort of "vain curiosity" having no relationship or relevance to the workings of the social world, he contends. The uniformity and constancy of the celestial world have no analogue in the variable world of human affairs. Neither the calculations of the mathematicians nor the experiments of the naturalists afford one the knowledge or capacity for civil life. An infatuation with the universal order of nature diminishes one's legitimate love for his own country. A philosopher who is a citizen of the world cannot passionately and ethically support his own nation against its enemies.[73]

Nature for Timon is neither the source of human prudence nor of moderation. Hippias's analogies from nature to the social realm are artificially contrived and fallacious. Nature does not always reveal its harmonious and beneficent face, nor is it always a proper teacher of human prudence. "The school of nature" also teaches depraved customs—belligerence and violence, infidelity and irreverence. It is also vanity to believe that natural philosophy makes people more pious. On the contrary, Timon argues, philosophy is like bloodletting: both good and bad humors are evacuated from the body. While philosophy claims to root out only superstition and not true religion, it often succeeds in expelling both. Timon also objects to the philosophical notions of *prudenza* and *virtù,* and to the lack of consensus about the ultimate meaning of life. While doctors strive to make the body healthy and soldiers seek victory in war, the moral philosophers offer no clear answer about the goal of human life and the notion of the good.

---

della dietà, à guisa d'animali irragionevoli dalla classe delli homini distratti e ecclusi . . . . [The kind of knowledge to which he refers is not scholastic] [275]: che nulla di certo da tanto laborioso mentale esercitio si conseguisce, essendoci, la verità inattingibile & inaccessabile, tuttavia negare non puoi che grande noia arrecaresti all'humano genere in descreditarli il suo sapere . . . ma il contemplativo diletto senza noia & iattura di alcuno sempre ci si appresenta agevole & pronto. Il gran teatro dell'universo al senso & intelletto di tutti li homini tanto nobili come plebei, ricci come poveri egualmente è aperto & spalancato & con liberale indiferenza li suoi mirabili spettacoli esponse & offerisce . . . ."

72. Ibid., pp. 277–78.
73. Ibid., pp. 279–82.

Contrary to Plato, philosophers should never be kings. They lack the passion to lead, the ability to have their constituencies notice and appreciate them.[74]

Timon finalizes his message by citing an eminent man "not born in Greece nor educated in our customs, expressed in his divine monuments."[75] The eminent man is once again Solomon and the citation is from Ecclesiastes 7:29: "God has made men plain but they have engaged in too much reasoning." As Timon puts it, it epitomizes "that condition of excellence" to which human beings should strive. Surely Timon's appeal to the Hebrew sage underscores for Luzzatto the Jewish source of this sentiment. That Socrates considers both the speeches of Hippias and Timon but, in the end, "is inclined to his [Timon's] useful instruction"[76] suggests not only the dénouement of *Socrate* but the fact that this position is ultimately that of Rabbi Simone Luzzatto himself.

Timon makes one more critical point before concluding his speech. Despite the uncertainty of knowledge and contingency of human experience, a person need not despair of functioning constructively in this world. Timon's address closes as it began, with the advice to live with the probable, to make ethical choices with the limited capacity human beings are endowed, and to embrace nature, which does not call out the truth in a loud voice but whispers with faint signs, offering humanity a course to follow—and one to avoid.[77]

Socrates' accusers remain dissatisfied with his conclusion that ultimate truth

74. Ibid., pp. 283–305. For example, p. 286: "Nella scola della natura imparò il suoi depravati costumi . . . li violatori della amicitia sostegno & condimento della humana vita . . . havendo anco nelli irragionevoli animali osservato l'infame concubito di figlioli con le madri . . . ." On the false assumption that philosophy leads to piety, he writes on p. 287: "anzi credo che alla filosofia sia avenuto ciò che sovente accade alla pratica della medicina, che mentre, imprende scacciare dall'infermo li depravati humori ch l'offendono insieme con essi detrude l'istessa vita; così anco questa temeraria sapienza non diretta da maggior lume, pretendendo distrugere la superstitione, fuga la istessa religione."

75. Ibid., p. 307: "Procurand'io ridurli a quella conditione di eccellenza, chi già egregio homo non nella Grecia nato nè con nostri costumi educato nelli suoi divini monumenti espresse, 'Deus fecit hominem rectum, & ipsi requiserunt cogitationes multas.'"

76. Ibid., p. 309: "& conferendo l'uno con l'altro ad esso Timone, & alla sua proficua instruttione inclinae."

77. Ibid., p. 310: "che tacitamente la istessa natura ci sussura & con invisibile cenno ci addita quello che convenga tracciare & scansare."

remains inaccessible to man and that he can still uphold a faith in God. His answer is elusive: He remains an enemy of the "wise" but not a friend of the vulgar and ignorant. He refuses to concede that his course of probability undermines moral virtue and religion. He concedes that the human soul has a strong propensity toward religion and the divine cult. Thus he would never scorn religious observance and the legitimate modes of public sacrifice. He only opposes the superstitions of the ignorant that appear in the guise of the divine beings in Job (2:1) who sought to destroy the saintly man. Rather, he seeks to procure those virtues that uplift the soul "from those scornful concepts that deface the beauty and shapeliness of the true religion." He approves of the rites "ordained by the urban magistrates in honor of God" but will not countenance the ridiculous beliefs and vain ceremonies of the plebeians.[78] With Plato not prepared to condemn him, the decision to execute Socrates is suspended; he is neither damned nor scorned. The vulgar continue to suspect him, but some scholars continue to hold him in esteem.[79]

Luzzatto's remarkable reconstruction of the trial of Socrates deserves a full examination of its sources, literary devices, and intellectual and political context. Having been virtually ignored by scholarship, it needs to be rehabilitated and integrated within the vast literature bearing Socratic influence from late antiquity to the twentieth century.[80] It should be examined as a primary text in the history of Jewish skepticism from Ecclesiastes to Santob de Carrion, Sanchez, La Peyrère, Spinoza, and beyond. And it requires elucidation as a text reflecting

78. Ibid., p. 313: "circa l'osservanza della religione giamai dispregiai, nè omessi. ma sempre conforme li riti patrij, nelli lochi convenevoli, tempi opportuni, & con modi legitimi publicamente sacrificai. . . . non perciò a guisa di giganti attentai detrudere Giove dal cielo, ma si bene procurai levarli dall'animo quelli dispregiabili concetti che deturpano la bellezza & formosità della vera religione . . . ma che però li riti da urbani magistrati ordinati in honoranza di Iddio, con ogni maggior esterno culto si devono osservare; & nondimeno le ridicole credenze, & vane cerimonie della plebe patientare si dovessero . . . ."

79. Ibid., pp. 315–16.

80. On this, see H. Spiegelberg, ed., *The Socratic Enigma* (New York and Kansas City, 1964), as well as the interesting essay of J. Bergmann, "Socrates in der Jüdischen Literatur," *Monatsschrift für Geschichte und Wissenschaft des Judentums* 44 (1936): 1–13, who briefly mentions Luzzatto's work.

the special cultural ambiance of Venetian Jewry in the middle of the seventeenth century.

Such an inquiry is obviously beyond the scope of this chapter. Yet even a cursory reading of *Socrate* indicates the broad erudition and wide range of ancient philosophical sources with which Luzzatto was familiar. Most significant for our purposes was his knowledge of ancient Stoicism and skepticism, both experiencing major revivals in the sixteenth and seventeenth centuries.[81] In all likelihood, he was familiar with Seneca and Cicero, either from their own works or from reading the major Neostoic of early modern Europe, Justus Lipsius, who is mentioned by Luzzatto in the *Discorso*.[82] His reading on skepticism also represented a combination of ancient and modern authors. Among the sources with which he was definitely familiar was, first and foremost, Sextus Empiricus, the author of *The Outlines of Pyrrhonism,* which he cites twice in the *Discorso*.[83] With its rediscovery in the sixteenth century and subsequent publications in 1562, 1569, and 1601, it became the most significant source of Greek skepticism in this period.[84] Luzzatto also mentions Gianfrancesco Pico della Mirandola's *Examen vanitatis doctrinae gentium,* published in 1520, which was clearly inspired by Sextus Empiricus some forty years before the first publication of his writing. Luzzatto proudly indicates Gianfrancesco's reliance on Ḥasdai Crescas in reject-

81. On Stoicism in early modern Europe, see J. L. Saunders, *Justus Lipsius: The Philosophy of Renaissance Stoicism* (New York, 1955); M. Morford, *Stoics and Neostoics: Rubens and the Circle of Lipsius* (Princeton, 1991); A. Grafton, "Portrait of Justus Lipsius," *The American Scholar* 1987: 382–90; G. Oestrich, *Neostoicism and the Early Modern State,* ed. B. Ostreich and H. G. Koenigsberger, trans. D. McLintock (Cambridge, 1982); and esp. W. J. Bouwsma, "The Two Faces of Humanism: Stoicism and Augustinianism in Renaissance Thought," in *A Usable Past: Essays in European Cultural History* (Berkeley and Los Angeles, 1990), pp. 19–73 (first published in *Itinerarium Italicum: The Profile of the Italian Renaissance in the Mirror of Its European Transformations,* ed. H. A. Obermann and T. A. Brady, Jr. [Leiden, 1975], pp. 3–60). On skepticism, the classic work remains R. Popkin, *The History of Scepticism from Erasmus to Spinoza,* 2d ed. (Berkeley and Los Angeles, 1979). See also, M. Burnyeat, ed., *The Skeptical Tradition* (Berkeley and Los Angeles, 1983).

82. See n. 19 above.

83. *Ma'amar,* pp. 125, 145.

84. See Popkin, *History of Scepticism,* chap. 2.

85. *Ma'amar,* p. 143. See C. B. Schmitt, *Gianfrancesco Pico della Mirandola (1469–1533) and His Critique of Aristotle* (The Hague, 1967). Schmitt and Popkin disagree over the extent of

ing Aristotelian science.[85] Although he does not mention it, Luzzatto may also have been familiar with *De incertitudine et vanitate scientiarum declamatio invectiva*, written in 1526 by Henry Cornelius Agrippa von Nettesheim. Leone Modena, Luzzatto's colleague, was familiar with the work; so were Jacob Ẓemaḥ and probably other Jewish intellectuals of the period.[86] I have yet to determine conclusively whether Luzzatto read other contemporary writers on skepticism, such as Francisco Sanchez,[87] Michel de Montaigne, and Pierre Charron. Whether or not he knew of Montaigne, Luzzatto's composition exhibits several features that present interesting parallels to his work, as we shall see below. In addition to Stoicism and skepticism, Luzzatto was quite well read in contemporary political thought, as Abraham Melamed has mentioned. Besides Tacitus, which Luzzatto might have known through Lipsius's recent edition and commentary, he had probably read Machiavelli, Botero, Boccalini, and More.[88] It also seems possible that he knew the writings of the Jesuit political writers of the second half of the sixteenth century: Antonio Possevino, Robert Bellarmine, Luis de Molina, and Francisco Suarez, particularly their attacks on Machiavelli and the *ragione di stato* and their attempts to defend the connection between positive human law and the laws of nature.[89] Be that as it may, it seems clear that Luzzatto's knowledge of philosophical tastes and political theories was relatively up-to-date. The implication that Jewish thought was somehow retarded or out of step with contemporaneous thinking does not appear to fit at all the case of Simone Luzzatto.[90]

Like Montaigne, Luzzatto was inclined to couple the rediscovery of ancient

---

Gianfrancesco's influence. (Cf. Popkin, *History of Scepticism,* pp. 20–22.) If Popkin is right about his minimal influence, then Luzzatto's use of this book is all the more significant.

86. On this work, see C. G. Nauert, Jr., *Agrippa and the Crisis of Renaissance Thought* (Urbana, Ill., 1965). On its influence among contemporary Jewish thinkers, see M. Idel, "Differing Conceptions of Kabbalah in the Early Seventeenth Century," *Jewish Thought in the Seventeenth Century,* pp. 168–74.

87. On Sanchez, see my remarks in chap. 10 below.

88. A. Melamed, "Simone Luzzatto on Tacitus: Apologetica and Ragione di Stato," in *Studies in Medieval Jewish History and Literature,* ed. I. Twersky (Cambridge, Mass., 1984), p. 154.

89. See Q. Skinner, *The Foundations of Modern Political Thought* 2 vols. (Cambridge, 1978), II: 135–173.

90. Cf. Septimus, "Biblical Religion," p. 432, n. 143, based on Melamed, "Aḥotan ha-Ketanah," p. 346.

theories with the discovery of the "New Heavens" and the "New Worlds." He consistently embellishes his skeptical arguments with references to these discoveries. Most dramatic is his succinct summary of Galileo's *Sidereus nuncius,* including the description of the telescope, the moon, and planets. In this he was preceded by Abraham Yagel and Joseph Delmedigo.[91] He also summarizes accurately the views of the Paracelsians, specifically their three primary elements instead of four.[92] I have already mentioned his most impressive discussions of contemporary optical theory, of Euclidian geometry, of topography and navigation, apparently stemming from his personal experiences in the port city of Venice.[93] His few and infrequent references to medicine suggest that his primary scientific interests lay elsewhere.

When one examines Luzzatto's narrative from beginning to end, it is the skeptical voice of Socrates that predominates. From the precise formulations of the preface and summary of the book's argument in the beginning to the final suspension of Socrates' trial, the author stresses time and again the futility of attaining epistemological certainty, the unreliability of the senses, and the diversity of human customs and judgments, thus effectively demolishing the pretensions of unaided human reason to ascertain the truth. The most dramatic parts of the book are the extended discourses of Hippias and Timon, their utter disagreement, Socrates' weighing of their respective positions, and his final decision in favor of Timon. Since both men ponder the relationship between human society and the natural world, their speeches are not only central to Luzzatto's book; they are also most relevant to the primary focus of this chapter.

Luzzatto's naming of these two interlocutors after two relatively minor intellectual figures in the ancient world is hardly fortuitous. Hippias of Elis was the subject of two dialogues attributed to Plato: *Hippius major* and *Hippias minor.*

---

91. See n. 46 above. See S. Drake, *Discoveries and Opinions of Galileo* (Garden City, N.Y., 1957) on Galileo's work. Yagel's summary is discussed in D. B. Ruderman, *Kabbalah, Magic, and Science: The Cultural Universe of a Sixteenth-Century Jewish Physician* (Cambridge, Mass., 1988), chap. 6; Delmedigo's summary is discussed in I. Barzilay, *Yoseph Shlomo Delmedigo (Yahar of Cardia): His Life, Works, and Times* (London, 1974), p. 150. See also Delmedigo, *Sefer Elim* (Odessa, 1865), pp. 300–301, 417, 432, 433.

92. *Socrate,* p. 22.

93. See nn. 47, 48, and 55–57 above.

Hippias was a diplomat with a high reputation as a sophist and practical crafts-man. He had also attained considerable expertise in mathematics, astronomy, and harmonics. In both dialogues, Hippius is vain and boastful. He considers himself knowledgeable in all matters and proves to be testy and impatient when Socrates badgers him with questions about the nature of beauty. He lamely pro-tests "the scrapings and shavings" of Socrates' arguments as pure rubbish. In the end, Hippius the renowned know-it-all is shown to be ignorant, caught in a delusion of possessing wisdom which Socrates must break down in order that he may ultimately recognize the radical finitude of his human intelligence.[94]

Timon of Phlius, on the other hand, was known as an early skeptic who wrote lampoons abusing the dogmatic philosophers. As Pyrrho's faithful disciple, Timon denied the possibility of self-evident general principles; all arguments were either circular or represented an endless chain hanging from nothing. Ac-cording to Sextus, Timon rejected the pursuit of philosophy and returned to the practical affairs of life. He maintained that the world had a twofold nature: the phenomenal and the real. While human beings can grasp the former through sensory perception, the true nature of the latter is never disclosed, either through the senses or the mind.[95] The Hippias and Timon of Luzzatto's dialogue were thus truly in character. Hippias, the self-assured and arrogant sophist, ignored completely the skeptical arguments that had preceded his address in propound-ing an orderly and harmonic universe accessible and comprehensible to the human senses and intelligence. When Hippias had completed his presentation, Timon wasted no time in demolishing his argument point by point.

The two speeches constitute two distinct concepts of nature: an older teleo-logical view, according to which nature embodies ideals and standards for all created species, conformity to which is beneficial, even necessary, for the pres-ervation of human society; and an opposing view that categorically denies any such universal harmony linking the natural with the good.[96] Another way of

94. See *The Dialogues of Plato,* trans. B. Jowett, 4 vols. (Oxford, 1953), 1:557–95, 603–23; and J. Beckman, *The Religious Dimension of Socrates' Thought* (Waterloo, Ontario, 1979), p. 95.

95. Diogenes Laertius, *Lives of Eminent Philosophers,* 2 vols. (Cambridge, Mass. 1958), ix. 109–15 (pp. 519–25); and C. L. Stough, *Greek Skepticism: A Study in Epistemology* (Berkeley and Los Angeles, 1969), pp. 16–34.

96. I am indebted to the formulation of D. L. Schaefer, *The Political Philosophy of Montaigne* (Ithaca, N.Y., 1990), p. 127.

categorizing the difference between the two would be to designate the first as an essentially Stoic position while the second constitutes a Pyrrhonist skeptical one. Ancient Stoicism, as William J. Bouwsma has noted, is not easily defined, representing part of a tangled bundle of Hellenistic ideas. Stoicism, in both its ancient and more modern forms, represents a kind of natural theology which assumed that a single cosmic order, rational and divine, pervaded all things. Its principles operate equally in physical nature, human society, and in the human personality. By grasping the general rationality of nature, man could discover the rational laws of his own society and psyche, and by following them, perfect himself. The Stoics also taught the notion of disciplining the body through *apatheia,* a cultivated indifference to physical needs and passions and to external circumstances. Whether a person was directed to improve the conditions of his existence or to accept them as necessary, whether to lead an activist life or to favor a contemplative withdrawal from society, points to a critical ambiguity and tension which is never fully resolved in Stoic thought.

From the sixteenth century on, Stoicism experienced a new lease on life, particularly as a force for order in a period of prolonged religious wars. The most important center of Neostoicism in the seventeenth century emerged in the Netherlands surrounding the writings of Justus Lipsius, who edited the works of Seneca. Lipsius advocated a system of ethics based on physics, whereby human beings were expected to follow the rules of conduct laid down by nature, the wise man became a true citizen of the world, and abstract reflection was devaluated in favor of the practical art of living.[97] While Luzzatto's Hippias does not espouse every strand of the Stoic philosophy, ignoring completely the notion of passive contemplation and societal withdrawal, the general lines of his approach and that of the Stoics patently conform with each other. The artificial analogies between the physical and social realms are neither novel nor a reflection of seventeenth-century Cartesian or Hobbesian philosophies, as one recent scholar has labeled them.[98] They are instead an older view of nature, dissenting

97. My summary is based on Bouwsma's essay and the other works mentioned in n. 81 above. On the commonplace seventeenth-century notion of the state duplicating the order of the macrocosm, see E. M. W. Tillyard, *The Elizabethan World Picture* (New York, 1944), pp. 79–89.

98. Melamed, "Aḥotan ha-Ketanah," pp. 397–98.

from the old scholastic position but equally dogmatic and teleological. Most important, this is a view which Luzzatto's Socrates considers, even flirts with, but ultimately rejects.[99]

Timon's position is easily identified with the Pyrrhonian argument in both its ancient and more modern manifestations. Luzzatto presents this position as the central theme of his book. The only reversal is expressed by Hippias. Timon's role is to reiterate the argument against the pretensions of dogmatic philosophy, to rebut Hippias's alternative epistemology, to overcome Socrates' hesitations, and ultimately to win his approval. It is not clear to what extent Luzzatto, through Timon's speech, employs doubt as a rhetorical device or actually stakes out a thoroughly Pyrrhonian position of indecision and suspension of judgment. From the last pages, it appears that Socrates does not oppose reason altogether but merely the dogmatic variety. He acknowledges that human beings are capable of functioning with tentative and probable knowledge in the social and political realms. Moreover, he seems to advocate a pragmatic secularism opposing the Stoic belief in the universal principles of nature required to validate governments. The Machiavellian ragione di stato appears to replace the eternal reason of Hippias and the Stoics.

Although there is no evidence to suggest that Montaigne's *Apology for Raymond Sebond* influenced Luzzatto's *Socrate,* there are several intriguing parallels between the two works, highlighted most clearly by David Lewis Schaefer's recent reading of Montaigne's classic essay.[100] According to Schaefer, Montaigne's putative defense of Sebond's work is undertaken to present his own view of

---

99. As I have already indicated, this is the basic problem in Melamed's analysis. By focusing almost exclusively on this speech of Hippias without placing it in the context of the entire book, especially Timon's critique and Socrates' ultimate acceptance of it, Melamed concluded that this position was that of Luzzatto. A more careful reading of the entire book does not support this conclusion.

100. Besides Schaefer, *The Political Philosophy* and the up-to-date bibliography he includes, I have benefited from the classic work of D. C. Allen, *Doubt's Boundless Sea: Skepticism and Faith in the Renaissance* (Baltimore, 1964); D. Frame, *Montaigne* (New York, 1965); P. Burke, *Montaigne* (New York, 1981); and V. Kahn, *Rhetoric, Prudence, and Skepticism in the Renaissance* (Ithaca, N.Y., 1985), chap. 5. I have used the English edition of *The Apology for Raymond Sebond* by M. A. Screech (London and New York, 1987).

the grounds and limits of human belief and knowledge. The work embodies a consistent "system of thought and a unifying political intention that belie its surface appearance of randomness and lack of public concern." [101] The *Apology* recalls the apology of Socrates; in the case of Montaigne, both Christian theology and classical philosophy are again "on trial." Despite his Stoic references in the *Apology* and elsewhere, Montaigne's allegiance is with Pyrrhonism. He advocates freedom to doubt and questions all opinion, excoriates the vanity of the philosophers' pretensions, and upholds the fundamental obscurity of nature. He is also critical of popular religious belief, arguing that God is a figment of the imagination, since human beings possess no knowledge of what lies beyond their world.[102]

But Montaigne's skepticism is fundamentally constructive, as Schaefer demonstrates. Once we are aware of our ignorance, our minds become free in a certain sense. Unlike the Pyrrhonians, who suspended all judgment, Montaigne contended that probable experience constitutes the only reasonable guide for human actions, that controlled experimentation is desirable, and that we should see nature as yielding not truth but utility. When Montaigne parenthetically mentions Copernicus, it is not to prove him right or wrong but only to argue for an open, nondogmatic basis for scientific theorizing. Copernicus suggests for him the possibility that "a third opinion, a thousand years from now will . . . overthrow the preceding two [Ptolemy and Copernicus]." [103]

As Schaefer puts it, Montaigne pays lip service to the older teleological view of nature but ultimately rejects it. When he makes his well-known comparison between humans and animals, he is even satirizing that position. In the end, Montaigne sought to divorce science from metaphysics, and likewise from theology. Despite the weighty skepticism of the essays, his project was a constructive and optimistic one, laying the theoretical and political foundations for scientific advance upon which Descartes and Bacon would build.[104]

Anyone reading Montaigne with this reconstruction in mind cannot miss

101. Schaefer, *Political Philosophy,* p. 39.
102. Ibid., pp. 39–113.
103. Ibid., pp. 115–133; the quotation is on p. 124.
104. Ibid., pp. 131–33.

the similarities to Luzzatto's work.[105] He too is infatuated with the account of Socrates' death and reconstructs a modern version of the *Apology*, putting "on trial" the philosophical pretensions of his age. He refers to Stoic doctrines in the *Discorso* and gives the Stoics a full hearing through the voice of Hippias, but in the end he too is persuaded by the Pyrrhonian arguments. Like Montaigne's, his break with the older teleological view of nature is neither radical nor dramatic. Socrates listens intently to Hippias but is "inclined" to follow Timon, just as Montaigne listens intently to Sebond and his hierarchical view of God and nature, along with the voices of the Stoics, but subtly adopts another view of nature and religious faith in his *Apology*. Luzzatto, like Montaigne, views skepticism as ultimately liberating and constructive rather than debilitating and destructive. Nature is not always harmonious, nor does it always embody the good. On the contrary, it can be chaotic and harmful unless human beings attempt to use and control it for their own benefit. It offers no ultimate guidelines to adapt to the political realm. Only the practicality and resourcefulness of ragione di stato can benefit the ruler. Luzzatto also advocates the course of probability ("the glimmer of the probable") in order to conduct normal human affairs. His interest in the sciences, particularly in the new theories of the universe, suggests an openness to experiment without preconceived notions. He also mentions Copernicus's theory in passing (in describing observations through the telescope) merely as a possibility, another opinion that challenges the orthodoxy of the regnant Ptolemaic view.

Yet there is another possible parallel between the two thinkers that is the most troublesome of all. I have already alluded to the misleading title page; as we have seen, there is no explicit discussion of divine revelation in Luzzatto's tome. Like Montaigne, Luzzatto, through his hero, Socrates, attempts to reassure his readers about his piety and support of public religious observance. According to Schaefer, despite Montaigne's appeal to religiosity and to a conventional fideism, his critique is directly aimed at Christianity and conventional religious faith; in his heart of hearts, he is anti-Christian and antireligious.[106]

---

105. While probably irrelevant, Montaigne's "Jewish" connection comes to mind. On this, see Popkin, *History of Scepticism*, p. 264, n. 48; Schaefer, *Political Philosophy*, pp. 204–8; and, most fully, R. Trinquet, *La Jeunesse de Montaigne* (Paris, 1972), chap. 5.

106. Schaefer, *Political Philosophy*, p. 42.

What can be said about Luzzatto in this regard? Does he use skepticism to embrace faith, as his title page implies, or to denigrate it?

A second look at the last pages of *Socrate* is in order. Timon, we recall, effectively explodes Hippias's claim that his type of philosophizing leads to greater piety. However, when Socrates finally accepts Timon's position, he too is confronted by the challenge of reconciling his philosophic position with his faith. His answer is evasive and hardly reassuring. He admits that the human soul is psychologically attracted to religious and public observance. Thus he can accept legitimate public sacrifice and rites "ordained by the urban magistrates in honor of God," but not the ridiculous beliefs and vain ceremonies of the common men. But he offers no clear definition of legitimate beliefs and ceremonies. And if there is no secure truth but only the "glimmer of the probable," on what basis does one decide? The subject is quickly dropped. Socrates goes free despite the suspicions of the vulgar and the esteem of some but not all the scholars.

Are we to assume that Socrates and Luzzatto are one? In some respects, this seems plausible. Socrates' consistent interest in the sciences and especially in mathematics coincides with the image Luzzatto cut among his Jewish contemporaries and with several explicit statements in the *Discorso* about the positive role of these fields within Jewish culture. His skepticism in *Socrate* has no analogue in the *Discorso,* although the latter explicitly refers to authors on the subject, including Sextus Empiricus and Gianfrancesco Pico della Mirandola. Most importantly, his Pyrrhonian attack on the arrogance of dogmatic philosophy is ultimately constructive in embracing a practical mode of dealing with the fallacies of the senses and the mind and encouraging scientific exploration of the natural world. Such a position could easily have been pushed in the direction of a constructive or mitigated fideism, as in the case of several of his Jewish and Christian contemporaries who denied scholastic philosophy while extolling the physical sciences.[107] It could have been shaped as a kind of Jewish version of Augustinianism, stressing the biblical understanding of creation, God's transcendence, and man's utter dependence on him, as the Maharal and other Jewish

---

107. I discuss the latter position among several contemporary Jewish thinkers in chaps. 6, 7, 9, and 11 below.

thinkers had articulated.[108] Luzzatto might also have spoken about God as David Nieto did, as a universal assumption *(De consensu gentium)* of all the major religions.[109] At the very least, he might have placated his Catholic readers in this regard, but he makes no such gesture.

Bernard Septimus, without the advantage of reading *Socrate,* offered an insightful but necessarily tentative intellectual portrait of Luzzatto, comparing him with Maimonides and Spinoza. Before closing this chapter, we might consider his profile more closely in relation to that emerging from our examination of *Socrate.* Septimus quotes Luzzatto's preface to a Hebrew book extolling the freedom of the human intellect and the decision of man "to consider and explore any subject he desires."[110] He emphasizes the *Discorso*'s repeated concern for legitimate worship of God free of superstition. While he acknowledges the Renaissance background of his thought, Septimus emphasizes Luzzatto's indebtedness to Maimonides. This is especially apparent in the battle he wages against superstition, in his concern with the power of scientific knowledge, and in his demoralized frustration with the decline of Jewish intellectual life in his era. Septimus even suggests that Luzzatto's pointed reference to superstition ("because of the familiarity it presumes to have with the higher causes, [it] frequently has little reservation about abusing men")[111] might easily refer to the mystical messianism of his day. In this respect, he shared the perspective of the older Modena and the younger Frances brothers.[112]

Septimus's portrait to this point correlates quite well with that of *Socrate.* Luzzatto is certainly no Maimonidean in his radical critique of scholastic epistemology. Nevertheless, his elitism, his disdain for the customs and superstitions of the "plebeians" are equally apparent in both his Italian works. But Septimus goes farther in suggesting a somewhat problematic relationship for Luzzatto between rationality and rabbinic tradition. I have already mentioned Luzzatto's

108. On the Augustinian position, see Bouwsma, "Two Faces of Humanism"; on the Maharal's position, see chap. 2 above.

109. See chap. 11 below.

110. Septimus, "Biblical Religion," pp. 399–400, taken from the beginning of Samuel ha-Kohen's commentary to Ecclesiastes and Job entitled *Zofnat Pane'ah* (Venice, 1656), pp. 2a–4b.

111. Quoted by Septimus, "Biblical Religion," p. 415.

112. See chap. 4 above and chap. 7 below

reference to Philo as a Jewish philosopher obliged to teach Gentiles and not Jews, and its possible application to Luzzatto himself.[113] The implication is that for Luzzatto the philosophical tradition has its own authoritative ethical-political teaching, which sometimes diverges from that of Jewish tradition. Septimus finally underscores the strong element of historicist relativism in his overall conception of Jewish law, a posture reminiscent of the author of the contemporaneous *Kol Sakhal* and of the medical writer Tobias Cohen, and perhaps Modena himself.[114] This leads Septimus to summarize Luzzatto's position as "a Jewish jurisprudence and policy informed by the precepts of practical reason and sensitive to changing historical realities."[115] But the new is tempered by the old for Septimus: in Luzzatto, "the new historical awareness and the old Jewish rationalism are still combined."[116] And when compared with Spinoza, whose critique of Jewish historical experience assumes a natural causation lacking divine providence, Luzzatto appears not to have crossed the line. Providence still operated for him, albeit minimally, and his Maimonidean vision remained intact.[117]

Our closer look at *Socrate* suggests the need to modify Septimus's image of a ghetto thinker balanced somewhere between Maimonides and Spinoza. In view of Luzzatto's radical skepticism—surely unprecedented among Jewish thinkers other than those of converso ancestry outside the boundaries of organized Jewish life—it is not so clear how the Maimonidean vision survived intact in the person of Luzzatto, unless one interprets Maimonides as a secret radical dressed in orthodox clothing, in the image suggested by Leo Strauss.[118] Skepticism by the seventeenth century was a potent force for either a constructive

113. See n. 4 above.

114. Septimus, "Biblical Religion," pp. 419–20, esp. n. 97, where he cites *Ma'amar*, p. 143. On Tobias's similar position, see chap. 8 below. On Modena's historicism, see B. Safran, "Leone da Modena's Historical Thinking," Twersky and Septimus, *Jewish Thought in the Seventeenth Century*, pp. 381–98.

115. Septimus, "Biblical Religion," p. 421.

116. Ibid., p. 428.

117. Ibid., pp. 429–31.

118. See, for example, L. Strauss, "How to Begin to Study *The Guide of the Perplexed*," in Moses Maimonides, *The Guide of the Perplexed*, trans. S. Pines (Chicago, 1963), pp. xi–lvi.

or destructive theology. Ultimately, skepticism could be redirected from targeting scholastic philosophy to targeting established religious faith and praxis, as happened covertly in the case of Montaigne and quite openly in the cases of La Peyrère and Spinoza. Was Luzzatto's grand omission of seriously treating revelation in *Socrate* an attempt to portray Socrates in the most accurate fashion, or an admission that revelation is neither demonstrable nor worthy of serious intellectual discourse? The inclusion of the doctrine in the title and its exclusion from the text suggest Luzzatto's ambivalence about treating it. Socrates' qualified acceptance of rites ordained by the urban magistrates (that is, the halakha?) and his rejection of scornful concepts that deface the true religion (the kabbalah?) also suggest the author's ambivalence. In view of the radical potential of *Socrate*'s critique when transferred from the forum of ancient Athens to the Jewish ghetto and rabbinate of seventeenth-century Venice, one might more accurately characterize Luzzatto's stance as a foreshadowing of the lens-grinder of Rijnsburg than as an afterglow of the sage of Fustat.

6

Between High and Low Cultures

ECHOES OF THE NEW SCIENCE IN THE WRITINGS OF

JUDAH DEL BENE AND AZARIAH FIGO

The assumption that rabbis Judah Assael del Bene (1615?–1678) of Ferrara and Azariah Figo (1579–1647) of Pisa and Venice were allies in promoting the study of the sciences and in appreciating the natural world might appear ludicrous at first blush. Until recently, the only scholar to make an in-depth comparative study of their writings focused on their severe criticism of rationalism. Isaac Barzilay, writing in 1967, understood "the uncompromising and negative attitudes of Figo and del Bene . . . against the growing *éloignement* between Christians and Jews, and the increasing hopelessness and despair among Italian Jews which had set in since the days of the Counter-Reformation."[1] Such staunch defenders of the faith, seemingly fixed in the traditionalist camp, would not appear to have flirted with the sciences at all. Neither was reputed for his scientific acumen; neither was known to have formally studied at a university level;[2] and neither devoted any of his writing to any scientific subject per se. Figo's major book, a collection of sermons entitled *Binah le-Ittim,* was published in Venice in 1648, while del Bene published his learned book of essays, the *Kissot le-Veit David,* two years earlier in Verona.

1. I. E. Barzilay, *Between Reason and Faith: Anti-Rationalism in Italian Jewish Thought, 1250–1650* (The Hague and Paris, 1967), p. 15.

2. I do suggest below, however, the possibility that Figo formally studied medicine.

There is no evidence to suggest that del Bene and Figo knew each other. Whatever their relationship, Barzilay was correct in viewing them as ideologically related, albeit for the wrong reasons. In actuality, Figo saw himself as a faithful student of Leone Modena. Del Bene may have been influenced by the apologetic writing of Modena, Azariah de' Rossi, and Simone Luzzatto; at the very least, he appears to identify with their general pro-Catholic orientation.[3] Moreover, neither man displays any interest whatsoever in the kabbalah and its sources—a position very much against the grain of their contemporary Jewish culture and apparently consonant with the ideology of Modena and Luzzatto.[4] Finally, although Figo and del Bene defend the Jewish faith against the corrosive influences of philosophical speculation, both remain open and even enthusiastic about scientific discovery. Despite their lack of scientific expertise, both display a keen awareness of the dramatic revelations of nature in their day and of the potential these revelations offered to human creativity and progress. For both men, such a recognition represented an exciting resource for bolstering Jewish faith in God and divine providence. Both convey their religious message in language informed by a new intellectual style characteristic of religious thinkers of the seventeenth century, both Jewish and Christian.

As Jewish leaders displaying no specialized training in the natural sciences, del Bene and Figo allow us to move beyond the elite circles of Jewish physicians and their students in assessing the impact of science and medicine on the larger Jewish community. But Figo offers us more in this respect than del Bene. Del Bene's composition was not written for a wide readership; it is esoteric in both style and content; and it is unambiguously a product of elite culture, albeit not a scientific one. Figo had a larger constituency in mind. A gifted preacher, he allows us a glimpse beyond the intellectual leadership to a congregation that supposedly absorbed and appreciated his message. From the perspective of their respective audiences, the two books are thus considerably different.[5] But be-

3. The evidence for Figo's relation with Modena is discussed below. The possibility that del Bene was influenced by Figo and Modena is suggested by Barzilay, *Between Faith and Reason*, pp. 213–14.

4. See chap. 4 above.

5. Robert Bonfil has discovered several sermons of del Bene which he compares with *Kissot le-Veit David*. See R. Bonfil, "Preaching as Mediation between Elite and Popular Cultures: The

cause of their common agenda, they offer a useful indicator of the awareness of and interest in the sciences across a relatively broad spectrum of the Italian Jewish community.

Joseph Sermoneta and Robert Bonfil have recently explored different aspects of del Bene's scholarly writing from a perspective quite different from that of Barzilay.[6] Whereas Barzilay concluded that del Bene's "style was awkward, his composition confused, and his work a clear indication of cultural decline,"[7] Sermoneta and Bonfil have underscored its complex baroque style, its radical break with medieval preconceptions, and its remarkably modern intellectual agenda. My sympathies clearly lie with the latter appraisal, and what follows is indebted to Bonfil's incisive portrait.

The real significance of del Bene's work lies in his rethinking of Jewish-Christian relations, his antagonism to Islam, and his total identification with Catholic spiritual and political ideals. His interest in the natural world is only a secondary theme of the book and, to a considerable extent, a natural byproduct and extension of his religious-political loyalties. Nevertheless, because this concern emerges in a context ostensibly unrelated to nature and the sciences, it is all the more interesting. It demonstrates how a Jewish religious thinker, in defending traditional ideals, could find in scientific observation and discovery a useful auxiliary and support. Moreover, it reveals how the new accessory of nature study subtly transformed traditional thinking into a new configuration that some might even label as "modern."

The key to understanding del Bene's new orientation, as Bonfil has pointed out, is his appreciation of Socrates and his disciple Plato, and his strong hos-

---

Case of Judah del Bene," in D. B. Ruderman, ed., *Preachers of the Italian Ghetto* (Berkeley and Los Angeles, 1992), pp. 67–88.

6. Barzilay, *Between Faith and Reason,* pp. 210–17; G. Sermoneta, "Aspetti del pensiero nell'ebraismo italiano tra Rinascimento e età barocca," *Italia Judaica,* vol. 2 (Rome, 1986), pp. 17–35; Bonfil, "Preaching as Mediation." On Judah's father, David, see D. Kaufmann, "The Dispute about the Sermons of David del Bene of Mantua," *Jewish Quarterly Review,* o.s. 8 (1896): 413–24. According to Bonfil, "Preaching as Mediation," p. 86, n. 86, Dr. Ariel Rathaus is preparing a study of del Bene's literary theory.

7. Barzilay, *Between Faith and Reason,* p. 210.

tility to Aristotle and his followers, whom he repeatedly labels "simple phi-losophers."[8] Socrates is mentioned in *Kissot le-Veit David* on three occasions. The first follows a long critique of the "simple philosophers who utilize the same methods by which they investigate nature in their investigations of the Divinity."[9] Furthermore, they question the reality of the first prophets and they deny all that follows from them—the Holy Scriptures.[10] In this respect, del Bene singles out "the head of the philosophers [Aristotle], who is mistaken without limit and restraint in everything he touches regarding the pipeline of the divine Torah and Moses, his servant."[11]

However, del Bene immediately makes it clear that all pagan philosophers, even atheists, are not necessarily pernicious to Jewish faith. His first example is Cornelius Tacitus, "who is honored by them [the Christians] more than any other ancient writer because he speaks the truth regarding the administration of government."[12] One can profitably read his works without absorbing his alien beliefs. In contrast, "the snares and vain syllogisms" regarding the divine realm of the false philosophers are to be avoided.[13] Del Bene's second example is Soc-rates, "who judged correctly that we have no knowledge and understanding of many of the investigations that entail the holy things of heaven."[14] Although Socrates was the teacher of Plato, who was the teacher of Aristotle, the latter did not follow Socrates, who declared "that every science and study has a boundary and a limit to which a person can reach but cannot surpass."[15]

The distinction between good and bad philosophers, then, is critical for del

8. Bonfil, "Preaching as Mediation," pp. 77–79. He explains the possible connotations of the term *pilosof pashut* as referring to Simplicius, Aristotle's commentator, or to the nickname of Galileo's interlocutor in his *Dialoghi dei massimi sistemi.* On del Bene's association of this term with black magic, see Bonfil, "Preaching as Mediation," p. 79, n. 32.

9. *Kissot le-Veit David,* 1:4, p. 10b.

10. Ibid.

11. Ibid.

12. Ibid. On Tacitus in Luzzatto's thought, see A. Melamed, "Simone Luzzatto on Tacitus: Apologetica and Ragione di Stato," in *Studies in Medieval Jewish History and Literarue,* ed. I. Twersky (Cambridge, Mass., 1984).

13. *Kissot le-Veit David,* 1:4, p. 11a.

14. Ibid.

15. Ibid.

Bene. Socrates and Tacitus were capable of observing the limits; both philoso-phized within the natural order of human society. Aristotle and the "simple philosophers" appropriated the methods of studying the material world for studying the divine. The results were not only wrong; they served to undermine the truths of the established religion of the prophets, of even the Bible itself. Del Bène ends the chapter by quoting Judah Ha-Levi's derision of the Aristo-telians of his day who clung to the "Active Intellect" deficient in the blessings of the Torah.[16]

In a later chapter, del Bene refers again to Socrates, claiming that although he did not understand the divine knowledge of the people, he would never deny its veracity.[17] In contrast, Aristotle—"the wise man in his own eyes"—denied it, declaring falsely that "God does nothing except reveal his secret to the one who philosophizes."[18] In light of this contrast, del Bene reaffirms his belief in the distinction between divine and naturalistic studies, quotes the sixteenth-century rabbi and exegete Eliezer Ashkenazi that creation ex nihilo can only be under-stood by the faithful, and blames Aristotle for encouraging perfidious notions of the world's eternity stemming from the inadequacy of his human investiga-tions.[19] Elsewhere, del Bene mentions Socrates and his sin against the pagan deities, but only to underscore his teaching relationship with Plato. Plato's good name was thus established through his connection with his distinguished teacher.[20]

Bonfil has correctly emphasized the bald contrast between Aristotle on the one hand and Socrates and Plato on the other: "The official culture granted to Aristotle the seal of approval associated with learned, illuminated, and sound analytical rationalism, in contrast with popular, obscurantist, mythological thought associated with Plato. . . . For avant-garde anticonformists . . . Aristotle would, of course, represent the tyranny of authority over reason . . . Plato would symbolize fertility of imagination, creative stimulus leading to an illuminating

16. Ibid., p. 12b.
17. *Kissot le-Veit David,* 1:8, p. 19b.
18. Ibid.
19. Ibid., pp. 19b–20a.
20. *Kissot le-Veit David,* 2:12, p. 33a.

free use of freedom."[21] Bonfil adds that Socrates better fit the latter image than Plato; thus he "became a hero for some in Del Bene's time."[22]

For Luzzatto, as we have seen, the avant-garde image of Socrates and Plato as liberators of human knowledge from the servitude of Aristotelian metaphysics fits quite well. And, to a certain extent, this holds true for del Bene as well. Both del Bene and Plato openly excoriate the "head of the philosophers" and extol Socrates for his efforts to concentrate on human society *(prudenza)* rather than on the unattainable questions of the universe, beyond which the mind cannot fathom with any certainty. Del Bene's approval of Tacitus is also analogous to that of Luzzatto. Luzzatto's attempt to respond to Tacitus's slanderous accusations against the Jewish people emerges out of the high esteem in which Tacticus was held among the political theorists of ragione di stato.[23] Luzzatto would have agreed wholeheartedly with del Bene's positive evaluation of the ancient theorist in general, his misrepresentations of the Jews notwithstanding.

Although del Bene and Luzzatto are similar in praising Socrates and Tacitus while criticizing Aristotle, there remains a critical difference in their approaches. Luzzatto's Socrates, as we have seen, ultimately follows the path of Timon, a complete skepticism regarding all human knowledge in both the material and divine realms. He is able to function in human society only because he repudiates the human claim to know anything with certainty in favor of the practical "glimmer of the probable." Regarding religious observance and ritual, he grudgingly grants his approval, as long as it remains unpolluted by the superstitious fantasies of popular religion.

One can detect in del Bene a strong tinge of that same skepticism about the security of human knowledge. Like Luzzatto, he acknowledges the fallibility of the senses,[24] the human incapacity to distinguish clearly an illusion from the real thing. Also like Luzzatto, he points out the limits of human investigation and the continual disagreements over what philosophers actually know.[25] As Luzzatto had described the wide spectrum of opinions regarding the origin of the

21. Bonfil, "Preaching as Mediation," pp. 77–78.
22. Ibid., p. 78.
23. This point is made well by Melamed in "Simone Luzzatto on Tacitus," esp. pp. 145–52.
24. *Kissot le-Veit David,* 1:2, p. 9a; 3:19, p. 46a.
25. Ibid., 1:7, p. 18b.

universe as well as theories of knowledge, del Bene elaborates on the manifold theories of the soul as articulated by the ancients from Empedocles to Pythagoras, Plato, and Aristotle.[26] Perhaps in the context of his skeptical tendencies, we should understand the interesting statement of del Bene that "the science of nature is a craft, not a science"[27]—that is, an acknowledgment that all we know is tentative and uncertain. Complete knowledge, the ultimate goal of true science, is unattainable to our senses and intellect.

Del Bene's Socrates, however, ultimately cannot dwell in "the glimmer of the probable," as Luzzatto's does. He requires the assurance of a secure faith in God and in his revelation. His skepticism is never an end in itself but a means for underscoring the need for divine sapience and for deriding those who claim that their own rationality is sufficient. In fact, del Bene's brief references to Socrates do not emphasize his skeptical probings at all. On the contrary, Socrates is complimented for not allowing his human speculations to contradict divine truth, for appreciating the boundaries of human knowledge so as to define explicitly the legitimate space in which faith is to function. Del Bene's Socrates liberates men from the authority of reason in order to subjugate them to the dictates of faith. Unlike Luzzatto's, his skepticism leads inevitably to a conventional fideism.[28] The destructive skepticism implicit in Luzzatto's Socrates, challenging all knowledge and all belief, is bridled by del Bene. Ultimately, Aristotle and pretentious human knowledge are challenged so as to elevate and protect the unassailable truths of traditional faith.

Within the boundaries of the permissible and the forbidden, human investigations of the natural world have their rightful and appropriate place. Quoting Maimonides and Isserles, del Bene distinguishes clearly between the licit investigation of physics and the inadmissible study of metaphysics.[29] Thus, he writes: "A Jew who has within him the spirit of God will desert that science which

26. Ibid., 3:19, p. 45b.

27. Ibid., 1:1, p. 6a; also cited by Bonfil, "Preaching as Mediation," p. 79. The statement underscores the practical aspect of understanding the usefulness of nature and its economic benefit for humankind.

28. R. Popkin, *The History of Scepticism from Erasmus to Spinoza*, 2d ed. (Berkeley, 1979), calls this position "a mitigated scepticism." See the discussion of Figo below.

29. *Kissot le-Veit David,* 3:19, pp. 45a–45b.

is not his inheritance."[30] But the observation of the lower world is acceptable and even enhances one's faith in God and in his creation out of nothing. The study of the processes of nature, like the remarkable limits between the sea and the land, testify to God's design and providence.[31] While Luzzatto might have underscored the irregularity and chaos of nature, its independent and unpredictable manner, del Bene stresses "the boundary of the sea, an eternal law never broken" which evokes wonder and exaltation, "songs and praises to God, thanksgiving to the master of wonders!"[32]

I might add parenthetically that del Bene's reference to Moses Isserles on the study of nature should be seen in the context of a later chapter of his book, where he praises the Ashkenazim for their sharp intellects while pointing out their limitations regarding rhetorical style and grammar. He mentions one exception: the talented preacher of Prague, Ephraim of Lunshitz.[33] That del Bene would refer to this student of the Maharal's, and earlier to his close colleague, Isserles, suggests that he too knew the Maharal's writings directly—particularly his demarcation of the boundaries of natural and divine study, which surely approximated del Bene's approach.[34]

When nature can be seen to yield the proper religious message, del Bene encourages its study and exploration. For him, the proper message is the notion of divine creation out of nothing. He returns to this theme more than any other, even when it appears forced and out of context.[35] He berates the ancient philosophers who tried "to bring the creation of the world closer to nature" by denying its unique and divine nature.[36] He appeals to the testimony of all monotheistic faiths that accept God's existence, ability, providence, and creation out of nothing. Only a small remnant of ancient or modern heretics might deny these assumptions.[37] Elsewhere, unlike Luzzatto, del Bene stresses that creation

30. Ibid., p. 46a.

31. Ibid., p. 46a. Cf. 5:32.

32. Ibid., pp. 46a–46b.

33. *Kissot le-Veit David,* 8:50, pp. 94b–95a.

34. See chap. 2 above.

35. He highlights the theme of creation in the introduction to the work (p. 6b). It is also the primary focus of chaps. 1:1, 1:2, 1:7, 3:16, 5:32, and 7:43.

36. *Kissot le-Veit David,* 1:1, p. 5a.

37. Ibid., p. 6a.

is the act of a purposeful God, not of an autonomous nature. The incompatibility of the four elements illustrates this point: "The law of nature does not deal with contraries but with similar parts that relate and approach each other. God's intelligence is unlike man's, since He knows how to overturn His division and to do as He pleases."[38] Nature acknowledges that "He is God to whom I am a student and of whom He is my teacher. . . for He carefully determines and contracts the boundaries and regions of the world's creation and [issues] its orders and not me."[39] Miracles are part and parcel of the natural order, since they emerge from God who intervenes in nature. God "acts as is his custom to make great miracles."[40] Citing Baḥya ibn Pakuda and Galen, del Bene concludes that human observation of the dynamic relations of the elements instills the proper religious attitude.[41]

There is little evidence of any technical mastery of the sciences in *Kissot le-Veit David*. The examples of natural processes are, for the most part, conventional and unspectacular. Del Bene still refers to the earth as the center of the universe and describes the sun's course, despite his knowledge of the heliocentric universe described in Delmedigo's *Sefer Elim,* which he cites.[42] He descants on the natives discovered in far-off lands,[43] on the usefulness of speculative astrology as opposed to the deterministic judicial variety,[44] on atoms and elements,[45] and on sea currents and land barriers.[46]

Del Bene's two most unusual chapters that touch on the study of nature, albeit indirectly, appear to be based on first-hand experience. The first is his remarkable description of the monastic life of Catholic clergy, who, unburdened by economic insecurity and family responsibility, can devote themselves exclusively to spiritual and cultural matters.[47] The participant in the collective life

38. *Kissot le-Veit David,* 1:7, p. 14b; see also 1:2, p. 8a.

39. Ibid., p. 17a.

40. Ibid., p. 17b.

41. Ibid., p. 18a. On Baḥya, see chap. 1 above.

42. *Kissot le-Veit David,* 3:16, pp. 41b–42b.

43. *Kissot le-Veit David,* 3:17, p. 42b.

44. Ibid., pp. 42b–43a.

45. *Kissot le-Veit David,* 3:19, p. 45b; 1:2, p. 9a; 1:7, pp. 14b–17b.

46. *Kissot le-Veit David,* 5:32.

47. *Kissot le-Veit David,* 7:42.

of the monastery "has time day and night to prolong his study in comfort and contentment while his books are open before him, since they belong to the entire fellowship."[48] Moreover, such a community honors and rewards those who devote themselves to the life of the mind, and thus "one should not be surprised by their predominance in the scholarly disciplines and sciences and by their achievements, by which they are praised."[49]

There is clearly a bitter note of jealousy in del Bene's account of the advantages these Christian scholars have over their Jewish counterparts: "In contrast [to them], one must surely wonder how the poverty and lowliness of the conditions of exile of a nation far and remote [see Is. 18:2.7] left us with any memory of Torah wisdom whatsoever, a twig from the stock [see Is. 11:1] of any science or wisdom for our ancestors and us."[50] Bereft of leisure and economic security and burdened with excessive taxes and penalties, Jews were seldom able to read books, let alone write them.[51] Del Bene's excursus on the sociology of knowledge should be seen in the context of other contemporary Jewish testimonies on the decline of Jewish culture in comparison with that of the Christians, such as those of Luzzatto, Modena, Delmedigo, and Cohen.[52] What distinguishes del Bene's lament is his profound understanding of the relationship between material well-being and cultural creativity; his realization that, lacking the optimal conditions for creativity afforded Christian clerics, Jewish scholars cannot hope to compete with them. Given the advantages of monastic life, Christian scholars produce scholarship—both religious and secular—under the proper conditions of detachment and tranquility, within an environment rich in libraries and colleagues.

In the next chapter del Bene appears to return to his familiar theme of creation, this time, however, with an unusual twist.[53] He launches into an elaborate and detailed account of seafaring in his day and of the extraordinary risks incurred by sailors, along with the obvious economic and political benefits oceanic

48. Ibid., p. 79a.
49. Ibid.
50. Ibid.
51. Ibid.
52. See chaps. 4 and 5 above and chap. 8 below.
53. *Kissot le-Veit David,* 7:43.

voyages entail. He speaks with considerable familiarity about the dangers of navigation: boats adrift in the midst of the sea, water and wind currents, storms and pirates. That men accept all these dangers to sail the seas and thus benefit European civilization in untold ways must be seen as an act of divine providence and beneficence. Seafaring has miraculously opened up international markets, whereby "all parts of society benefit each other, and what is deficient God provides, so that each person receives the fruit of another land by which he gains from two tables—from his own and from one readied by an associate of a people of his choosing."[54] Del Bene then provides an inventory of exotic products that have entered the European market through the sea trade.[55]

Besides the economic benefit, there is also a spiritual one for him. By the new connections opened up through sea travel, the truths of "our holy Torah" are publicized throughout the world. He is aware that the Catholic missionaries spreading the gospel are not teaching the Jewish faith, but he does not quibble about this distinction: "Even if they also do not observe the words of this Torah as we do today, nevertheless, they still believe that it is the Torah from heaven that was given at Sinai by Moses. . . . For it was God's holy will to awaken a spirit of men of very good virtues, masters of a language spoken according to the Torah today who are called Christian to spread out afar a fence to those distant islands and to succeed in their purpose."[56]

The discovery of the new worlds, the exploitation of the new markets, and the success of the new missions are among "the miracles of the science of nature."[57] While hunters and fishermen take precautions to protect themselves from harm, the seafarers, rich or poor, take to the ships to stimulate and advance their civilization. There is no rational explanation for this behavior, del Bene contends, except for divine intervention that propels them, that stimulates their faith in a universal world where there will be "one nation and one shepherd for everyone, a faith by which we and our loved ones are judged alike. Thus we believe and thus we agree that it will come about in the end of days."[58]

54. Ibid., p. 80a.
55. Ibid., p. 80b.
56. Ibid., p. 81a.
57. Ibid., p. 82a.
58. Ibid., p. 82b.

Sermoneta and Bonfil have noted the extraordinary lengths to which del Bene goes in identifying with the spiritual and political aspirations of his Catholic benefactors. His ugly portrait of the Ottoman Turks, the enemies of the Venetian republic during the prolonged battle over Crete, and his loyalty to the Catholic government in which he resides are unparalleled in contemporaneous Jewish literature. Luzzatto's conventional flattery of the Doge and his support for the Venetian war effort in the opening of *Socrate* pales in comparison to del Bene's gushing enthusiasm. This is more than simple political strategy; it is an authentic expression of the internalization of Catholic attitudes by a seventeenth-century Jewish writer who is still proud of his unique heritage and committed to its linguistic and doctrinal purity,[59] but who nevertheless considers his Jewish identity intimately linked to the spiritual and political fate of his Catholic neighbors. He sees their faith as almost identical with the Jewish one; he sees their mission to "the far-off islands" as a form of teaching Torah to the world; he views their enemies as his own; and he is even envious of the way they educate themselves and produce their culture. Bonfil has further noted the parallel between del Bene's mind-set and that of the Jesuits: "In a sense," he writes. "rabbis such as Del Bene accomplished a function within Jewish society similar to that accomplished by Jesuits among Christians. They strove to cope with the inception of modernity and secularism without causing any damage to religious faith. They even acted as vehicles of modernity and secularism within Jewish society."[60]

The above summary of del Bene's chapters on monastic education and on the spiritual mission of the discoveries should dispel any doubt about his "Jesuit" mentality. We might take Bonfil's notion a step further by specifically considering the unique Jesuit commitments to the study of nature and the sciences and their possible applicability to del Bene and to other Jews like him. In recent years, Jesuit science has received considerable scholarly attention.[61] The Jesuits,

59. I refer to del Bene's concern for maintaining standards of Hebraic literacy among Italian Jews in *Kissot le-Veit David,* 2:9.

60. Bonfil, "Preaching as Mediation," p. 84.

61. See esp. W. B. Ashworth, Jr., "Catholicism and Early Modern Science," *God and Nature: Essays on the Encounter between Christianity and Science,* ed. D. C. Lindberg and R. L. Numbers (Berkeley and Los Angeles, 1986), pp. 136–66; R. Feldhay, "Knowledge and Salvation in Jesuit Culture," *Science in Context* 1(1987): 195–213; R. Feldhay and M. Heyd, "The Discourse of

especially in Italy, were the most scientifically oriented group among Catholics but were hardly the most prominent contributors to the scientific revolution. In Rivka Feldhay's words, they offer a context where the new science was diffused and propagated rather than created and advanced.[62] Their significance lay in creating a new discourse, a rhetoric of theological justification, that enabled traditional Catholicism to reformulate its teachings in light of the new sciences. There were also obvious limitations to their scientific pursuits: the constant need to reconcile observation and experiment with a traditional, even mystical metaphysics; their methods of educational control in organizing knowledge; their often indiscriminate eclecticism; and a distrustful reticence on larger theoretical questions. Scholars have offered a number of suggestions as to why the Jesuits were particularly drawn to scientific activity. They include the ideal of apostolic spirituality, which sanctified the values of labor and learning in this world, and the significance attached to experiment and collaboration. These religious values in turn are strikingly parallel to the Puritan ideals of diligence and utility already noticed by students of Protestant science. They also offer interesting parallels to Jewish ideals.

Of course, del Bene's scientific concerns and knowledge are quite limited, especially in relation to those of several of his more erudite contemporaries, such as Delmedigo, Luzzatto, and Tobias Cohen. But even his narrower interest suggests several obvious parallels with the Jesuits. He too viewed nature as a reflection of God's providential design. He, like the Jesuits, saw the new discoveries as divine promise and opportunity to missionize the world. He strongly admired the methods of learning and collegial collaboration of the Jesuit model. Most significantly, he could integrate scientific progress, along with the new economic and political realities, into his own traditional way of thinking.

When one looks beyond del Bene to other Jewish religious thinkers of this era, the parallels with the Jesuit approach abound: a this-world orientation, an esteem for learning, an effort to diffuse and popularize scientific culture, a prac-

---

Pious Science," *Science in Context* 3 (1989): 109–42; and S. Harris, "Transposing the Merton Thesis: Apostolic Spirituality and the Establishment of the Jesuit Scientific Tradition," *Science in Context* 3 (1989): 29–65.

62. Feldhay and Heyd, "The Discourse of Pious Science," p. 110.

ticality and eclecticism eschewing larger theoretical questions, and a preference for unsystematic exposition in the context of biblical commentary. There are obvious differences, chief among them the lack of institutional support, particularly on the university level, to carry out advanced scientific activity in a supportive spiritual environment. As we have seen, the few structures, chiefly among Paduan students, where Jewish and scientific studies could be integrated were hardly comparable to the enormous success and diffusion of the Jesuit colleges. Nevertheless, it is fair to conclude that just as del Bene, Modena, Luzzatto, and countless other Italian Jews admired some of the ideals of the Counter-Reformation Church, particularly those of the Jesuit order, they could similarly identify with doctrines that viewed nature as a cherished source of spirituality and promoted the study of mathematics, the biological, and physical sciences as a vital part of a religious education.

In turning from Judah del Bene's esoteric tome to Azariah Figo's more popular sermons, another kind of question needs to be addressed. No doubt, as we have already seen, the most intense interaction between Judaism and the new sciences was felt primarily by Jewish intellectuals, particularly rabbis and physicians. This situation mirrored that of the Christian community, where science was nurtured essentially by political and church leaders. To what extent, however, were scientific matters the concern of the many within the Jewish community rather than the few? The cultural historian faces a daunting challenge in estimating the wider impact of ideas beyond the elite circles described by the extant sources. A search through expository texts, scientific handbooks, biblical commentaries, and philosophical and kabbalistic writing leaves no doubt that there was a restricted public which was both sufficiently motivated and capable of reading and digesting such esoteric and complex materials. How many Hebrew readers could comprehend the long excurses on mathematics and astronomy in Joseph Delmedigo's *Sefer Elim,* or even the more simplified explanations of the heavens and the earth in David Gans's *Neḥmad ve-Na'im?* Even Tobias Cohen's and Jacob Ẓahalon's handbooks of contemporary medical practice,[63] despite the intentions of the authors, could hardly be called "popular"

---

63. To be considered in chap. 8 below.

compendia in the sense that Dr. Spock's volumes on baby care are today. No evidence suggests that such Hebrew textbooks were to be found in the libraries of many Jewish households.

The voluminous literature of Jewish sermons preached in this era in every community might enable us to identify a wider audience interested in scientific accomplishment. As Marc Saperstein has argued, "for scholars concerned with the development of Jewish thought, sermons containing philosophical or kabbalistic teachings removed from their technical sources and addressed to ordinary congregations provide a crucial means for measuring the impact of ideas not merely on a small circle of original minds but also on a whole community."[64] The central place assigned to questions of scientific import in the sermons of Christian preachers, especially in England, is well known and has allowed historians to draw distinct connections between the practitioners of science and both religious radicals and religious establishments.[65] No such undertaking has ever been attempted with respect to Jewish sermons, a source still relatively untapped by Jewish historians, as Saperstein's discussion makes clear.

Sermons reveal less than one would like to know. The printed sermon is never identical with the oral original. There is little sense of who heard the sermon, how the congregation responded to it, and whether the preacher succeeded in communicating his message.[66] Many printed sermons appear so convoluted and dense that one wonders how they could have been delivered in the first place, let alone understood by a laity, even a highly educated one.[67] And in the case of scientific subjects, what preacher would be moved even to introduce such a topic when exclusively preoccupied with religious and spiritual matters?

64. M. Saperstein, *Jewish Preaching, 1200–1800: An Anthology* (New Haven and London, 1989), p. 1.

65. See, for example, R. S. Westfall, *Science and Religion in Seventeenth-Century England* (New Haven, 1958); M. C. Jacob, *The Newtonians and the English Revolution* (Ithaca, N.Y., 1976); C. Webster, *The Great Instauration: Science, Medicine, and Reform* (London, 1975); and chaps. 11 and 12 below.

66. These issues are discussed by Saperstein in the introduction to *Jewish Preaching*. See also the essays in D. B. Ruderman, ed., *Preachers of the Italian Ghetto* (Berkeley, 1992).

67. This is especially the case for Figo's contemporary, Judah Moscato. See Moshe Idel's judgment on his corpus in his essay in Ruderman, *Preachers of the Italian Ghetto.*

Figo, though renowned as a preacher, was hardly known for his scientific interests or accomplishments. At first glance, he appears to be the most unlikely candidate to teach "science" in the course of his religious homilies. But this is precisely why his sermons are intriguing. If I can make a case for the penetration of scientific attitudes into the domain of his seemingly traditional and even "antirational" teachings, the likelihood of finding other candidates with similar attitudes seems high.

Azariah Figo (or Picho), the rabbi of Pisa and later Venice, is primarily known through his two major printed works: his commentary *Giddulei Terumah* (Venice, 1643), an extensive commentary on the *Sefer ha-Terumot* of Samuel Sardi (1185/ 90–1255/56), the first comprehensive code of Jewish law devoted exclusively to civil and commercial law; and his collection of sermons entitled *Binah le-Ittim,* printed in Venice in 1648, a year after Figo's death, and republished some fifty times.[68]

In recent years, Figo's claim to fame as a preacher (at least the academic kind) has been largely due to the sympathetic portrait painted by Israel Bettan in his classic work on Jewish preachers.[69] Bettan placed Figo in the company of such luminaries as Isaac Arama, Jonathan Eybeshitz, and Figo's contemporary Judah Moscato. But even without Bettan's stamp of approval, Figo undoubtedly commanded the attention of many readers of sermons, especially Jews in eastern Europe. Figo's sermons still evoke interest among traditional Jews, as evidenced by the attractive new edition published in Jerusalem as recently as 1989.[70]

68. A number of Figo's sermons were published in Samuel Aboab's *Devar Shemuel* (Venice, 1702).

69. I. Bettan, *Studies in Jewish Preaching* (Cincinnati, 1939), pp. 227–72.

70. *Sefer Binah le-Ittim* (Jerusalem, 1989), 2 vols. My citations below are from this volume. It is worth noting that among all the Italian preachers of his age, Figo was surely the most popular. While the more colorful and prolific Leone Modena published a single volume of sermons that was never reprinted after his death, Figo's own collection went through some fifty editions. Such extraordinary popularity as a preacher, particularly among eastern European Jews, requires a historical explanation. Part of the answer is obviously related to the elegant simplicity of Figo's style, the relevance of his ethical messages, and his effective affirmation of traditional Jewish concerns. Part of his effectiveness and popularity might also be due to the language of science he adduces in conveying his message. Surely the message resonated

Figo's image as a traditionalist, antirationalist, and renouncer of "Gentile wisdom" is reinforced by Bettan's assessment of him as a man who "violently wrenched himself away from the intellectual pursuits of an earlier day and calmly retreated within the four ells of the law."[71] Bettan's portrait is virtually the same as the earlier descriptions of Abba Apfelbaum and Israel Zinberg.[72] The latter even labeled Figo a typical preacher of the old Franco-German type who wished to know nothing of secular matters. Harry Rabinowicz offered a similar appraisal of Figo's fundamentalist image: "[He] leaned toward a strict interpretation of Jewish law. He opposed the establishment of a theater in the ghetto of Venice and criticized the members of his community for usury, flaunting their wealth, internecine wrangling, laxity in ritual observances, and sexual irregularities."[73] Finally, Isaac Barzilay devotes an entire chapter of his book to Figo, underscoring his critique of rationalism as a danger to Jewish uniqueness and his consciousness of exile and longing for national redemption.[74]

One important piece of information that appears to challenge this standard evaluation of Figo's intellectual leanings is his close relationship to Leone Modena. Figo had composed a sonnet to adorn Modena's Hebrew collection of sermons published in 1602, and Modena had actually listed Figo among his students.[75] Modena had again enlisted him in 1624 to flatter Joseph Ḥamiẓ through his poetry in celebration of Ḥamiẓ's completion of his medical studies.[76] Figo's participation in this event not only suggests his ongoing relationship with Modena but also points to his identification with Modena's long-felt commitment to the study of medicine and the sciences among Italian Jews. That

---

among eastern European congregations of the nineteenth century, as well as among Italian ones of the seventeenth.

71. Bettan, *Studies in Jewish Preaching*, p. 228.

72. A. Apfelbaum, *Rabbi Aʒariah Ficcio [Fichio]* (Drohobycz, 1907); I. Zinberg, *A History of Jewish Literature* (Cincinnati and New York, 1974), 4:175–77

73. H. Rabinowicz, "Figo, Azariah," *Encyclopedia Judaica*, 6:1274. See also his *Portraits of Jewish Preachers* (in Hebrew) (Jerusalem, 1967), pp. 150–58.

74. Barzilay, *Between Reason and Faith*, pp. 192–209.

75. See Apfelbaum, *Rabbi Aʒariah Ficcio*, pp. 87–91.

76. See Leibowitz, *Seridim Mikitvei ha-Pilosof ha-Rofe ve-ha-Mekubbal R. Yosef Ḥamiẓ* (Jerusalem, 1938), pp. 50–51; and chap. 3 above.

Figo never refers to the kabbalah in any of his sermons (unlike his contemporary Judah Moscato, but like del Bene) also suggests his tacit agreement with Modena's emphatic criticism of the place of mysticism in Jewish culture.[77] Figo's aversion to the kabbalah also stands in sharp contrast to Joseph Ḥamiẓ's subsequent passionate embrace of it, Modena's disapproval notwithstanding.

The characterizations of Figo's spiritual proclivities mentioned above are based on a reading of Figo's sermons, and especially on his introduction to *Giddulei Terumah*, where he wrote: "I went . . . after the vanity of a love of 'the children of strangers,' secular studies of various kinds. But immediately upon reaching the beginning of the harvests of the time of my adolescence, the Redeemer had compassion on me . . . for the eyes of my ignorance were opened. . . . So I beheld and recognized the shame of my youth, whereby I had made the principal thing unimportant and the unimportant the principal thing. I was exceedingly ashamed that my hands were weakened from the essential words of the Torah, the study of the Gemarah and all related to it."[78]

By Figo's own account, then, he had once involved himself in secular pursuits but soon realized their vanity and turned to the exclusive study of rabbinic sources. All of the historians mentioned above plainly accepted Figo's declaration at face value. They apparently never considered that such an acknowledgment may have been no more than a literary device in the sixteenth century and that such a standardized opening made good "political" sense in winning the favor of readers of an original commentary on a relatively unstudied legal text.[79] Both Bettan and Barzilay reluctantly acknowledged traces of Figo's earlier pursuits of the "children of strangers" in his later sermons, and particularly his preoccupation with the essence and method of philosophy vis-à-vis Judaism and his frequent use of medical analogies. Bettan even admitted that

77. On Modena's attitude to the kabbalah, see Moshe Idel, "Differing Conceptions of Kabbalah in the Early Seventeenth Century," *Jewish Thought in the Seventeenth Century,* ed. I. Twersky and B. Septimus (Cambridge, Mass., 1987), pp. 137–200.

78. Azariah Figo, *Sefer Giddulei Terumah* (Zolkiev, 1809), p. 3b.

79. Compare, for example, the introduction to Abraham Portaleone's *Shilte Gibburim* (Mantua, 1612), where he similarly acknowledges and renounces his youthful sins in studying the secular sciences. Yet any reader of his book will readily notice that this renunciation was hardly complete!

Figo's "grand renunciation" of his secular interests was either made too late or was not quite complete enough to affect the essential character of his preaching.[80] Commenting on Bettan's description, Yosef Yerushalmi considered this inner contradiction an "oscillation between attraction and resistance to gentile wisdom" that was also typical of other thinkers of Figo's day.[81]

Yet acknowledging the paradoxical coexistence of attraction and resistance to secular pursuits in the thought of a Jewish preacher is not the same as explaining it. To what degree Figo renounced his intellectual past and retreated into Talmudic studies remains an open question and invites a fresh reading of his sermons. Moreover, it behooves the historian to ask which intellectual pursuits Figo considered legitimate, why he was offended by certain rational involvements while apparently approving of others, and how it is possible to understand Figo as a consistent (as opposed to "oscillating") religious thinker with a clear pedagogic agenda for the Jewish constituency he served. In answering these queries about Figo's thinking through a study of his sermons, one is also offered the rare opportunity to characterize more broadly the mental universe he shared with members of the Sephardic congregation of Venice who listened to and may even have been moved to concur with the message of his skillful homilies.

I begin an examination of Figo's sermons with one delivered in Venice on a Rosh ha-Shanah that happened to fall on the Sabbath. After quoting a midrashic passage about God's raising his voice on the New Year, he opens with the following remark:

> The human being was given intelligence by [God] . . . who endowed him
> with great strength . . . until He filled his heart on numerous occasions with
> the capacity to make artificial inventions analogous to the actions of nature.
> Because of the weakness of matter or the deficiency in its preparation . . . man
> tries to correct and replace it by some discovery or invention drawn from
> his intelligence, to the point where he will not appreciate what is lacking in
> nature. We have indeed noticed weak-eyed persons who, out of a deficiency
> of the matter of their eyes, were unable to see at a distance or [even] close

80. Bettan, *Studies in Jewish Preaching,* p. 230.
81. Y. H. Yerushalmi, *From Spanish Court to Italian Ghetto* (New York, 1971), pp. 373–74.

up and were thus very nearsighted. Yet human intelligence was capable of creating eyeglasses placed on the bridge of the nose which aid in magnifying the strength of vision for each person, depending on what he lacks, either a little or a lot. This was similarly the case for the eyeglass with the hollow reed [the telescope] of Rabban Gamaliel [where it is stated] in chapter 4 of Eruvin: "Whereby as soon as I looked, it was as if we were in the midst of the [Sabbath] boundary."[82]

One wonders what a congregation of worshippers might have thought of so bizarre an opening for a sermon on the first of the high holy days. But Figo must have appreciated the mental universe of his audience, so he chose to begin with something familiar to them. He would introduce his lesson on Jewish religious values by espousing an ideal which he and his congregants apparently shared: that of the human mandate to replicate, intervene in, and improve upon nature. The products of nature often appear deficient or unfinished; they invite human craftsmen and inventors to correct and improve God's handiwork. The examples of eyeglasses and the telescope (which Figo explicitly claims as an originally Jewish invention that long preceded the invention of Galileo) unambiguously place the rabbi's remarks in their seventeenth-century context of scientific invention and discovery, especially in the fields of optics and astronomy. By beginning in such an unconventional manner, Figo undoubtedly assumed that he would gain the attention of his audience more readily than by plunging into a more typical rabbinic discourse.

Figo pauses to illustrate his point about correcting inadequate vision with two illustrative biblical phrases.[83] But then he proceeds to enlarge upon his original insight: "One can draw analogies to other deficiencies like lameness and broken legs. Not only such cases but even that which is lacking from one's intelligence can be repaired, as in the case of enhancing one's memory. One can make an effort to remember things, as is well known from the invention

82. *Binah le-Ittim,* 1:72–73. On the "telescope" of Rabban Gamaliel and Galileo, see D. B. Ruderman, *Kabbalah, Magic, and Science: The Cultural Universe of a Sixteenth-Century Jewish Physician* (Cambridge, Mass., 1988), p. 98. Figo refers to B. T. Eruvin 43b.

83. *Binah le-Ittim,* 1:73.

of spatial memory [memory systems]."[84] He illustrates this invention by reference to Joseph's request to the cupbearer to remember him to Pharoah (Genesis 40:14). According to Figo, Joseph asked him "to engrave the impression in his imagination . . . so that he will conceive and relate the thought of Joseph to that of some well-known object that often occurs to him. By visualizing the object, he will remember Joseph." Of course, the cupbearer "did not employ [the technique] of spatial memory on his behalf. Accordingly, he forgot to mention him to Pharoah."[85]

Where Figo is leading his curious listeners with this unusual slant on the familiar biblical story is now made clear: "It follows that if by natural means related to material things, a person can try to correct his deficiencies by substitutions, by exchanging one thing for another, what might one do regarding spiritual things and with matters related to the perfection of one's soul dependent on the fulfillment of the divine commandments? With the latter example, a person is obliged, in any respect, to make signs and inventions in order not to forget them, as in the case of *ẓiẓit,* about which it is stated: 'And you shall see them and remember.' "[86] If the fringes on the prayer shawl can be perceived as a technique of enhancing memory, the need to create an artificial sign to remember the sound of the shofar on a sabbath day, when it cannot be sounded, might logically follow: "God gave our hearts something to replace the sounds of the shofar on this holy day of Shabbat and Rosh ha-Shanah . . . but the commandment was not completely abolished since the memory evoked by the biblical verses that speak about the shofar . . . is sufficient to cause an impression of replacement exemplifying the commandment of the sounding itself."[87]

Such a strategy of stimulating his listeners to conjure up the memory of the sound of the shofar on a day when they needed to hear it but could not, might be dismissed as a clever rhetorical device if not for the fact that the preacher was taking for granted something that the historian cannot take for granted.

84. Ibid. On memory systems in the sixteenth century, see J. Spense, *The Memory Palace of Matteo Ricchi* (New York, 1987).

85. *Binah le-Ittim,* 1:73.

86. Ibid., 1:73–74.

87. Ibid., 1:75.

What was familiar to and what appealed to his congregation was the notion of human beings gaining mastery over the natural world. Illustrating this notion by reference to the manufacture of eyeglasses and telescopes, to the creation of artificial limbs and memory systems, and finally to *ẓiẓit* and the biblical passages that recall the sound of the shofar, might appear to be a convoluted way of making his point, but to Figo's mind he was teaching his Jewish message by appealing directly to the immediate cultural context of his listeners. He was not teaching contemporary science to his coreligionists; rather, he assumed that this knowledge was a commonplace in their experience of the world. As any wise preacher would do, Figo appropriated that experience to make his point about the religious message of the Jewish holy day. His assumptions about what his congregants knew and liked offer us some sense of the impact that "scientific" modes of thinking were having on rabbi and congregation alike.

Bettan and Barzilay have noted Figo's frequent employment of medical analogies to convey his spiritual message. Barzilay concluded that such references do not warrant the inference of an intimate acquaintance with either science or philosophy; rather, they should be attributed to "the impact of the spirit of the time."[88] Of course, Figo's sermons do reveal a particular spirit or mentality—a scientific one—characteristic of his age. But Figo's preoccupation with the functioning of the body and human illness, in light of his connection with Modena, Ḥamiẓ, and Padua, suggests more: an informal or even formal contact with medical education. Be that as it may, it is apparent that he proudly displayed his medical knowledge and was fond of utilizing it when preaching.

A good example of Figo's utilization of medical analogies is in a sermon delivered on Shabbat Teshuvah (the sabbath falling during the high holy day period). Figo opens by referring to the line in Jeremiah (3:14, 3:22): "Turn back O rebellious children, I will heal your afflictions."[89] The connection between repentance and healing in the verse and in a rabbinic elaboration on it offers Figo the appropriate opportunity to descant on the treatment of a sick patient. Following a conventional Galenic therapy, Figo suggests two approaches to healing a person overtaken by "the evil humor which sickens the body and

88. Barzilay, *Between Faith and Reason,* p. 193.
89. *Binah le-Ittim,* 1:81.

brings a person to the danger of death": either by natural means, "whereby he will fortify himself to fight with his illness and defeat it," or by artificial means, that is, "evacuations and bloodletting and the like." Echoing his point in the sermon described above, he adds: "Thus a person will try by human industry to help nature and to gain what it lacks."[90]

The connection between healing the body and healing the soul is now made explicit: "This evacuation is none other than the essence of repentance that discharges and removes all sin and guilt and crime and restores a person to health." Just as there are two avenues of healing the body, so there are two avenues of repentance: "repentance out of love, whereby the strength of one's intelligence will grow by itself . . . or repentance out of fear, which is truly an external healing."[91]

Although artifical healing is licit, it is inferior to natural healing in at least three ways. First, artifical remedies are uncertain, since the physician can only estimate the proper dosage to be offered the patient. Often he misdiagnoses, evacuating insufficiently or excessively and causing more harm than good. Second, artificial remedies such as bloodletting weaken the body and diminish the patient's strength, for good humors are eliminated along with the evil one. Finally, artificial remedies are usually administered under coercion, often causing pain or other discomfort. In contrast, natural evacuation transpires pleasantly without undue agitation. All three advantages of natural healing correlate with the realm of the spirit. A repentance out of love is always superior to one gained through the fear of chastisements. Like the doctor who misdiagnoses and causes his patient harm, a person might repent solely out of fear of punishment while ignoring the sin which is the principal cause of his moral deficiency. Just as evacuation might cause the elimination of good humors along with the bad, so too the removal of a bad quality by external means might also encourage a person to distance himself from a good quality. Finally, repentance out of love is never accompanied by the stress and inner turmoil that accompany repentance out of fear.[92]

90. Ibid., 1:81–82.
91. Ibid., 1:82.
92. Ibid., 1:84–87.

Figo adds a fourth and most significant advantage of natural over artificial healing: healing that is dependent upon external drugs is usually not totally effective; the bad humor is not completely removed and the illness eventually returns. This is not the case with natural healing, where the body is cured conclusively. The distinction between voluntary repentance and that effectuated under duress can also be correlated in this respect.[93]

In other sermons, Figo similarly favors such comparisons between moral and medical therapy. In one passage, he differentiates between an immoral person who can still repent and one whose condition is hopeless by drawing an analogy between a patient who still feels pain, even excruciating pain, and one whose limb is dead and insensitive to pain, and whose condition is hopeless.[94] In another passage, he enumerates four steps in maintaining a regimen of good health and demonstrates how moral sin can virtually be prevented by the same prescriptions.[95] Once he compares the gradual increase of dosage to a sick patient with the gradual educational process of teaching Torah.[96] He even expresses his uncertainty about whether to make a funeral oration long or short by reference to the analogy of a doctor who finds contradictory symptoms in his patient, making his diagnosis extremely difficult.[97] None of these analogies exhibits highly specialized knowledge of medicine or the biological sciences. They are easy to comprehend, appropriately for the forum in which they were meant to be presented. They do reveal, however, an intimate sense of the practice of medicine, the dilemmas the doctor faces daily, the uncertainty of his cures, and the dangers and inadequacies of standard medical treatment. In sum, they suggest the perspective of a person who fully appreciated the meaningful connection between the medical and rabbinic professions—that is, of a physician who also happened to be a doctor, a common coincidence in the Italian Jewish community that Figo served.

Barzilay has pointed out Figo's constant emphasis on the dangers of rationalism and its corrosiveness to the Jewish community's faith in its unique reve-

93. Ibid., 1:87.
94. Ibid., 1:90–105.
95. Ibid., 1:105–24.
96. *Binah le-Ittim*, 2:16–23.
97. Ibid., 2:388–97.

lation.[98] In a fully conventional way, Figo seeks to demonstrate the inadequacy of human reason in contrast to revealed truth on two counts: it is inaccessible to the majority of people and it lacks moral concern. In the first place, since only the few have the capacity to acquire natural knowledge, a belief in miracles and divine intervention in the natural order is necessary, since miraculous occurrences impress the uninitiated more than the mere uniformity and regularity of nature.[99] In the second place, the Gentile astronomer who searches the heavens does so merely to fulfill the needs of his intellectual appetite, not his moral or spiritual one.[100] For the Jew who masters astronomy, his knowledge leads him to perform divine commandments and to serve his Creator. Such arguments suggest for Barzilay a fundamental antirationalism, which he perceives as part of an emerging mentality of "Jewish nationalism" in the late sixteenth century.[101]

There is no doubt that Figo's utterances reflect an antagonism to philosophical speculation and a deep belief in the superiority of the revealed wisdom of the Jewish sages (though not necessarily kabbalistic ones). But Barzilay's analysis remains deficient in ignoring the language and conceptual underpinnings of Figo's defense of Jewish revelation and in failing to appreciate the scientific context informing his criticisms of philosophy.

Figo's sermon on the second day of Shevuot offers a convincing illustration of the preacher's underlying assumptions.[102] His theme is precisely the difference between the knowledge of the philosophers and the revelatory experience of Sinai. "It is well known," he writes, "that the sciences based on foundations of learning and built on rational assumptions are dangerous and unreliable, since human intelligence is limited, small, and weak." They are liable to error and omission and lack the assurance of complete truth. In contrast, "those things to which the senses and experience testify are truthful; no doubt will arise regarding them or fear of error or false knowledge. . . . Regarding the latter, the sage in Ecclesiastes [7:23] stated: 'All this I tested with wisdom: I thought I could fathom it but it eludes me.'" Figo interprets the line to mean that all that was

98. Barzilay, *Between Faith and Reason,* esp. pp. 195–202.
99. See esp. *Binah le-Ittim,* 1:267–75.
100. Ibid., 2:110–27, esp. 110–14.
101. Barzilay, *Between Faith and Reason,* p. 197.
102. *Binah le-Ittim,* 2:85–94.

acquired 'through experience which I gained through the experiential faculty of knowledge" can be known truthfully. But "theoretical knowledge denuded of sensual knowledge is certainly far from me."[103] The student of seventeenth-century culture will recognize this distinction—between the scholastic philosopher and the natural philosopher and empiricist—as a commonplace which we have already noted in del Bene. One can know the heavens and the earth only by observation and experiment, not by a theoretical construct of their apparent reality in the mind's imagination.

For Figo, the epistemological basis of the new empiricism is equivalent to that of the Torah: "The Divine Wisdom [God] understood that the holy Torah would not be accepted by the Israelite nation on the basis of knowledge stemming from investigation and research . . . but rather with things felt and familiar through seeing and hearing. . . . No man can acquire an idea except by way of the senses. . . . The Torah gives strength and vitality to what the senses acquire."[104]

Figo's argument regarding the superiority of the experiential knowledge of the Torah to the theoretical and inevitably finite knowledge of the philosophers patently echoes Judah Ha-Levi's medieval critique of Spanish Jewish philosophy and that of earlier thinkers.[105] Equally unoriginal is his argument that although the knowledge of the Torah is complete and stands on its own, that of the secular sciences is interdependent: "Someone cannot be an astronomer without prior knowledge of mechanics and mathematics, nor a doctor without prior knowledge of natural philosophy. Nor can a person acquire any knowledge unless he is accustomed to logic. . . . It happens that one [field] justifies and prepares for the other, for without the prior one, the latter would have no reality. But our Torah does not require any other wisdom nor any external knowledge, for everything is in her; she guides and informs herself with her own conclusions, principles, and ideas."[106]

I have quoted at length in order to propose that Figo was more than a

103. Ibid., 2:85.
104. Ibid., 2:85, 88.
105. See, for example, Judah Ha-Levi, *Sefer Ha-Kuzari,* 2:56, 63–66; 3:53, 4:24–25.
106. *Binah le-Ittim,* 2:88.

mere borrower of Ha-Levi's classical antiphilosophical arguments. His description of the interrelatedness of all sciences betrays an unmistakable familiarity with these arguments. He leaves the distinct impression that he knows what it takes to be an astronomer or a physician and that he has studied the fields he enumerates. More important, although he argues for the insufficiency of the sciences, he clearly does not dismiss their validity altogether. What he finds reprehensible is a knowledge lacking empirical foundations, based solely on intellectual constructs, and arrogantly claiming to perceive of reality and of the truth. It is no mere coincidence that the language of "hearing and seeing" of the Torah and the rabbis was also the hallmark of his own era, the rallying cry of Galileo, Bacon, and other virtuosi. I contend that Figo was fully aware of the seventeenth-century associations of this language when he evoked it, and, more important, that the convergence of its traditional and modern meanings resonated unmistakably in the ears of his listeners. By couching his advocacy of Torah learning in the contemporary language of experience and empiricism, he was clinching his argument for the relevance of Judaism in a way Ha-Levi never could have achieved. In Ha-Levi's time, such language was surely perceived as anti-intellectual, fundamentalist, and conservative. To an audience fully attuned to seeing and hearing rather than cogitating, Figo's defense of Judaism must have sounded modern and up-to-date.

A succinct description of Figo's intellectual style based on a correct reading of his sermons would thus emphasize a clear and consistent understanding of the relationship between Judaism and the larger cultural space he inhabited. Figo did not oscillate whimsically between rationalism and irrationalism, between study of the Talmud and of the secular sciences. His sermons, written after his apparent renunciation of the sciences in the introduction to his halakhic commentary, bespeak a man supremely cognizant and confident of his knowledge of medicine and the sciences. They are unmistakably part of his universe of discourse and that of his congregants, and he boldly appropriates their conceptual framework in teaching Judaism. Figo deplored the useless speculations of philosophers of the old scholastic style, and particularly their pretensions to understand the world better than those who placed their trust in divine revelation. But such criticism was not synonymous with antirationalism. For him and those he addressed, the value of empiricism, a firm reliance on the senses, and the human mandate to create and improve upon nature were to be taken for granted.

Figo's position—a kind of "mitigated or constructive scepticism,"[107] which he shared with del Bene, the Maharal, and others—was becoming extremely fashionable among Jews and Christians alike by the middle of the seventeenth century. In the new discourse of pious science as articulated by such luminaries as Mersenne and Gassendi,[108] science was a hypothetical system based on and verified through experience alone. It never claimed to possess absolute truth, but merely to describe the appearance of things, and thus it did not compete with the sacred, indubitable verities of divine revelation. By separating physics from scholastic metaphysics, and by establishing a legitimate "division of labor" between the natural sciences and Judaism, Figo had fashioned a formidable argument by which to defend the legitimacy of Jewish revelation in his day. By skillfully incorporating this argument into the rhetoric of his sermons, he had discovered an effective strategy to project the compelling image of "a wise and discerning people"[109] into the minds and hearts of his discriminating congregation.

107. The term is Richard Popkin's, as discussed in his *History of Scepticism*, chap. 7.

108. Besides Popkin's work, see P. Dear, *Mersenne and the Learning of the Schools* (Ithaca and London, 1988) and L. Sumida Joy, *Gassendi the Atomist: Advocate of History in an Age of Science* (Cambridge, 1987). Cf. R. Bonfil's similar conclusions regarding David del Bene in his "Preaching as Mediation."

109. See Deut. 4:6.

7

Kabbalah, Science, and Christian Polemics

THE DEBATE BETWEEN SAMSON MORPURGO AND

SOLOMON AVIAD SAR SHALOM BASILEA

Well into the first half of the eighteenth century, the issues regarding the place of the kabbalah in Jewish culture, argued so
vigorously by Leone Modena against Joseph Ḥamiẓ and Joseph
Delmedigo a century earlier, continued to evoke acrimonious debate among Jewish intellectuals of the Italian ghettos. As in the
case of Modena's rigorous assault, the matter of the kabbalah was
never considered in isolation but was often interlaced with other
intellectual and social concerns, not the least being the emerging
prominence accorded the study of the sciences, and especially
medicine, within the Jewish community.

In this chapter I will consider another controversy between
two distinguished Italian rabbis and writers of the late seventeenth and early eighteenth centuries, Samson Morpurgo of
Ancona (1681–1740) and Solomon Aviad Sar Shalom Basilea of
Mantua (c. 1680–1749).[1] By examining the complex web of issues

1. On Morpurgo, see E. Morpurgo, *La Famiglia Morpurgo de Gradisca
sull'Isonzo 1585–1885* (Padua, 1909); M. Benayahu, "R. Samson Morpurgo:
Some Information and Sources of His Life" (in Hebrew), *Sinai* 84 (1978–
79): 34–165; idem, *Sefer Eẓ ha-Da'at* of R. Samson Morpurgo" (in Hebrew),
Alei Sefer 6–7 (1978–79): 129–44; idem, "The Polemic of R. Samson Morpurgo with the Priest Benetelli" (in Hebrew), *Alei Sefer* 8 (1979–80): 87–
94. On Basilea, see S. Simonsohn, *History of the Jews in the Duchy of Mantua*
(Jerusalem, 1977), index.

raised by the rabbis' disagreement, their larger social and intellectual contexts, and their common assumptions, I hope not only to locate the role of scientific discourse within their cultural world but also to underscore its symbiotic relationship to other primary expressions of Jewish religious thought: to philosophy, to Jewish-Christian dialogue and debate, to messianic heterodoxy, and especially to kabbalistic theosophy.

At first glance, the disagreement between the rationally inclined Morpurgo and Basilea, "the great eighteenth-century apologist of the authenticity of kabbalistic tradition," as Gershom Scholem once called him,[2] appears to be a case of déjà vu. Once again we appear to be confronted by the rational philosopher crossing swords with the traditional kabbalist over the definition of spirituality in Judaism. In 1704 Morpurgo, a twenty-three-year-old rabbi and recent medical graduate of the University of Padua, published a modest commentary on the popular ethical work *Sefer Beḥinat Olam* (The Book of the Examination of the World) by Jedaiah ben Abraham Bedersi ha-Penimi (c. 1270–1340).[3] Morpurgo's commentary, *Eẓ ha-Da'at* (The Tree of Knowledge), attempted to elucidate this small lyrical treatise on the futility and vanity of the world and on the rewards of the intellectual and religious life. On the surface Bedersi's work seems to contain little to upset even the staunchest traditionalist. It had been published in Italy as early as the late fifteenth century and had been republished frequently, accompanied by a variety of commentaries.[4] Bedersi, of course, was well known as an apologist for Maimonidean philosophy, but only in the last lines of *Sefer Beḥinat Olam* does his allegiance to the sage of Fustat become overt.[5] Most of Bedersi's text commendably nurtures ethical and religious sensibilities.

---

2. G. Scholem, *Sabbatai Ṣevi: The Mystical Messiah* (Princeton, 1973), p. 517.

3. *Sefer Eẓ ha-Da'at* (Venice, 1704); on Bedersi and his writing, see A. Halkin's essay in *Encyclopedia Judaica* (Jerusalem, 1971), 9:1308–10 and the bibliography he cites.

4. The work was first published in Mantua by Estellina, wife of Abraham Conat, between 1476 and 1480. Morpurgo, in his introduction, mentions the commentaries of Moses ibn Ḥabib and Jacob Frances. Other commentators include Yom Tov Lipmann Heller, Isaac Moncon, Jacob (of Fano?), Leone of Mantua, and Immanuel Lattes the Younger. (See I. Broydé, "Bedersi, Jedaiah Ben Abraham," *The Jewish Encyclopedia* (New York and London, 1907), 2:626.)

5. I quote from the English translation of Broydé, "Bedersi," p. 626: "Finally, turn neither to the left nor to the right from all that the wise men believed, the chief of whom was the

Nevertheless, Basilea denounced Morpurgo's work some twenty-six years later in *Sefer Emunat Ḥakhamim* (The faith of [or in] the Sages), published in Mantua in 1730.[6] He was particularly infuriated by Morpurgo's introduction, extolling philosophical investigation in general and in particular the achievements of Abraham ibn Ezra and Maimonides; and by the inclusion in Morpurgo's treatise of a poem by the notorious seventeenth-century Hebrew poet Jacob Frances criticizing the excessive study of the kabbalah by Italian Jews.[7]

The publication of Frances's poem was surely Morpurgo's most provocative gesture in Basilea's eyes.[8] Morpurgo was undoubtedly aware of the controversy his action was bound to stir up among the many devotees of the kabbalah: he published the *Eṣ ha-Da'at* anonymously, although other writers alluded to him by his first name at the end of the work.[9] The brothers Jacob and Emanuel Frances were well known for satirizing the movement surrounding the messianic figure of Shabbatai Ẓevi. Jacob not only opposed the Sabbatian movement but appeared uncompromisingly hostile to all students of the kabbalah, messianic enthusiasts or not. In 1661 he published the satirical poem against the kabbalah which immediately aroused the anger of the Mantuan rabbis, especially the kabbalist Solomon Formigini, who tried to confiscate all copies of the poem. Having evaded the rabbis' recriminations by moving to Florence, Jacob died in 1667—a sure sign of divine justice in the mind of his enemies. Although Emanuel lived until the end of the century, Jacob's death quieted one of the most vociferous voices against the kabbalah in seventeenth-century Italy.[10] In republishing Jacob's obnoxious poem in 1704, Morpurgo must have been aware that he was reviving painful memories among a rabbinic establishment that was committed to the study of the kabbalah cleansed of the antinomian and hereti-

---

distinguished master Maimonides, of blessed memory, with whom no one can be compared from among the wise men who have lived since the close of the Talmud."

6. *Sefer Emunat Ḥakhamim* (Mantua, 1730), pp. 16b, 17a, 22a, 27a, 29b–31b.

7. See esp. ibid., pp. 29b–31b.

8. *Sefer Eṣ ha-Da'at*, pp. 35b–36a.

9. Ibid., pp. 36b, 37a.

10. On the Frances brothers, see G. Scholem, *Sabbatai Ṣevi: The Mystical Messiah* (Princeton, 1973), pp. 516–18; S. Bernstein, *Diwan le-Rabbi Emanuel ben David Frances* (Tel Aviv, 1932); P. Naveh, *Kol Shirei Ya'akov Frances* (Jerusalem, 1969); and see the strong criticism of Naveh's work by E. Fleisher in *Kiryat Sefer* 45 (1969–70): 177–87.

cal tendencies of the previous century. The nasty controversy had long been over, so why not let Jacob Frances's satire remain buried with its author? But Morpurgo went ahead impetuously, so it seemed, and republished the despised poem. Even as late as 1730 Basilea could not forgive Morpurgo for maligning the sacred traditions of Judaism, just as Jacob Frances had done some seventy years earlier.

What then meets the casual eye of the twentieth-century observer is a classic confrontation between a rationalist disciple of the "infidel" Frances and a kabbalist committed to defending the centrality of mysticism within Jewish culture. Yet a closer examination of Morpurgo's composition and Basilea's condemnation reveals certain anomalies. In the first place, there exists the cordial, even friendly relationship between Basilea and Morpurgo, even at the time of Basilea's stinging critique. Basilea opened his condemnation of Morpurgo's work by emphasizing the good character of the author, who "is known as a sage, a fearer of heaven and an expert in the books of the Torah."[11] And throughout his caustic remarks he refrains from mentioning Morpurgo by name. Even more revealing is a legal query that Basilea had addressed to Morpurgo some fifteen years earlier. Despite Morpurgo's "indiscretion" in publishing Bedersi and Frances, Basilea was obviously not averse to consulting Morpurgo as a rabbi and medical specialist on the legality of using a certain medicine for curing heart patients that consisted of wine of questionable religious sanctity.[12]

Furthermore, although Morpurgo had no interest in the kabbalah, he was not hostile to it. In fact, he married the daughter of an illustrious kabbalist of his day, Joseph Fiametta—a fact not overlooked by Basilea, who mentioned Fiametta in his defense of the moral character of the kabbalist leaders of his generation.[13] Morpurgo's good relations with Basilea and Fiametta, despite their seeming adversarial positions, invites comparison with those of several other contemporaries who were supposedly engaged in bitter ideological dispute. Simon Bernstein was surprised to discover a cordial relationship between the kabbalist R. Mahalel Haleluyah, Morpurgo's predecessor in the Ancona rabbinate and an

11. *Sefer Emunat Ḥakhamim*, p. 30a.

12. Samson Morpurgo, *Sefer Shemesh Ẓedakah* (Venice, 1740) on *Yoreh De'ah*, n. 28, pp. 78a–79a.

13. *Sefer Emunat Ḥakhamim*, p. 31a.

acknowledged follower of Shabbatai Zevi, and Jacob Frances, the arch-enemy of the Sabbatians in Italy.[14] Jacob Frances was also on good terms with the kabbalist Moses Zacut, and Emanuel Frances apparently held a positive view of the kabbalah throughout his life.[15] How often the historical evidence conspires against our neat categories of who should be antagonistic to whom and gives the lie to the notion that rationalists and kabbalists usually dislike each other. Even the normally judicious Gershom Scholem categorically proclaimed that Jacob Frances's rationalism was "sufficient explanation for his uncompromising rejection of Sabbatian messianism."[16] Yet were all "rationalists" (a term which Scholem never carefully defined) automatically anti-Sabbatians? And should we automatically call such formidable "rationalists" as physicians Benjamin Mussafia or Benedict de Castro irrational simply because they enthusiastically endorsed Sabbatian messianism?[17] Again we are confronted with seeming paradoxes that require close scrutiny and utmost caution in interpretation.

When we turn to the content of Morpurgo's commentary and Basilea's critique, this conventional wisdom about rationalism and irrationalism is further exploded. To be sure, Basilea would have liked his readers to believe that his position and Morpurgo's were irreconcilable. He enlists the homily of his mentor Moses Zacuto on the distinction between "wise [ḥakham] and "discerning" [navon] as they appear in two biblical passages: Genesis 41:39 and Deuteronomy 4:6. In the first passage describing Pharoah, the adjective "discerning" precedes "wise," while in the second passage, referring to the Jewish people, "wise" precedes "discerning." According to Zacuto, the position of the two words teaches the absolute difference between a Jew and a non-Jew regarding the acquisition of knowledge. The latter "understands why a thing is like this or that, comprehends something from something else, and afterwards from these assumptions, he acquires knowledge; and if the assumptions are true, then the inferences [based on these assumptions] will be true. But for the children of Israel, all their wisdom is received from tradition, and from the latter they comprehend some-

14. See S. Bernstein, "The Letters of Rabbi Mahalel Halelujah of Ancona," *Hebrew Union College Annual* 7 (1930): 513.

15. Naveh, *Kol Shirei,* p. 34; Bernstein, *Diwan,* pp. xxiv–xxviii.

16. Scholem, *Sabbatai Ṣevi,* p. 517.

17. On Benedict de Castro, see chap. 10 below.

thing from something else . . . for 'wisdom' *[ḥokhmah]* is what a person learns from his teacher, and 'discernment' *[binah]* is what he understands by himself." In Basilea's view, this fundamental difference explains the fallibility of "Gentile" wisdom in contrast to that of the Jewish kabbalistic tradition. Because the Gentile philosophers relied exclusively on their own intellectual resources, their rational assumptions were eventually proven wrong. Hence by the time of Morpurgo and Basilea, all of Aristotle's pronouncements about the universe have been rejected, contemporary philosophers "have completely denied" his entire cognitive system, and philosophy in these times "has become something else never anticipated by Aristotle in the first place." Thus to resurrect Bedersi's outmoded philosophical ruminations for a present generation of Hebrew readers, and to extol the flawed insights of such students of the discredited Aristotle as Maimonides and ibn Ezra, as Morpurgo had seemingly done, was to ignore a fundamental existential reality of the eighteenth century, according to Basilea.[18]

Basilea's persuasive rhetoric notwithstanding, Zacuto's stark contrast between wise kabbalists and discerning philosophers did not faithfully represent the positions of Morpurgo or Basilea at all, as the latter well knew. In reality, Morpurgo's "philosophy" showed little appreciation for Aristotelian metaphysics and Basilea's kabbalah was hardly reducible to the mere transmission of a sanctified tradition. When one identifies their real positions, it is the remarkable confluence of their views that is striking.

Let us examine more carefully the intellectual posture of Samson Morpurgo. What was the nature of his "rationalism" and how would he have defined himself in relation to his philosophic forebears—Aristotle, Maimonides, and Bedersi? From the opening of his introduction, it is clear that he seeks to locate a median between the excesses of philosophic speculation that have led to heresy, and a Jewish intellectual life absorbed in mystical theosophy. He excoriates those "evil and sinning men" among the philosophers who have deviated from traditional beliefs.[19] Yet he is unwilling to discard the baby with the bathwater; there remains a tradition of honest and faithful philosophical speculation in Israel

18. *Sefer Emunat Ḥakhamim*, pp. 30a–30b.
19. *Eẓ ha-Da'at*, pp. 3a–3b.

exemplified by Maimonides and ibn Ezra. And it is that tradition he seeks to defend and perpetuate. "If the divine kabbalah is precious, so too is philosophy," he contends.[20] He has no objection to the kabbalah per se, despite his inclusion of Frances's satire; he merely pleads for coexistence for both streams of Jewish spirituality.

Morpurgo also has in mind a particular emphasis in espousing the virtues of the philosophical quest. His primary concern, from the beginning to the end of his work, is "natural philosophy"—exploring the secrets of the natural world, the wonders of the heavens and the earth. He writes:

> In every direction man turns, he will comprehend and be enlightened with wisdom, understanding, and intelligence. . . . If he turns his face to the west to see the sun setting in its majesty . . . he will understand the secrets of wisdom. If he gazes to the sky to count the stars and to know the laws of heaven and their constellations, he will . . . be made wise in everything. If he looks in the depths of sheol to fathom what is in the water under the earth . . . even there his eyes will observe that the ordinances of God are just. . . . In everything where [God's] spirit dwells, man will go until his intelligence and the spirit of his discernment will carry him easily among all creatures above and below, from one extremity to the other, so that from everything, he will learn intelligence and acquire understanding.[21]

Morpurgo also refers specifically to the quality of discernment, approaching the definition Moses Zacuto had used but giving it a more focused meaning in relation to investigating the physical world: "A discerning heart *[lev navon]*", Morpurgo writes, "has no limit to its movements by which a person may wander the way of the earth to its length and breadth. For he loves and desires to investigate and trace the roots of his existence whence he was hewn."[22] For Morpurgo, such an ideal investigation is the one he plans and enthusiastically shares with the readers of his introduction: a treatise on the laws of ritual purity of beef and fowl based on the science of surgery and medicine.[23] It is also ex-

20. Ibid., p. 3a.
21. Ibid., p. 5b, commenting on Bedersi's text, chap. 2, pt. 1.
22. Ibid., p. 5a.
23. Ibid., p. 3b.

emplified by his learned responsum to R. Joseph Cases, another physician from Mantua, in 1716, on feeding an ill person snake meat. His learned analysis of the various types of medical remedies, including that of serpent meat, according to the views of the "ancient doctors" as well as the "modern doctors," is based throughout on a thorough empiricism.[24]

Morpurgo's naturalism reflects a commitment to the new sciences of his day and stands in direct opposition to the dogmatic metaphysics of Aristotle and his commentators. In a striking departure from his previous reverence for Maimonides, he openly disputes Bedersi, who had called for full adherence to all of the philosopher's positions. Morpurgo would countenance his views on religious law but nothing more. A new generation of researchers of nature had emphatically rejected Maimonides' notion of the Active Intellect based on Aristotle, of formless matter, of forms and accidents, of the four elements and the fifth essence, and of heavenly motion, as well as his medical know-how.[25] For Basilea, Morpurgo's negation of Maimonides' philosophical assumptions was sufficient proof ("as a hundred witnesses") of the emptiness of all philosophical investigation.[26] But he had surely missed Morpurgo's point. The specific answers that philosophers provided were not at issue. Each generation investigates nature through its own devices and discloses something its predecessors missed. What was critical was the search itself, the process of disclosure, the commitment to using one's discernment to penetrate the divine mystery as deeply as possible. For Morpurgo, self-discovery was surely of greater value than mere acceptance of revealed truth.

If Morpurgo's empiricism informs his philosophical commitments, a similar empiricism informs Basilea's kabbalistic commitments A short Latin compendium on the rules of geographical measurements strangely appended to Basilea's Hebrew defense of the kabbalah is as good a sign as any of his passionate interest in the processes of nature. But Basilea's entire *Emunat Ḥakhamim* offers an even more eloquent testimony of how the study of nature, unencumbered by the assumptions of Aristotelian metaphysics, could be properly integrated with

24. *Sefer Shemesh Ẓedakah* on *Yoreh De'ah*, pp. 80a–81b, n. 29; H. J. Zimmels, *Magicians, Theologians and Doctors* (London, 1952), pp. 122–24.

25. *Sefer Eẓ ha-Da'at*, p. 34b.

26. *Sefer Emunat Ḥakhamim*, p. 30b.

kabbalah. It is not the kabbalist, claims Basilea, but the Aristotelian philosopher who remains blinded by his own metaphysical dogmas.

Take the following remarkable anecdote about an old man from Mantua who taught in the *yeshivah:*

[He was considered a great scholar] in the wisdom of the Torah, philosophy, and medicine, and was one of the leaders of our congregation. Because of his great knowledge, he would categorize as impossible anything which his intelligence deemed so, since he could not fathom its cause. One day he sat and taught "the enlightened" of our people, wearing eyeglasses on the bridge of his nose as old men were accustomed to do. I said to him: "Master, the spectacles on your nose can make people appear so that their heads are below and their feet are above; that they extend their heads to the ground and their lower extremities toward heaven, so that when a person walks to the east, it will appear to him that he goes to the west. So all things might appear to be opposite of what they actually are." All the "enlightened ones" standing there laughed; all of them readily agreed that this is certainly not true and anyone who so believes is counted among the fools. The wise old doctor declared: "You 'astronomers' [naturalists, scientists] say nothing more than nonsense, because such a thing is impossible." He wanted to make his words compelling by offering clear proofs, taken from philosophy and appropriate to the intelligence, which I will not enlarge upon here. I then asked him to hand me his glasses and I placed them far from his eyes at the point where the image breaks up [the focal point] and beyond it. He then observed along with the others standing there what was impossible for them to believe. This was because he had not studied the science of optics even though he was a great scholar, and he did not understand how the lens works and how the rays [entering] the eyes or any rays are bent. . . . On the contrary, he always imagined the opposite to be the case, for with the spectacles on his nose he read a book and perceived everything to be in order. Maimonides' case is similar, since he learned only the doctrines of Aristotle in these matters and could not understand that our voice from below works above; thus he denied the power of using God's names.[27]

27. Ibid., p. 17a.

Like the Mantuan scholar, Maimonides had understood the world through the lens of a scholastic conceptual scheme. Despite his intellectual accomplishments, Maimonides could not be expected to understand the cultural and scientific world of the eighteenth century, a world where the potency of forces not understood by the intellect was deemed possible and even regularly observed. It wasn't that "the great eagle" was dead wrong; he was simply wearing the wrong lens.

Having disclosed the myopia of the Aristotelian philosophers limited by their own metaphysical dogmas, Basilea could champion the scientific knowledge of rabbinic and kabbalistic sages once thought to be tragically out-of-date, as Maimonides himself had admitted.[28] The empirical study of nature could now become a tool to subvert the rational orthodoxies of the past while reconfirming the previously discounted sapience of ancient Jewish traditions.

Basilea's commitment to experimentalism in substantiating rabbinic opinions on nature is best revealed by two marvelous examples he supplies. In the first instance, he upbraids the Aristotelian philosopher Gersonides for questioning the rabbinic understanding of a biblical verse (1 Kings 6:4), assuming the rabbis lacked a precise understanding of Basilea's obviously favorite science of optics. He proceeds to offer his readers a long discourse on the refraction of light rays, explains how light is dispersed through a wide aperture and shines more brightly through a narrow one, and closes his discussion by describing an experiment he performed with the aid of a rabbinic colleague. The scenario of the kabbalist Basilea, crouched in a darkened room with one of Venice's most distinguished rabbis, R. Jacob Aboab, examining the effect of light rays through a narrow opening in the window, performing a scientific experiment to reaffirm the truth of their sacred tradition, is as revealing a snapshot as any regarding the complexity of the Jewish intellectual ambiance in the Italian ghettos in the eighteenth century and the place of science in that setting.[29]

In the second instance, Basilea attempts to defend a seemingly odd position of the rabbis in the Talmud (B.T. Rosh ha-Shanah 24b), where two witnesses contend that they saw the old moon in the morning sky in the east and the

28. See chap. 1 above.
29. *Sefer Emunat Ḥakhamim,* p. 6a.

KABBALAH, SCIENCE, AND CHRISTIAN POLEMICS

new moon in the evening sky in the west. Although R. Johanan ben Nuri had declared such testimony false, since the old moon could never be visible twenty-four hours before the appearance of the new one, Basilea was not prepared to dismiss this observation out of hand. He enlists the evidence of recent explorers of the New World, even mentions the writing of Johann Kepler, and then attempts to calculate the course of the moon in relation to the earth as it might appear in Jerusalem. Uncertain of his own tentative conclusions, he turns to two Christian astronomers in the city of Bologna, including the well-known Eustachio Manfredi (1674–1739). Both men confirm his judgment and the testimony of the Talmud; Manfredi even writes a long responsum with many proofs, according to Basilea. No doubt testimony confirming rabbinic sapience from so unlikely a source would have fully justified Basilea's exhilaration in proclaiming the words of the psalmist (Psalm 144:15): "Happy the people who have it so; happy the people whose God is the Lord."[30]

Recent scientific information thus became for Basilea both a formidable ally in denigrating dogmatic philosophy and a conceptual framework in which to enhance and elevate the esoteric dimension of his Jewish identity. He offers a most elaborate testimony of how nature study unrelated to Aristotelian metaphysics could properly be integrated with the kabbalah. He frames his remarks within a critique of Maimonides' classical definition of the rabbinic esoteric pursuits called *Ma'aseh Bereshit* and *Ma'aseh Merkavah,* which Maimonides had labeled physics and metaphysics, respectively. For Basilea, however, *Ma'aseh Bereshit* is divided into two parts: "The first includes what human investigation can evaluate and the second is that which is only known by the tradition of the prophets." In the first category, Basilea places the legitimate and praiseworthy occupations of the naturalists, who observe, describe, and classify the multitude of natural things. In the second category, the naturalist is provided an understanding of the actual causes of natural occurrences by reflecting on the higher power that generated them. Thus, plants grow up by "what Plato called an idea . . . and what naturalists did not know and therefore called an occult quality . . . and these are the secrets of the Torah." In the final analysis, Basilea concludes, "a

30. Ibid., pp. 8b–9a. On Manfredi, see G. Tabarroni, "Eustachio Manfredi," *Dictionary of Scientific Biography* (New York, 1974), 9:77–78.

person will understand the natures of created things in their root causes through the kabbalah and not through doubtful [human] investigation . . . and these two inquiries, that which is known by human investigation and that known by the kabbalah of our forefathers, is called inclusively *Ma'aseh Bereshit.*" What remains is *Ma'aseh Merkavah,* the ultimate reflection of the kabbalists on the divine world, the diety, and his celestial hosts. By disassembling physics from Aristotelian metaphysics and reassembling the former with kabbalistic metaphysics, Basilea not only promoted the study of the natural world in Judaism but underscored the supreme importance of kabbalistic revelation.[31]

Accordingly, the positions of Morpurgo and Basilea were indeed closer than either of them might have admitted. Morpurgo appreciated the kabbalah even though he was no kabbalist. And he, like Basilea, had repudiated Aristotelian philosophy firmly and unambiguously. Both enjoyed the startling insights of the new sciences and each, in his own way, embraced the new mood of Baconian empiricism. The scientific revolution of the seventeenth century had engendered a full restructuring of the relationship between what was rational and what was not, and the intellectual responses of these two rabbis were surely products of that realignment.

If the two men had more to agree than to disagree on, why was there a controversy? Why so emotional an outburst against Morpurgo from Basilea more than a quarter-century after Morpurgo's modest book had appeared? Why did Morpurgo reopen the wounds of the Sabbatian controversy in the first place with the republication of the Frances poem, and why did he conceal his identity if he believed his small publication would attract such little notice? Morpurgo usually shunned controversy, as his modest letters to the fanatical defender of the faith against heresy, R. Moses Ḥagiz, reveal.[32] To act consciously in so provocative manner was surely out of character for him.

I would argue that the debate had to do less with substance than with appear-

31. *Sefer Emunat Ḥakhamim,* pp. 20b–21b.

32. See I. Sonne, "An Exchange of Letters between R. Moses Ḥagiz and R. Samson Morpurgo Concerning Nehemiah Ḥayon and His Faction [1703–05]" (in Hebrew), *Koveẓ al Yad* 2 (12) (1937): 157–96. On Ḥagiz, see E. Carlebach, *The Pursuit of Heresy: R. Moses Hagiẓ and the Sabbatian Controversies* (New York, 1990).

ances—that is, the fear of a Jewish leadership projecting an image of communal weakness, of intellectual and moral depravity in the eyes of the non-Jewish world. Morpurgo's provocation and Basilea's belated outburst reflect a deep-seated anxiety and insecurity about the viability of Jewish communal life, the authority of the rabbinate, and the ability of the Jewish community to withstand the continual social, economic, and intellectual pressures exerted by the Christian majority. Certainly the internal debate over the messiahship of Shabbatai Zevi had taken its toll in dividing the community into antagonistic factions. But, as we have seen, a semblance of mutual respect and tranquility between individuals in both camps still prevailed. By the beginning of the eighteenth century, the controversy over Nehemiah Hayon, the disciple of Abraham Cardoso, and his public pronouncements about the nature of Jewish belief engendered new acrimony and mutual recriminations from all sides.[33] But the main issues of the Hayon debate, as recent scholarship has shown, had little to do with Sabbatian messianism and much to do with upholding rabbinic authority, containing heresy, and maintaining the proper public profile of the Jewish community within Christian Europe.[34] In the many documents of the Hayon affair,[35] the pervasive need to maintain the correct public face of the Jewish minority is the major concern of the writers, including the peace-loving Morpurgo.

Upholding the proper image of Jewish life was an obsession shared by Morpurgo and Basilea, and it seems to have set them on a collision course despite their shared religious and intellectual values. Both had something else in common: a long and bitter encounter with Christian missionaries and polemicists. A large portion of each rabbi's intellectual output was devoted to defending the faith and good name of Judaism. At about the same time that *Ez ha-Da'at* was published, Morpurgo became entangled in a bitter polemic with the friar Luigi Maria Benetelli. In 1703 Benetelli had published a highly learned treatise against

33. The most recent treatment of the Hayon debate is found in Carlebach, *Pursuit of Heresy*. On David Nieto's critique of Hayon, see chap. 11 below.

34. In addition to Carlebach, see Y. Liebes, "The Ideological Foundation of the Hayon Debate" (in Hebrew), *Proceedings of the Eighth World Concress of Jewish Studies,* Division C (Jerusalem, 1982), pp. 129–34; and see chap. 11 below.

35. See esp. M. Friedman, "Letters Relating to the Nehemiah Hiya Hayon Controversy" (in Hebrew), *Sefunot* 10 (1966): 482–619.

the Jews, citing an enormous variety of classical and contemporary Hebrew sources. In 1705 he published a summary of the responses of two rabbis, one of whom was Morpurgo, with his own rejoinder.[36] Among the most critical points made by the rabbis against the Christian, two stand out: that the kabbalah was not essential to Jewish faith and that it does not describe the Christian God.[37] Morpurgo's attitude toward the kabbalah was undoubtedly shaped by such Christian manipulation of Jewish sources. There was nothing wrong with the kabbalah per se; only when it rose to dominate and stifle other expressions of Jewish spirituality, Jewish faith became unbalanced, irrational, and subject to the kind of Christian missionizing in which the shrewd Benetelli excelled. And when Nehemiah Ḥayon arrogantly revealed kabbalistic secrets reminiscent of Christian dogma, the trinity in particular, the dangerous excesses of kabbalistic enthusiasm, the loss of rational anchors of Jewish faith, and the undermining of traditional rabbinic authority became blatant. The sanity and healthy skepticism of Bedersi's lyric message were surely appropriate to such a situation, and even the sarcasm of Jacob Frances was in place in countering the too powerful influence of the kabbalists, who had exposed a vulnerable Jewish community to dangerous enthusiasts like Ḥayon and to persistent missionaries like Benetelli.

Basilea's encounter with Christian polemics was no less intense. His teacher and fellow Mantuan rabbi Judah Briel had long engaged in debates with Christians, and Basilea too composed a treatise defending the sanctity of the Jewish Passover against Christian aspersions.[38] Yet the encounter for which he became a cause célèbre of the Mantuan ghetto occurred only three years after *Sefer Emunat Ḥakhamim* appeared. As he was making his regular visit to the Mantuan

36. On Benetelli, see Benayahu, "The Polemic of Samson Morpurgo"; F. Parente, "Il Confronto ideologico tra l'ebraismo e la chiesa in Italia," *Italia Judaica*, vol. 1 (Rome, 1983), pp. 359–62. The two works of Benetelli are: *Le Saette di Gionata scagliate a favor degli Ebrei da padre lettore F. Luigi Maria Benetelli Vicentino dell'ordine de' Minimi* (Venice, 1703) and *I Dardi rabbinici infranti dal padre lettore F. Luigi Maria Benetelli Vicentino dell'ordine de' Minimi* (Venice, 1705).

37. *I Dardi rabbinici*, pp. 8–9. This follows Benetelli's "Breve trattato della cabbala degli Ebrei."

38. On Basilea's work, see Simonsohn, *History of the Jews of the Duchy of Mantua*, p. 84; on Briel's, see *Encyclopedia Judaica* (Jerusalem, 1971), 4:1372–73, and W. Horbury, "Judah Briel and Seventeenth-century Jewish Anti-Christian Polemic in Italy," *Jewish Studies Quarterly* 1 (1993–94): 171–92. Briel is also mentioned in chap. 9 below.

prison on a Friday afternoon in May 1733, he bent over to put money in the alms box, as was his custom, when suddenly a Christian hooligan painted a large cross on his rear. As he left the prison, he was mocked by the commoners of the neighborhood, to whom he retorted angrily: "You should not laugh if you notice where the cross has been placed." His response so infuriated the Church authorities that he was thrown into prison and held for almost a year despite his failing health. Even after his release, he remained under house arrest until 1739 and was restricted to the ghetto until his death in 1743.[39]

The incident of the rabbi's defiant rear end and the publication of his *Sefer Emunat Ḥakhamim* are surely both related to Basilea's profound sensitivity to Judaism's beleaguered status in the mind of an often hostile Christian majority. It was certainly not the time for Jews to be seduced by the blandishments of scholastic philosophy that undermined their sacred calling. He scolds Morpurgo for extolling philosophy as a means of gaining favor in the Christian world and quotes Joseph Delmedigo about the dangers of exposing Jewish youth to the corrosive intellectual atmosphere of Paduan university life.[40] How inappropriate to publish Frances's criticism of Jewish sages and communal leaders when their authority is challenged and undermined daily! Rather it is a time to reaffirm "the faith *in* the sages" (my emphasis), in the unique teachings of Judaism, and in the blessed legacy of kabbalistic tradition.[41] So formidable a tool as science can reconfirm the relevance and reliability of the kabbalists and their teachings. Basilea's spirited defense of the kabbalah and its teachers, including his cutting remarks about Morpurgo's writing, were surely motivated by the emphatic need to bolster the image of the kabbalistic scholar both within the Jewish community and outside of it, to demonstrate anew, in Moses Zacuto's words, the superiority of Jewish "wisdom" to mere Gentile "discernment."

In sum, a relatively minor series of events, the endorsement of the ideal of philosophizing by one Italian rabbi and the displeasure it evoked in another, tells us a good deal about the intellectual world of Italian Jewry at the begin-

39. Simonsohn, *History of the Jews,* p. 158.

40. *Sefer Emunat Ḥakhamim,* pp. 30a, 30b; cf. chaps. 3 and 4 above.

41. Compare Carlebach, *Pursuit of Heresy,* p. 482; S. Rosenberg, "Emunat Ḥakhamim," *Jewish Thought in the Seventeenth Century,* ed. I. Twersky and B. Septimus (Cambridge, Mass., and London, 1987), pp. 285–341.

ning of the eighteenth century. What at first appears to be the familiar jousting between a philosopher and a kabbalist reveals instead a more nuanced and dynamic cultural environment, one in which Jewish intellectual life was deeply affected by new attitudes toward nature and science, but also one in which the stark reality of Christian belligerence and intolerance still intruded oppressively into the enterprise of Jewish self-reflection and self-affirmation.

8

On the Diffusion of Scientific Knowledge within the Jewish Community

THE MEDICAL TEXTBOOK OF TOBIAS COHEN

Padua's most distinguished Jewish medical graduate, with the possible exception of Joseph Delmedigo, was Tobias Cohen. Certainly, his *Ma'aseh Tuviyyah* was the most influential early modern Hebrew textbook of the sciences, especially medicine. First published in Venice in 1707 after a delay of some six years, it was reprinted in the same city in 1715, 1728, 1769, and 1850, in Jessnitz in 1721, in Lemberg in 1867 and 1875, in Cracow in 1908, in Jerusalem in 1967 and 1978, and in Brooklyn in 1974. No other Hebrew work dealing exclusively with medical and scientific matters, and unrelated directly to concerns of religious law, was so widely read and appreciated.[1] A close examination of the text, its author, and their cultural context is in order.

Tobias and his book have not gone unnoticed by earlier scholars.[2] On the basis of several documents published in the last

1. I refer to other Hebrew texts comparable to this work later in this chapter.

2. Some of the earlier studies of Tobias include M. Bersohn, *Tobisz Kohn lekarz polski* (Cracow, 1872); D. Kaufmann, "Trois docteurs de Padoue," *Revue des études juives*, 18 (1889): 293–98; idem, *Dr. Israel Conegliano und seine Verdienste um die Republik Venedig bis nach dem Frieden von Carlowitz* (Budapest, 1895); L. Lewin, "Die jüdischen Studenten an der Universität Frankfort an der Oder," *Jahrbuch der jüdisch-literarischen Gesellschaft* 14 (1921): 217–38; A. Levinsohn, *Tuviyyah ha-Rofe ve-Sifro Ma'aseh Tuviyyah* (Berlin, 1924); E. Carmoly, *Histoire des médecins juifs anciens et modernes* (Brussels, 1844), pp.

century, the outline of Tobias's biography has been told and retold. Born in Metz in 1652, Tobias Cohen grew up in the home of a physician-rabbi who had fled from Narol, Poland, in 1648, during the Chemelnicki persecutions. Tobias studied in a yeshivah in Cracow before entering the University of Frankfurt an der Oder in 1678. Tobias and his close companion, Gabriel Felix of Brody,[3] were among the first Jews to be allowed to study medicine at the university. Their exceptional status was the result of the intervention of the Great Elector of Brandenburg, Friedrich Wilhelm, who even supplied both of them with an unprecedented governmental stipend. But even the Great Elector's extraordinary efforts were insufficient to overcome the mounting opposition to their presence at the university on the part of the faculty, who were unwilling to authorize Jews to practice medicine by awarding them university degrees.

Gabriel and Tobias subsequently traveled south to the more tolerant surroundings of the University of Padua, with its long-established custom of welcoming Protestants and Jews into its nominally Catholic medical school. Joining the significant number of Jewish students already enrolled at the university, the two Ashkenazic Jewish students found substantial support from Solomon Conegliano, himself a distinguished graduate of Padua's medical school and a rabbi, who offered them tutorial work to supplement their formal coursework and rabbinic studies to enrich their spiritual lives.[4] Both students matriculated with doctorates in philosophy and medicine in 1683.

Upon his graduation, Tobias's medical career apparently flourished. He was

---

247–51; D. Margalit, *Ḥakhme Yisrael ke-Rofim* (Jerusalem, 1962); J. O. Leibowitz, "Tobie Cohen: Auteur medical de langue hébraïque (1652–1729)," *Revue d'histoire de la médecine hébraïque* 17 (1964): 15–24; and D. A. Friedman, *Tuviyyah ha-Cohen* (Jerusalem, 1940). The late William W. Brickman of the University of Pennsylvania had begun a major research project on Tobias before his death, which included plans for an English translation of *Ma'aseh Tuviyyah*. He graciously shared with me some of his preliminary research notes written in 1982.

3. On Felix, see R. Briel, "Une Lettre de Gabriel Felix Moschides," *Revue des études juives* 32 (1896): 134–37.

4. On the importance of Padua as a center for training Jewish medical students and on Conegliano's school in particular, see chap. 3 above and my essay "The Impact of Science on Jewish Culture and Society in Venice," in *Gli Ebrei e Venezia*, ed. G. Cozzi (Milan, 1987), pp. 417–48.

called to the Ottoman Empire, where he served as a personal physician to several sultans in Adrianople and Constantinople. He composed his medical encyclopedia in Turkey and arranged for its publication in Venice through the good offices of Conegliano, who lavishly praised his former student in a lengthy foreword to the work. Tobias lived in Jerusalem from 1715 until his death in 1729.

The above outline hardly illuminates the many faces of this fascinating author and medical practitioner. From Poland to Germany to Italy, the Ottoman Empire, and Jerusalem, Tobias's life and career appear to embody an enormous and variegated cultural landscape. Regrettably, the life cannot be fully and amply described. Besides a few documents located at Frankfurt and Padua, and several other insignificant writings of Tobias, we are left only with the author's own modest account of his struggles and good fortunes in the pages of *Ma'aseh Tuviyyah*. Like that of Joseph Delmedigo, his older contemporary, to whom he should inevitably be compared,[5] Tobias Cohen's peripatetic career can be only faintly reconstructed from the extant sources of his life, primarily his own writing.

Previous scholars have summarily described the contents of Tobias's major work, with its traditional divisions dealing first with matters of the divine world, the heavens, the earth, and the human species, and then with medicine: physiology, pathology, and therapy. They have readily pointed out that the most significant part of the book, both in size and in sophistication, is that dealing with medicine. The earlier chapters on God, divine providence, cosmography, the contemporary subjects of Copernican astronomy and the possibility of multiple worlds, on strange creatures and physiognomy, the elements, and even the seemingly misplaced discussion of the notorious false messiah, Shabbatai Zevi, all provide a broad introduction and backdrop for the critical essays on medicine that follow. Although Tobias has been considered relatively conservative and traditional for having labeled Copernicus "the firstborn of Satan,"[6] he has fared better as a medical writer, particularly for his able description of Harvey's discovery of blood circulation[7] and for his own observations on the Polish skin

5. See chap. 4 above.

6. See, for example, A. Neher, "Copernicus in the Hebraic Literature from the Sixteenth to the Eighteenth Century," *Journal of the History of Ideas* 38 (1977): 219–21.

7. See J. O. Leibowitz, "Harveian Items in Hebrew Medicine," *Ha-Rofe ha-Ivri* 2 (1957): 74–79 [Hebrew]; 134–38 [English].

disease, *Plica Polonica*.[8] Yet despite a sizable bibliography on specific subjects of the book, there exists no overall evaluation of the author's goals in writing the work, no accurate sense of his scientific knowledge, and little appreciation of his ultimate accomplishment.

To understand the novelty of Tobias's composition, we would do well to compare it with a similar work of his older Jewish contemporary, Jacob Zahalon, the *Oẓar ha-Ḥayyim,* published in Venice in 1583, the year of Tobias's graduation from Padua. Although Tobias never refers to it explicitly, he could hardly have failed to take notice of this ambitious text, written by an illustrious Jewish physician and rabbi, a graduate of the University of Rome and an eye-witness to the horrendous plague of 1656 that swept through the city's neighborhoods, including the ghetto itself.[9] It too is a massive textbook covering all the main fields of medical knowledge and purporting to provide therapeutic advice to doctors and laymen alike. Zahalon, like Cohen, was a highly educated doctor, not a boorish magical healer or a charlatan of the sort that Tobias caustically debunked for claiming to possess sophisticated knowledge available only to university graduates like himself.[10] Zahalon's compendium lacked the elaborate ruminations on the metaphysical and physical worlds which accompanied Cohen's work, but this deficiency was apparently the result of lack of funds alone. The *Oẓar ha-Ḥayyim* seems to have been only part of a much more comprehensive undertaking—an encyclopedia of all knowledge, including a discussion of divine matters. But it was never published and, except for one section that exists in manuscript, was either lost or left incomplete.[11]

8. See D. Sadan, "Plica Polonica," in *The Field of Yiddish: Studies in Language, Folklore, and Literature,* 4th Collection, ed. M. I. Herzog et al. (Philadelphia, 1980).

9. On Zahalon and his work, see J. O. Leibowitz, "R. Jacob Zahalon, Man of Rome and his Poem in Honor of the Sabbath of Hanukah 1687" (in Hebrew), in *Scritti in Memoria di Enzo Sereni,* ed. D. Carpi et al. (Jerusalem, 1970), pp. 167–81; H. Friedenwald, *The Jews and Medicine,* 2 vols. (Baltimore, 1944), 1:268–79; H. A. Susland, *A Guide for Preachers on Composing and Delivering Sermons: The Or ha-Darshanim of Jacob Zahalon* (New York, 1987).

10. On Tobias's debunking, see *Ma'aseh Tuviyyah* (Cracow, 1908; repr. Brooklyn, 1974), p. 82b. All page references are to this edition.

11. *Oẓar ha-Ḥayyim* (Venice, 1683), title page: "*Sefer Oẓar Ha-Ḥayyim* on the profession of medicine, which is part III of *Sefer Oẓar Ha-Ḥokhmot . . . .*" See also MS Budapest-Kaufmann

Although Zahalon and his writing have been the subject of a number of recent essays, the work merits further scrutiny, particularly to elucidate the author's motivation in composing the text and in seeing it printed.[12] We shall pause to consider the book here only to compare it with Tobias's work, but even this cursory examination might allow us to enrich our appreciation of Zahalon's achievement as well as that of Cohen's.

The Roman physician opens his work with a theological and legal justification of the practice of medicine in Judaism. Having demonstrated to his satisfaction that "the science of medicine is a commandment and a value," Zahalon elaborates on the utility of his medical dictionary. In a city where no doctor lives but where there is a "wise and enlightened student," apparently one of rabbinic law, the student will be able to comprehend the methods of healing the sick by utilizing this guidebook. When a doctor is located far from the city and temporary advice is required, or where a medical controversy arises among local doctors, the book can provide support, Zahalon claims. Even where no controversy exists, any physician will find the book useful as a kind of *Shulḥan Arukh*, "an ordered table," obviously analogous to the authoritative code of Jewish law of the same name, written by Joseph Karo more than a century before. As Zahalon puts it: "One is able to understand with this book the accepted and correct view . . . a *Shulḥan Arukh* before them [the disputing physicians] without any disagreement regarding what is written in medical works, for I have written in the most correct, accepted and tried manner." Finally, Zahalon adds that the book will be useful to those indigent (Jewish) sick who are unable to pay for the services of a "Gentile doctor." Any such person can "easily" master the art of healing using his handbook.[13]

The strongest impression one receives from this introduction, and from the entire book, is one of self-assurance, of the absolute certainty with which Zahalon tenders his medical prescriptions. There is no sense of hesitation, no unresolved therapy, no disagreement or proposal of alternatives about the cor-

---

A 293 (Institute for Microfilms of Hebrew MSS, National and University Library, Jerusalem, n. 14715), entitled *Sefer Oẓar Ha-Shamayim,* apparently another part of this larger work.

12. See n. 9 above.

13. *Oẓar ha-Ḥayyim,* introduction.

rect physiology or pathology. There is simply "the most correct, accepted and tried manner," and it is sufficient that both the doctor and the patient consulting this book know it and nothing more.

This unwavering confidence in classical medical therapy is consistent throughout Ẓahalon's text. He unhesitatingly quotes Galen, Hippocrates, and Aristotle on almost every subject treated. He is seemingly oblivious to alternative theories of matter other than the four elements of Aristotle.[14] From the latter, he conventionally derives the four primary qualities, four temperaments, and four humors.[15] His pathology is thoroughly Galenic, appealing to humoric balance as critical to good health and approving of evacuation of excessive humors through bloodletting.[16] He defines fever by paraphrasing the standard definition of Avicenna as heat contrary to nature (preternatural heat), extraneous to the innate heat of the body, kindled in the heart, and diffused through the arteries and veins by means of the spirit and the blood.[17] There is not even a faint echo of the well-publicized discussions of the subject among seventeenth-century physicians.[18] The ancients regularly have the last word on this topic and on others. Occasionally, Ẓahalon offers a fresh insight or refers to more recent sources. He is fond of quoting the physicians Abraham Zacutus and Amatus Lusitanus, perhaps because of their Jewish ancestry;[19] he also refers to Joseph Duchesne (Quercetanus), to Pietro Castelli's *Antidotario romano,* and to Girolamo Calestini.[20] But such occasional references to contemporary sources never serve to undermine standard treatments; on the contrary, they bolster previous positions. Ẓahalon's textbook vividly demonstrates the hold that classical medical procedures had on a respected university graduate and clinical physician well into the seventeenth century. In the light of such traditionalism Ẓahalon could pronounce, with full sincerity and innocence, that his medical handbook was authoritative, without the slightest hint that a storm of controversies was

14. Ibid., p. 28b.
15. Ibid., p. 29a.
16. See, for example, ibid., pp. 1a, 29a–32b, 37b.
17. Ibid., p. 9a.
18. On Tobias Cohen's discussion of fever, see below.
19. See, for example, *Oẓar ha-Ḥayyim,* pp. 15b, 17a, 19b, 56b, etc.; and see chap. 10 below.
20. Ibid., pp. 38b, 58a.

pean academic discourse.[25] Yet he chose to write in Hebrew, to underscore his link to his cultural past, and to encourage his coreligionists to believe that they still remained full-fledged participants in the exciting scientific culture emerging throughout the Continent.

On the other hand, Tobias wrote in a rich Hebrew style rather than in Yiddish. Unlike the popular medical manual of Issachar Teller, the *Be'er Mayyim Hayyim,* published about 1650,[26] or even the highly condensed Hebrew compendium called the *Sefer Dimyon Ha-Refu'ot,* written by Abraham Wallich, Tobias's fellow student at Padua, published in 1700,[27] *Ma'aseh Tuviyyah* remains a dense, challenging text to the uninitiated. Despite the didactic features of the text—its clear introductions, headings, and subheadings and its splendid diagrams and illustrations—it could hardly be studied by the indigent poor or by the untutored yeshivah student, as Zahalon had hoped. Tobias's compendium, with its exhaustive references to new and old scholars, to conflicting theories of knowledge, and to conflicting medical procedures, reads more like a Talmudic discussion than a *Shulhan Arukh,* a simplified code of prescribed procedures.

In fact, Tobias, in contrast to Zahalon, exhibited little sympathy for the "masses" and little confidence in their ability to acquire a discipline that had taken him a lifetime to master. The first words of his introduction to the medical sections of his textbook transparently reveal his true feelings on the matter:

> The field of medicine seems habitual and easy in the mouths of fools, yet how difficult it really is in the eyes of the true doctor. . . . The masses are mistaken in this notion that the [untutored] physician with experience alone is the best doctor who lacks analogic reasoning and reflection and who does not see the light of the Torah and science. . . . If there were no need for this [that is, for such academic credentials], why would a [Jewish]

25. I refer to such specialized medical writings of Marrano doctors as Amatus Lusitanus and Elijah Montalto or to the encyclopedia of Isaac Cardoso. See chap. 10 below.

26. Issachar Teller, *Be'er Mayyim Hayyim,* published with the Hebrew translation of Hippocrates' *Aphorisms* by Joseph Solomon Delmedigo, photocopied from Prague edition, ca. 1650, with introduction by J. O. Liebowitz (Jerusalem, 1968).

27. Abraham Wallich, *Sefer Dimyon Ha-Refu'ot* (=*Harmonia Wallichia Medica*) (Frankfurt, 1700).

physician waste his time and his finances to inflict his body with pain and to endanger himself through studying in the universities of the Gentiles, who abuse Jewish students? It would be sufficient accordingly for such a person to remain in his house or to serve [as an apprentice] for some state-appointed doctor . . . as is the custom in this land [Turkey]. . . . But don't the unintelligent realize that a person is not called a scholar without knowledge, nor a doctor without a doctorate, nor distinguished or ordained without rabbinical ordination? Moreover, no Jew in all of Italy, Poland, Germany, and France would ever consider studying the science of medicine without first stuffing himself with the written and oral Torah as well as the other sciences, as is the case for the large number of students of my teacher . . . Solomon Conegliano, as I can personally testify, among them those who become rabbis and physicians to kings and great nobles. And among all of them, I am the least significant.[28]

Tobias proceeds to lambaste those who claim to offer a variety of medical cures but who have never studied academic medicine and end up irresponsibly endangering their patients. To be a successful physician, for Tobias, involved years of painful devotion to study, intense exposure to rabbinics as well as to the secular sciences. And Tobias would be the last to claim, like Zahalon, that this kind of well-rounded education could be reduced to a single medical manual. On the contrary, a student utilizing Tobias's textbook would come to appreciate how imposing the field of medicine actually is, how complex and uncertain its findings, and how awesome the task of functioning as a good physician. The perspective of *Ma'aseh Tuviyyah*, in striking contrast to *Ozar Ha-Hayyim*, is elitist to the core. It is meant to extol and elevate the Jewish physician educated in the mold of the author himself, to castigate those who would presume to be doctors without proper qualifications, and to demonstrate the formidable challenges of mastering the discipline, but to argue, in the end, that Jewish students, with the proper training and commitment, can still rise to the top of their profession.

How might we explain the differences in perception between Zahalon and Cohen? Are they attributable only to differences of personal experience or out-

28. *Ma'aseh Tuviyyah*, p. 82b.

look, or are other social and cultural factors decisive in shaping their individual attitudes and the contents of their respective handbooks? Tobias's book offers additional clues in clarifying their diverging concerns.

Cohen's deep-seated sense of inferiority and insecurity appears to be shaped by forces larger than his unpleasant experiences as a student in Frankfurt. In the first place, he presents a revealing portrait of the theological challenges posed to Jewish faith in his era. He was fully aware of the potential dangers of pantheism or materialism brought about by the new sciences:

> There exist weak-minded men of deficient intelligence and understanding, not only from among the Gentile nations, who never observed the light of the Torah, but also among the members of our people, the nation that walks in the darkness of the exile, although the light of the Torah shines on them. Some of them deny God's existence completely in their hearts, thinking that the world has no originator, creator, or leader but only that everything is determined by nature and its custom. Some of them are skeptical of this position and remain uncertain and vacillating, since they lack true knowledge of it. For how can they believe something they do not know? Still others among them, although they believe that there is a God who created the world, do not understand what they believe. This is because they lack knowledge and intelligence to sketch and imprint God's reality in their own minds—as well as His unity, eternity, and essence—on a truthful basis, but rather do so on the basis of tradition alone, which they received from their forefathers.[29]

That Tobias's concern is not just a standard pronouncement about the corrosive effect of philosophy in general but reflects a specific problem of his own era is strongly suggested by two related discussions in the introductory sections of his book. First is his treatment of Copernicus and the arguments both in favor of and against the theory of heliocentricity and its ramifications for religious faith.[30] Second is his consideration of the notion of infinitely inhabited worlds

29. Ibid., pp. 1a–1b.

30. Ibid., pp. 42a–44b. This section has been discussed by Neher, "Copernicus," and by H. Levine, "Paradise Not Surrendered: Jewish Reactions to Copernicus and the Growth of Modern Science," in R. S. Cohen and M. W. Wartofsky, eds., *Epistemology, Methodology, and the Social Sciences* (Boston, 1983), pp. 210–12; M. Panitz, "New Heavens and a New Earth:

and its implications for Jewish faith regarding the unique status of the earth, mankind, and the singular revelation of the Torah to the Jewish people.[31] On both issues, Tobias is expansive enough to present both sides of the argument. There is no doubt that he is impressed by the refreshingly consistent and utterly simple arguments of Copernicus against the Ptolemaic universe. And although he labels Copernicus "the first-born of Satan" and is unwilling to accept his view because it literally contradicts the biblical verse, Tobias offers no more than a tepid defense of the traditionalist position. Similarly, his counterarguments against an infinite universe are neither rationally satisfying nor empirically compelling. It is sufficient to maintain a traditional position in order to conform with "the religion of our Torah."[32]

Despite Tobias's sincere effort to present himself as a staunch traditionalist, the evidence indicates that his exposure to the new sciences had affected his understanding of God and divine revelation. As we might expect in a book describing nature, the argument from design figures prominently among his proofs of God's existence. He waxes eloquent about the interconnected universe designed to serve human needs and about nature's harmonious order, which is synonymous with that of the Creator.[33] Elsewhere he dismisses the assumption of the eternity of the world because "almost no one in our day among all the nations could believe in the earth's eternity; rather, all acknowledge its creation [out of nothing]."[34] Moreover, Tobias typically places less credence in demonstrating the truth of religious belief through miracles than in the pub-

---

Seventeenth- to Nineteenth-Century Jewish Responses to the New Astronomy," *Conservative Judaism* 40 (1987–88): 37–38; and Ruderman, "The Impact of Science," pp. 436–37, and idem, *Science, Medicine, and Jewish Culture in Early Modern Europe*, Spiegel Lectures in European Jewish History 7 (Tel Aviv, 1987), pp. 20–21. My translation of Tobias's statement in both essays (p. 437 and p. 21, respectively): "These are the proofs . . . according to Copernicus' view . . . ; however, the counterarguments are easily confusing etc." should be corrected to read: "however, the counterarguments are easily proven etc." My thanks to Prof. David Berger for pointing out the error.

31. *Ma'aseh Tuviyyah*, pp. 58a–59a; and see Panitz, "New Heavens," pp. 31–32; Ruderman, *Science, Medicine, and Jewish Culture*, p. 21; idem, "The Impact of Science," p. 437.

32. *Ma'aseh Tuviyyah*, p. 59a.

33. Ibid., pp. 3a, 4a–4b.

34. Ibid., p. 58a.

lic attestation of God by an entire people.[35] Neither formulation is particularly original, but each recalls the arguments frequently employed by religious thinkers of the seventeenth century, particularly the argument *de consensu gentium.* Among contemporary Jewish writers on nature, David Nieto had explained his belief in God along similar lines.[36]

One might be tempted to disregard the significance of such theological affirmations, surely unspectacular in the broader contexts in which they are located. Yet before doing so, we might consider one other statement of Tobias that stands out for its seeming boldness and potential unorthodoxy. It emerges as a reaction to Maimonides' firm position that the Torah can never be changed. Tobias is unwilling to accept this categoric statement unless it represents a revealed tradition. But if it is not, Maimonides' formulation appears dubious to him:

> According to straight logic, we do not observe any proof for his arguments based on the verse [Deuteronomy 13:1]: "You should not add to it nor diminish from it." [Compare Maimonides, *Guide,* 3:41, 2:39.] That he cites . . . this verse only warns us not to add or subtract regarding the commandments on the basis of our own intelligence. But who would object to the Holy One, blessed be He? Can He never add or subtract? Regarding [Maimonides' argument] about the equibalance and perfection [of the divine commandments], all this relates to something which is equibalanced in the mind, that is, what a person's intelligence conjures up to be equibalanced. It is still possible that it can change according to the understanding of those who receive [the commandments]. An example of this is food, which is equibalanced for a baby as milk but for a young man as bread, meat, and wine. Similarly, the divine commandments need to change according to the times, as in the case of the command forbidding the consumption of meat from a living animal by the first man which was later allowed to Noah and his sons. . . . From this one learns that although the divine religion is never changed nor modified regarding everything, it is possible for one part to change from being forbidden to being permitted and vice versa.[37]

35. Ibid., pp. 7b–8a.
36. On Nieto's use of this argument, see chap. 11 below.
37. *Ma'aseh Tuviyyah,* pp. 8b–9a

Cohen concludes by noting the number of biblical and rabbinic passages utilized by those who scoff at Jews and Judaism and refers the reader to a short bibliography of appropriate defenses of the Jewish faith that focus on such misunderstood passages, including the works of Saadia, Ha-Levi, Kimḥi, Isaac of Troki, Abravanel, the Maharal, and even Azariah de' Rossi.[38] Defending Israel's good name while rebuking Maimonides and calling for moderate changes in Jewish law makes an interesting juxtaposition. Was Tobias actually suggesting modest "reforms" in Jewish law? Why was he raising the subject in the first place in his textbook of the sciences? And did he believe that Israel's good name and the proper defense of its sacred literature required certain alterations in Jewish law? Whatever the answers to these questions, one might argue that his unusual statement was shaped in part by his concern to present as rational and enlightened an image of Jews and Judaism as possible to his readership.

More than any other factor, however, Tobias believed that the image of Jews was degraded in the Gentile world by his coreligionists' pathetic obsession with false messiahs. A discussion of the messianic idea in Judaism, and of Shabbatai Ẓevi in particular, might appear out of place even in the theological sections of Tobias's compendium. That the author devotes so much space and displays so intense a reaction to this phenomenon should not be overlooked in evaluating his motives in composing the entire volume.[39]

Elisheva Carlebach has recently discussed the vindictive references to Sabbatianism by the close of the seventeenth century in Christian polemics against Judaism and the consequences of apostasies to Christianity on the part of individual Jews whose hopes were shattered by Shabbatai Ẓevi's own apostasy.[40] Several of Tobias's Jewish contemporaries fully appreciated the vulnerability of Jews to Christian missionizing in the wake of the Sabbatian debacle and forcefully pointed out the dangers of Jewish communal disintegration in their anti-Sabbatian writings. Tobias joined this group in underscoring the havoc that false messianic figures had wrought within the Jewish community both in the past and in the present. He especially noted the exploitation of Jewish messianic

38. Ibid., p. 9a.

39. See ibid., pp. 15b–19b.

40. E. Carlebach, "Sabbatianism and the Jewish-Christian Polemic," *Proceedings of the World Congress of Jewish Studies, Division C* 2 (1989): 1–7.

frenzy by Christian polemicists. In the context of the despair evoked by the failed Sabbatian movement, the Christians triumphantly argue: "And why do you continue to dream that [the messiah] will surely come and not tarry when in fact several false messiahs led you astray in your foolishness? . . . And now in this exile you already remain lowly and despised among the nations for so long a time, and you have become a proverb and a byword [compare Deut. 28:37 and elsewhere] among all of them. You have no king, no ruler, and no government, and this is only because of the great sin you committed regarding the true messiah . . . in killing him. He is Jesus Christ who came to this world to redeem you, but you killed him and did not accept him."[41]

This messianic deception, Tobias adds, "gave our enemies an opportunity to make fun of us and to defame us, almost providing a sword in the hands of the Gentiles to kill us."[42] After reviewing the history of messianic delusion, especially the recent episode of Shabbatai Zevi, Tobias again expresses his bitter despair over the dire ramifications of messianism and the sullied image of Judaism it projected in the eyes of the non-Jews.

Such an extraordinary outburst on the calamity of false messiahs allows us to appreciate most vividly the connection between medical and scientific discourse and feelings of cultural and religious inferiority in the mind of Tobias. Zahalon had also experienced the first phases of the Sabbatian movement in his own lifetime, but his medical work bears no reference to it. In the ensuing years, the negative consequences of Sabbatianism had dramatically left their imprint on Jewish life, as the writings of Moses Ḥagis, David Nieto, Jacob Sasportas, Isaac Cardoso, and several others testify.[43] As we have seen in the case of Samson Morpurgo and Solomon Basilea, Jewish leaders and thinkers at the turn of the eighteenth century had become increasingly preoccupied with the weakened state of European Jewry, its susceptibility to Christian missionary pressures, and the conspicuous erosion of their own traditional authority.[44] Tobias too felt acutely the crisis of Jewish communal life in his era and the sense of despair and insecurity it had engendered. His response was to direct his energies to restor-

41. *Ma'aseh Tuviyyah,* p. 17b.
42. Ibid., p. 19b.
43. See chap. 11 below and the references to Sabbatianism listed there.
44. See the previous chapter.

ing the intellectual image of the Jews by writing a sophisticated and updated scientific and medical textbook. Like Nieto, Morpurgo, Cardoso, and others, Tobias believed that a knowledge of contemporary science could profitably be employed to bolster and rehabilitate Jewish culture in an age of intellectual and religious turmoil exacerbated by frenetic messianic enthusiasm.

Ma'aseh Tuviyyah not only reveals an altered cultural perspective; it also discloses a radically transformed intellectual attitude on what constitutes the medical sciences. We have observed how Jacob Zahalon's *Ozar ha-Ḥayyim* presents a thoroughly traditional portrait of medicine based almost exclusively on classical sources. Upon opening the pages of Tobias's compendium, the contrast is immediately evident. The basic organizational structure of the two tomes is roughly equivalent. With minor variations, both works are constructed along the lines of similar seventeenth-century textbooks, often called "Institutions of Medicine," divided into the following sections: a definition of medicine, physiology, pathology, symptomology or semiotics, pharmacology, and finally therapy.[45] However, when one examines the content of the parallel sections of the two books, the differences are remarkable.

Tobias, at least initially, presents the views of Galen, Aristotle, Hippocrates, or Avicenna on the various topics he treats, but then he shifts openly to contemporary sources and opinions, often those that directly contradict the standard therapies of the field. Most prominent is his enthusiastic endorsement of the new chemical philosophy associated with the Paracelsian school. The Paracelsians, or iatrochemists, affirmed the union of chemistry and medicine; they were contemptuous of ancient medical authority, especially Galen and Aristotle; they advocated a new theory of disease that denied the Galenic system, based on the four humors and cure by "contraries," and replaced it with a cure by "similitude." Most important, they vigorously searched for chemical analogies in the biological realm. By regarding chemical processes such as decomposition and distillation as keys to understanding nature as a whole, the Paracelsians offered

45. On the fivefold division of these textbooks, see N. G. Siraisi, *Avicenna in Renaissance Italy: The Canon and Medical Teaching in Italian Universities after 1500* (Princeton, 1987), p. 101; L. King, *The Road to Medical Enlightenment, 1650–1695* (London and New York, 1970), pp. 15, 181–83.

a revolutionary perspective for understanding physiology and pathology as well as a flood of new medical remedies, chemically derived from minerals and plants.[46]

There is no doubt, from the frequent remarks of Tobias about the flowering "of a new medicine which dwells in the bosom of the physicians of our time,"[47] of his enthusiasm for iatrochemistry, particularly its medical applications. In fact, his interest in sharing his knowledge of chemical medicine with his Hebrew readers was undoubtedly a primary motivation for composing his textbook in the first place. To appreciate fully the extent of his indebtedness to this new school, as well as his selective utilization of its assumptions and discoveries, we need to consider more closely the sources upon which he relied.

Paracelsus is nowhere mentioned in Tobias's text, and for good reason.[48] The founder of the new chemical philosophy had not only vilified Jews; he had sought especially to negate the idea that the Jews possessed a particular talent for medicine superior to that of Christians:

> As regards medicine the Jews of old boasted greatly, and they still do, and they are not ashamed of the falsehood [involved]; they claim that they are the oldest and first physicians. And indeed they are the foremost among all the other nations—the foremost rascals, that is . . . . He [God] also put a curse on those who protect the Jews and who mix with their affairs, and yet they vindicate for themselves all praise of medicine. Let us pay no attention to all that, for if the Jews achieve anything in medicine, they have not inherited it from their forefathers but have stolen it from others, from strangers by robbery as it were . . . . Medicine has been given to the Gentiles, and therefore we revere and praise the Gentiles as the most ancient physicians.[49]

46. On the new chemical philosophers, see A. G. Debus, *The English Paracelsians* (London, 1965); idem, *The Chemical Philosophy: Paracelsian Science and Medicine in the Sixteenth and Seventeenth Centuries*, 2 vols. (New York, 1977); J. R. Partington, *A History of Chemistry*, 4 vols. (London and New York, 1961–70); W. Pagel, *Paracelsus: An Introduction to Philosophical Medicine in the Era of the Renaissance* (Basel and New York, 1958); idem, *Joan Baptista Van Helmont: Reformer of Science and Medicine* (Cambridge, 1982).

47. *Ma'aseh Tuviyyah*, p. 82b.

48. On p. 124a, however, he refers to the "sect of Paracelsus."

49. Quoted by H. Friedenwald, *The Jews and Medicine* (Baltimore, 1955), 1:55, from Paracelsus's *Labyrinthus medicorum errantium*, 1553. See also F. Kudlien, "Some Interpretative Remarks

Whether or not Tobias was familiar with Paracelsus's calumnies against Jewish physicians, such views would surely have irked him, given his sensitivity about the seeming decline of Jewish culture. He would have been uncomfortable with the Christian overtones of Paracelsus's chemical philosophy as well. Paracelsus's search for natural knowledge was colored throughout by a religious quest for God. For him, the search for divine "signatures" in nature, the unraveling of analogies and correspondences, was connected intimately with understanding the divine mystery of creation. He had also promoted the notion that the physician's calling was divine, for in his chemical search throughout the natural world, the Paracelsian physician-magician performed the pious duty of demonstrating to mankind the infinite love of the Creator to his creatures.[50] Although so elevated a ministry was conceived only for pious Christians, the fusion of medicine, magic, and scientific inquiry with mystical theology might potentially appeal to some contemporary Jewish physicians.[51] Yet it held little attraction for the more rational and pragmatic Tobias.

Tobias's reluctance to quote Joan Baptista Van Helmont, the most important iatrochemist after Paracelsus, was probably motivated by the same factors. Despite Van Helmont's own reservations regarding Paracelsian symbolism, his original chemical and medical innovations, especially his new notion of diseases that gain possession of the body like parasites, and his quest to understand the specificity of nature rather than the relational patterns of the ancients, must have made him appear bizarre to a Jewish physician like Tobias. He too was consumed with mystical spirituality, with the union of his mind with divine light, and with the notion that the truths he unveiled about nature were the result of his direct communication with God. Such prophetic claims of Helmontian medi-

---

on the Antisemitism of Paracelsus," in *Science, Medicine, and Society in the Renaissance: Essays in Honor of Walter Pagel,* ed. A. G. Debus (New York, 1972), 1.121–26.

50. Besides the references in n. 46 above, see W. Pagel, "Religious Motives in the Medical Biology of the Seventeenth Century," *Bulletin of the Institute of the History of Medicine* 3 (1935): 97–128, 213–31, 265–312.

51. Compare, for example, the parallel reflections of the sixteenth-century Jewish physician, Abraham Yagel, in D. B. Ruderman, *Kabbalah, Magic, and Science: The Cultural Universe of a Sixteenth-Century Jewish Physician* (Cambridge, Mass., 1988), although Yagel never refers to Paracelsus.

cine, as in the case of those of Paracelsus, were just as unappealing to Tobias as the enthusiasm of Shabbatai Zevi and his prophets.[52]

By the beginning of the seventeenth century, however, the iatrochemists had essentially split into two distinct groups: those like Roger Fludd who continued to link their observational data with a quest for religious truth, in order to construct a universal chemical philosophy of nature; and those like Sylvius de le Boe and Thomas Willis who exhibited little interest in the religious dimensions of the chemical philosophy, stressing instead the significance of chemical innovations in the field of medicine.[53] The latter group virtually secularized Paracelsian and Helmontian tendencies, trying to explain medical phenomena almost exclusively by the chemistry of the day, without recourse to metaphysics, Christian or otherwise. It is this group which attracted Tobias Cohen's attention. Indeed, among the many references he cites in *Ma'aseh Tuviyyah*, Sylvius and Willis are the most frequent and prominent.

Sylvius (1614–72) and Willis (1621–75) were the two most influential iatrochemists of the late seventeenth century. Sylvius practiced medicine at Leiden and Amsterdam and became professor of medicine at Leiden University. He openly rejected the mystical philosophy of Helmont, was one of the earliest proponents of Harvey's theory of the circulation of blood, and consistently attempted to explain medicine through the chemistry of his day. Thus he described digestion as a process of fermentation, explained disease in terms of an excess of either acid or alkali, and understood fever to be the result of an abnormal composition of lymph, pancreatic juice, and bile. Sylvius was neither a philosopher nor an experimentalist. His positions were based on conjecture and inference gained from the new discoveries of anatomists, physiologists, and chemists.[54]

Willis was the most important member of the Oxford circle of physiological chemists, a community of researchers deeply affected by Harvey's discovery of circulation who attempted to apply new modes of thinking influenced by atomism and the new chemical philosophy to the remaking of physiology. Willis's

---

52. On Van Helmont, see esp. Pagel, *Joan Baptista Van Helmont*.

53. See Debus, *Chemical Philosophy*, 1:205.

54. On Sylvius, see esp. Partington, *History of Chemistry*, 2:282–86; King, *Road to Medical Enlightenment*, pp. 93–108; Debus, *Chemical Philosophy*, 2:526–30; A. B. Davis, *Circulation Physiology and Medical Chemistry in England, 1650–80* (Lawrence, Kan., 1973), pp. 74–81.

first publication, *De fermentatione*, was published in 1659 and immediately left its impact on the field. It consisted of two parts: a theoretical discussion of the process of fermentation and a practical one of its application in explaining fevers. Willis rejected the Aristotelian notion of the four elements in favor of the iatrochemists' five principles: three active [spirit, sulfur, and salt] and two passive [water and earth]. For Willis, all change of natural phenomena could be reduced to the process of fermentation, which he defined as the internal motion of the particles or principles of any body, a kind of corpuscular rearrangement. All diseases were perversions of natural fermentation; fever was the result of the effervescence of sulfur and spirit in the circulating blood. The physician had to function like a vintner; like wine, blood and the humors had to be kept in well-tuned fermentation.[55]

Besides Sylvius and Willis, Tobias referred frequently to several other chemical physicians. He was fond of citing Michael Ettmüller (1644–1683), professor of medicine and botany at Leipzig, whom he often places together with Sylvius, although Ettmüller had reservations regarding Sylvius's acid-alkali theory. Nevertheless, he consistently prescribed chemical remedies and his writings were well known throughout Europe.[56] Tobias also quotes Daniel Sennert (1572–1637), a professor of medicine at Wittenberg. Sennert's massive *Institutionum medicinae*, first published in 1611, was a standard seventeenth-century textbook. Sennert clearly represented a middle-of-the-road position, attempting to harmonize Paracelsus with Aristotle and Galen. He adopted the three chemical principles of sulfur, salt, and mercury but also retained the four elements in a system where both principles and elements intermingle.[57] Other signifi-

55. On Willis, see esp. Debus, *Chemical Philosophy*, 2:519–26; R. G. Frank, Jr., *Harvey and the Oxford Physiologists* (Berkeley, Los Angeles, and London, 1980), pp. 164–69; H. Isler, *Thomas Willis (1621–1675): Doctor and Scientist* (New York and London, 1968); Davis, *Circulation Physiology and Medical Chemistry*, pp. 81–90, 154–58; L. J. Rather, "Pathology at Mid-Century: A Reassessment of Thomas Willis and Thomas Sydenham," in A. G. Debus, ed., *Medicine in Seventeenth-Century England* (Berkeley, Los Angeles, and London, 1974), pp. 71–112.

56. On Ettmüller, see Partington, *History of Chemistry*, 2:298–300; L. Thorndike, *A History of Magic and Experimental Science*, vol. 7 (New York and London, 1958), p. 237, and vol. 8 (New York and London, 1958), pp. 153–63.

57. On Sennert, see esp. Partington, *History of Chemistry*, 2:271–76; Debus, *Chemical Philosophy*, 1:191–203; L. King, "The Transformation of Galenism," in Debus, *Medicine in Seventeenth-Century England*, pp. 7–31.

cant chemists and anatomists cited by Tobias include Johann Hartmann (1568–1631), the first professor of iatrochemistry at Marburg and throughout Europe;[58] Thomas Bartholinus (1616–80) of Copenhagen, the discoverer of the thoracic duct and the lymphatic system;[59] Gaspare Aselli (1581–1625) of the University of Pavia, the discoverer of the chylous vessels;[60] Rembert Dodoens (1516–85) of the University of Leiden, a distinguished botanist and physiologist;[61] and Adriaan Van Den Spiegel (1575–1625) of Brussels and Padua, well known for his contributions to anatomy and embryology.[62]

It is clearly beyond the scope of this chapter to identify all of Tobias's medical sources.[63] What should be sufficiently clear from this brief profile is, first, Tobias's wide erudition in some of the most recent literature of his profession, and second, his particular interest in the therapies of chemical medicine. How he acquired such sophisticated learning and why he was so attracted to the chemists he studied still require further elucidation. Before suggesting an explanation, I would like to offer one good illustration of Tobias's utilization of the sources he read.

I already have mentioned Jacob Zahalon's traditional treatment of fevers, referring specifically to his paraphrase of Avicenna's definition.[64] In this, Zahalon was following the important part of standard university courses based on the fourth book of the *Canon,* where Avicenna first defined fevers, differentiated them into three types, and then presented a full exposition of the causes, diagnosis, and treatment of each type and subtype. According to this definition, fever was "heat contrary to nature" or "preternatural heat," as distinct from innate

58. See Partington, *History of Chemistry,* 2:177–81; R. Schmitz in *Dictionary of Scientific Biography (DSB),* vol. 6 (New York, 1972), pp. 145–46.

59. See C. D. O'Malley in *DSB,* 1 (New York, 1970), pp. 482–83.

60. See L. Premuda in *DSB,* 1 (New York, 1970), pp. 315–16.

61. See M. Florkin in *DSB,* 4 (New York, 1971), pp. 138–40.

62. See G. A. Lindeboom in *DSB,* 12 (New York, 1975), pp. 577–78.

63. For a recent evaluation of Tobias's sources on physics and mechanics, see S. Bolag, "A Selection of Scientific Sources in Hebrew Compositions from the 17th and 18th Centuries" (in Hebrew), *Koroth* 9 (1987): 137–40.

64. See n. 17 above.

heat, which was vital and natural to bodily functions. Galen further regarded all fevers, whether continuous or intermittent, as having a periodic pattern, each form depending upon the putrefaction or decomposition of a particular humor. In sum, this traditional view considered febrile heat as a substantial entity and causal agent in its own right, not as the consequence of physiological changes in the body.[65]

Van Helmont had already criticized this understanding of fevers. In the seventeenth century, the subject was a central issue for a large number of medical writers, especially the chemists. Willis and Sylvius both began their publishing careers with treatises on fevers. As we have seen, both rejected the traditional humoral physiology and explained fever as the result of physical and chemical processes. For Sylvius in particular, an abnormal composition of lymph, pancreatic juice, and bile gave rise to excessive effervescence and agitation that produced the febrile heat. The chemists' view was still transitional and indebted to classical analysis. Nevertheless, their position exemplified a shift from the Galenic physiology of humors and the definition of fever as substance to a new vocabulary of Cartesian corpuscles, chemical constituents, and Harveian circulation that facilitated an understanding of fever as an effect of physiological processes rather than as a causal agent.

Anyone reading Tobias's discussion of fever immediately senses his struggle to reconcile the controversy between the ancients and the moderns. He begins conservatively by attributing fevers to excessive humors and presents their traditional categories.[66] But he soon indicates "that the opinion of the latest doctors is not the same as the ancients'" since the former "consider [the cause of fever] to be dependent on ferments and digestion of the spirits in the body." Upon faithful investigation, Tobias "chooses Sylvius and those who follow him, and especially the great doctor known to me,[67] Ettmüller, who follows in his foot-

---

65. For a comprehensive study of the theories of fever in this period, see W. F. Bynum and V. Nutton, eds., *Theories of Fever from Antiquity to the Enlightenment,* supplement 1 of *Medical History* (London, 1981), esp. the essays of I. M. Lonie, "Fever Pathology in the Sixteenth Century: Tradition and Innovation," pp. 19–44, and D. G. Bates, "Thomas Willis and the Fevers Literature of the Seventeenth Century," pp. 45–70. Further discussions are also found in the literature on Sylvius and Willis mentioned above.

66. *Ma'aseh Tuviyyah,* p. 112a.

67. Perhaps Tobias meant by this that he had met Ettmüller.

steps . . . [all of whom] are possessed by a different spirit in attributing fever to boiling of the blood, that is, in Latin, *[de] fermentatione* . . . which [is called] in the *Gemarah* fermenting wine *[yayin toses]*." The moderns, he adds, recognize two kinds of ferments which result in continuous and intermittent fever.[68]

Before proceeding with his description of the moderns' view of fevers, Tobias inserts the following revealing lines:

> I would not be inclined, loving reader, to press your legs against the wall of my studies, to force you to follow in the path or in the steps of the latest doctors, without deviating to the right or to the left; however, the truth follows its own course. Those moderns, by virtue of perseverance and investigation by way of surgery, labored to make new discoveries in addition to those gained by iatrochemistry, through investigation by cooking, boiling, and the fermentation of wine and other liquids, and through the acidification of all acidy substances. [Accordingly], they established the correct way and enlightened our eyes, and in our generation they discovered the straight and easiest path for doing medicine. Moreover, the patient does not disdain or refuse to take [their medicines].[69]

Such enthusiastic support of the moderns against the ancients should not be taken for unreserved endorsement in all cases. In contrast, after presenting Thomas Willis's five principles as a "modern alternative" to the standard Aristotelian four causes, Tobias responds much more conservatively: "Since my only purpose is to select words from the philosophers that are appropriate for our holy Torah and that agree with the blessed sages, I will enlighten and instruct you with a definite proof and with true arguments that the elements are indeed four, not less and not more." Even "the noble one of the doctors," as he calls Willis, was capable of erring when matters of sacred tradition are concerned.[70] And even with respect to the controversial use of bloodletting in the treatment of fevers, Tobias is more circumscribed. He carefully points out that the ancients "placed their trust in bloodletting for any fever," while the moderns

68. *Ma'aseh Tuviyyah*, pp. 112a–112b.

69. Ibid., p. 112b.

70. Ibid., p. 71a. For an example of the moderns confirming a Torah view opposing Aristotle on the question of whether "women produce seed," see ibid., p. 118a.

(Sylvius, Ettmüller, and their followers) "distanced their path from bloodletting except when in great need."[71] In this instance, and in other places as well, he appears more ambiguous and tentative. The new learning was in the process of overtaking the old, but the latter had not been completely vanquished. It stood side by side with the new, transparently revealing this physician's difficulty in absolutely repudiating the one in favor of the other.

Having described Tobias Cohen's extensive background in contemporary medical literature, especially that written by the iatrochemists, we might finally ask how he acquired this impressive knowledge and what led him to pursue this particular line of inquiry in so conscientious and thoughtful a manner. The easiest way of answering the first question would be to attribute his broad mastery of books and authors to the invention of the printing press. No doubt, the wide diffusion of printed medical and scientific textbooks accounts in part for Tobias's vast and up-to-date knowledge. Moreover, the ability of the press to disseminate knowledge quickly and effectively most certainly accounts for Tobias's desire to publish his book and for its clear and coherent format, including the efficient use of diagrams and illustrations.[72]

Tobias could have also mastered what he did by simply being a good student at Frankfurt or Padua.[73] Although the study of the profession of university teaching in this period is still in its infancy, recent work suggests that Tobias's sophisticated medical knowledge was not so unusual. At Padua, for example, the traditional university statutes obliged professors to convey a clearly defined and unchanging body of knowledge to their students by presenting a standard group of classical texts with traditional commentaries. Thus professors of medical theory taught a three-year course consisting of the works of Hippocrates, Galen, and Avicenna.[74] However, as Nancy Siraisi has recently demonstrated,

71. Ibid., pp. 114a–b.

72. Cf. E. L. Eisenstein, *The Printing Press as an Agent of Change,* 2 vols. (Cambridge, 1979), vol. 2.

73. Note that the majority of his medical sources are northern European; he may have familiarized himself with several of them even before entering the University of Padua.

74. See B. Dooley, "Science Teaching as a Career at Padua in the Early Eighteenth Century: The Case of Giovani Poleni," *History of Universities* 4 (1985): 117–18.

Avicenna's *Canon* was not seen as the last word on the subject; on the contrary, it provided a mere framework for introducing new medical notions and proce-dures.[75] Lorenzo Baccetto, for example, the humble third extraordinary professor of theoretical medicine at Padua in 1687, met his obligations in teaching the *Canon* with extensive references to Gilbert, Bacon, Boyle, Gassendi, Harvey, Van Helmont, Mayow, and other modern authors.[76] And even the less radical but better-known G. Battista Morgagni, teaching medical theory at the univer-sity in the early part of the eighteenth century, successfully integrated modern approaches to physiology and pathology by lecturing on the classical texts. Thus he openly rejected Aristotle's four elements and four primary qualities, exposed his students to more recent work on blood, the lymphatic system, di-gestion, reproduction, and embryology, and frequently quoted the iatrochemical physicians. Among the authors he refers to in his lecture notes, Willis, Syl-vius, Ettmüller, Van Diemerbroeck, Sennert, Dodoens, and Van Helmont figure prominently.[77] Although the first chair in chemistry at Padua was not established until 1749, the opportunities to acquire specialized knowledge of the latest litera-ture in chemical medicine and in other more recent fields were readily available well before that date, and certainly during Tobias's student years.[78]

Such a method of learning had limitations as well as advantages, as Siraisi points out. The university medical student was expected to master his discipline by first familiarizing himself with a classical literature and with the historical contexts of disagreement over ancient theories; only then could he move on to acquire more detailed knowledge, more experience, and even new approaches. Such an educational arrangement fostered "a mental climate where syncretiza-tion and attempted reconciliation of the old and new" were more typical than any thorough or absolute repudiation of the past."[79] Tobias Cohen's textbook

75. Siraisi, *Avicenna in Renaissance Italy*.

76. Ibid., p. 122.

77. Ibid., pp. 213–17. Morgagni's lectures on Galen, Hippocrates, and Avicenna are avail-able in a modern edition of his *Opera postuma*, 7 vols. to date (Rome, 1969-), with modern introductions and indices of sources.

78. See V. Giormani, "I Precedenti dell'istituzione di un insegnamento chimico all'Uni-versità di Padova," *Quaderni per la storia dell'Università di Padova* 18 (1985): 43–91.

79. Siraisi, *Avicenna in Renaissance Italy*, p. 355.

reflects the level of scientific knowledge as well as the syncretistic and harmonizing climate of his university training. No doubt he was a more diligent and committed student than most,[80] overcoming severe hardships to reach his level of expertise. Nevertheless, it would be wrong to exaggerate his intellectual achievements. As *Ma'aseh Tuviyyah* amply testifies, he took full advantage of his educational surroundings to attain an understanding of his field available to the most willing and able of his classmates. Contrary to his own claims, his Hebrew manual was as good as, but not necessarily better than, similar medical textbooks written by non-Jews.

Yet Tobias Cohen's medical and scientific textbook was still unique among Hebrew books published in early modern Europe. As we have seen, other contemporary Jewish scholars attempted to write similar scientific compendia. Joseph Delmedigo and David Gans produced sophisticated and learned introductions to mathematics, physics, and astronomy. Joseph Zahalon, Abraham Wallich, and Issachar Teller wrote medical handbooks. Wallich, Cohen's classmate, similarly displayed his knowledge of chemical physicians like Ettmüller and Willis;[81] so did Isaac Cantarini, another distinguished Jewish graduate of Padua.[82] And there were, of course, recent printed versions of medieval Hebrew textbooks on astronomy and medicine, such as those of Abraham Bar Ḥiyya, Meir Aldabi, Isaac Israeli, and Moses Maimonides; and Hebrew translations of Latin texts, such as those of Avicenna and Peurbach. Yet the relatively limited impact of any of these works underscores the significance of Tobias's effort. Gans's astronomical text was never published in his lifetime and only once in 1743, while Delmedigo's was published in 1629 and only once more in the nineteenth century. Moreover, both were comprehensible only to the most sophisticated student of the sciences. The handbooks of Zahalon, Wallich, and Teller were also published only once and had limited readership. The modest achievements of the last two are hardly comparable, in any case, to the more massive undertaking of Tobias. Cantarini was probably the most erudite

---

80. On the lack of student interest in university study at Padua, see Dooley, "Science Teaching as a Career," pp. 120–22.

81. See, for example, Wallich, *Sefer Dimyon ha-Refu'ot,* pp. 47, 48, 73.

82. See M. Osimo, *Narrazione della strage compiuta nel 1547 contro gli ebrei d'Asolo e cenni biographi della Famiglia Koen-Cantarini* (Casale Monferrato, 1875), p. 74.

physician among Italian Jews in the seventeenth century, yet he wrote *consilia*, not a textbook.[83] And the earlier texts were proving to be hopelessly out of date, reflecting a retrograde body of knowledge and mental outlook, of serious interest primarily for their perceived intrinsic value as sacred literature. In contrast, Tobias's work was both readable—well organized and illustrated, filled with up-to-date and pragmatic information—and attractive, in a spiritual sense, in bolstering Jewish cultural pride. Its multiple editions testify to its enduring popularity.

Thus, by composing a medical textbook in Hebrew, Tobias took full advantage of his university training to address an educational and psychological need he keenly felt. He had discovered in seventeenth-century chemical medicine a body of information that was intellectually appealing and practically useful. By eschewing the mystical enthusiasm, the Christian coloring, and the hermetic and alchemical features of the Paracelsians for a didactic textbook; and by aspiring to train Jewish minds to identify knowledge with the layout of words on the printed page, rather than the divine hieroglyphics of the mysterious natural world, Cohen fully identified himself with an emerging field of study, a chemistry to be studied, methodized, and employed for purely utilitarian purposes rather than one to be experienced or religiously celebrated.[84] In this sense, Tobias had fully imbibed the secular and scientific spirit of his age.

83. The consilia are no longer extant. On Cantarini, see Osimo, *Narrazione,* pp. 76–93; H. A. Savitz, "Dr. Isaac Ḥayyim ha-Cohen Cantarini," *The Jewish Forum* 43 (1960): 80–82, 99–101, 107–8.

84. On the emergence of chemistry in the seventeenth century and its break from iatro-chemistry, see O. Hannaway, *The Chemists and the Word: The Didactic Origins of Chemistry* (Baltimore and London, 1975).

9

Contemporary Science and Jewish Law in the Eyes of Isaac Lampronti and His Rabbinic Interlocutors

The Jewish community of Ferrara in the first half of the eighteenth century, like the rest of Italian Jewry, was dominated by physicians and rabbis, who in most cases were the same persons.[1] No Jew better exemplified this fusion of Jewish legal and scientific expertise than Isaac Lampronti (1679–1756), Ferrara's most illustrious Jewish citizen, a "medico teologo tra i dotti celebratissimo," as a later generation of his fellow citizens once called him.[2]

1. See D. B. Ruderman, "The Impact of Science on Jewish Culture and Society in Venice," in G. Cozzi, ed., *Gli Ebrei e Venezia secoli XIV–XVIII* (Milan, 1987), pp. 417–48, 540–42; idem, *Kabbalah, Magic, and Science: The Cultural Universe of a Sixteenth-Century Jewish Physician* (Cambridge, Mass., 1988); and esp. chap. 3 above.

2. "A most celebrated physician-theologian among the learned." The reference is found on a stone tablet affixed by the citizens of Ferrara on April 19, 1872, to the house which he once occupied. On Lampronti and his work, see B. J. Levi, *Della Vita e dell'opera di Isaaco Lampronti* (Padua, 1871); also published in Hebrew (Lyck, 1871); I. Lampronti, *Paḥad Yiẓḥak,* ed. S. Ashkenazi, 5 vols. to date (Jerusalem, 1961–86), esp. the bibliography cited in 1:1, n. 1; I. Sonne, "Building Stones for the History of the Jews of Italy" (in Hebrew), *Ḥorev* 6 (1941): 76–114; M. Benayahu, "R. Isaac Lampronti and R. Shabbatai Elḥanan Min ha-Zekanim (Hebrew)," *Sinai Sefer ha-Yovel* (Jerusalem, 1957–58), 491–503; J. Klausner, "An Unknown Manuscript of Homilies by R. Isaac Lampronti" (in Hebrew), *Kiryat Sefer* 36 (1960–61): 123–36; B. Cohen, "A List of Authors of Responsa Printed in the *Paḥad Yiẓḥak,*" *Festschrift für Aron Freimann* (Berlin, 1935), 141–43; idem, "A List of Authors of Responsa Printed in the *Paḥad Yiẓḥak*" (in Hebrew), *Sefer ha Yovel*

Educated in both rabbinics and medicine, Lampronti had studied with the distinguished rabbi-physician Isaac Cantarini[3] and then completed his medical studies at the University of Padua. After Padua he resumed his rabbinic studies in Mantua, under the supervision of two other illustrious rabbis, Judah Briel and Joseph Cases. Cases was also a doctor and graduate of the University of Siena;[4] Briel had not formally studied medicine but was well versed in Latin literature and the natural sciences.[5]

Lampronti's career in Ferrara illustrates quite dramatically the successful implementation of the dual tracks of his vocational training. Beginning his career as a teacher in the Italian *talmud torah,* he taught his young pupils Hebrew grammar, Italian, and arithmetic, along with traditional Jewish subjects. His students also enhanced their language skills by translating Lampronti's weekly Italian homilies into Hebrew.[6] When he also employed them as research assistants to copy materials for inclusion in his planned talmudic encyclopedia, the directors of the community objected, claiming this project interfered with his teaching. Undaunted by this rebuff, he continued to work on his life-long project. He published the first journal devoted to issues of Jewish law, the *Bikkurei Kezir Talmud Torah.* Although the journal failed after the third issue, his monumental encyclopedia, the *Pahad Yizhak,* was published in part during his lifetime and

le-Aleksander Marks, ed. D. Frankel (New York, 1943), 41–57 (continuation of previous article); M. Wilensky, "Review Essay of *Sefer ha-Yovel le-Aleksander Marks*" (in Hebrew, with additions to B. Cohen's list), *Kiryat Sefer* 23 (1947): 193–200. The articles of Levi, Cohen, Wilensky, and Sonne were reprinted as an appendix to the edition of the *Pahad Yizhak* which appeared in Jerusalem in 1972–73. See also Y. Raphael, *Rishonim ve-Aharonim* (Tel Aviv, 1957), pp. 203–24; and S. Jarcho, "Dr. Isac Lampronti of Ferrara," *Koroth* 8 (1985): 203–6.

3. On Cantarini, see M. Osimo, *Narrazione della strage compiuta nel 1547 contro gli ebrei d'Asolo e cenni biografici della famiglia Koen-Cantarini* (Casale Monferrato, 1875), pp. 67–93; and H. A. Savitz, "Dr. Isaac Hayyim ha-Cohen Cantarini," *The Jewish Forum* 43 (1960): 80–82.

4. On Cases, see S. Simonsohn, *History of the Jews in the Duchy of Mantua* (Tel Aviv, 1977), p. 700.

5. On Briel, see Simonsohn, *History of the Jews,* pp. 698–99; Carlebach, *Pursuit of Heresy: Rabbi Moses Hagiz and the Sabbatian Controversies* (New York, 1990), pp. 125–33; and W. Horbury, "Judah Briel and Seventeenth-Century Jewish Anti-Christian Polemic in Italy," *Jewish Studies Quarterly* 1 (1993–94): 171–92.

6. See the Klausner article mentioned in n. 2 above.

completed after his death. While functioning as rabbi and head of the *yeshivah,* Lampronti continued to practice medicine and even corresponded on medical subjects with his former teacher Isaac Cantarini among others.[7]

Lampronti's talmudic encyclopedia provides ample evidence of his binary intellectual concerns. Lampronti never hesitates to comment on the medical and scientific aspects of the halakhic issues with which he deals. He refers to contemporary medical opinions, challenges accepted practice uninformed by medical knowledge, quotes medical texts, and enlists the medical opinions of some of his learned Jewish contemporaries.[8] But it is not only the substance of his lengthy rabbinic excursuses that demonstrates this dual allegiance to rabbinics and medicine; it is also indicated by the form of his immense composition, originally written in 120 volumes. Scholars have already noticed the striking resemblance between Lampronti's *yeshivah* and a secular academy for higher learning. One might even suggest that Lampronti's aborted periodical and his completed encyclopedia are both reminiscent of the products of a scientific academy, emerging within a community of scholars and their students working in concert to publish their papers and linking their collective findings together.[9]

In order for Jewish students to enter and succeed in medical schools, Jewish preparatory schools with dual curricula in rabbinic and scientific subjects, along with Latin language instruction, were obviously a necessity. Such institutions existed, at least in theory, from at least the mid-sixteenth century, as demonstrated by the plan of operation of the proposed school of David Provençal in Mantua.[10] Judah Messer Leon probably implemented a similar program of

7. This is all discussed by Levi in his work mentioned in n. 2. See also W. Bacher in *The Jewish Encyclopedia,* 7:601–4, which is based on Levi.

8. See the convenient anthology of such passages in D. Margalit, *Ḥakhmei Yisrael ke-Rofim* (Jerusalem, 1962), pp.152–74.

9. See my discussion on scientific societies in chap. 3 above, as well as in the epilogue below.

10. Provençal's proposal is printed in S. Assaf, *Toledot ha-Ḥinukh be-Yisra'el,* 4 vols. (Jerusalem, 1939–43), 2:115–20. On the education of Jewish physicians in earlier periods, see chap. 1 above.

studies for his own students as early as the late fifteenth century.[11] And similar schools existed in the seventeenth and eighteenth centuries, such as those of Isaac Cantarini and Solomon Conegliano in Padua.[12] Lampronti's academy was obviously shaped along the same lines, but because of its emphasis on imitating the accepted procedures of academic learning—publishing the results of research, compiling and organizing knowledge, and working cooperatively within a communal setting—the school and its literary products became the quintessential Jewish institution of learning in Italy, where Judaism and the biological sciences, along with the propaedeutic language training necessary to pursue both, were meaningfully fused.

In light of the stimulating intellectual environment in which Lampronti and his colleagues labored, it was natural that questions informed by contemporary scientific knowledge should be raised in clarifying and deciding matters of Jewish religious law. This was hardly the first time that Jewish authority based on divine revelation had been challenged by the competing authority of theories and values informed by contemporary scholarship. Indeed, the evolution of the *halakha* and of Jewish legal exegesis in general constitutes an ongoing encounter with such challenges.[13] Yet in Lampronti's day the challenge of contemporary science was especially acute both because of the extraordinary scientific achievements of the age and because, as we have seen, Jewish savants, especially in Italy, had been exposed to an unprecedented degree to formal university instruction and to the plethora of recently published texts in Latin and Italian that heralded the new scientific revolution. One might even state that by Lampronti's time the educated leadership of the Jewish community, like their Christian counterparts,

11. Cf. I. Rabinowitz, Introduction to his edition of Judah Messer Leon, *The Book of the Honeycomb's Flow* (Ithaca and London, 1983), esp. pp. xxvi–xxvii, l–liv.

12. Cf. the references to Cantarini in n. 3 above. Cantarini's school is suggested by his involvement with Lampronti's Paduan studies. On Conegliano's school, see chaps. 3 and 8 above.

13. On the challenge of science to Maimonides' halakhic position, for example, see I. Twersky, "Aspects of Maimonides' Epistemology: Halakah and Science," in J. Neusner, E. S. Frerichs, and N. Sarna, eds., *From Ancient Israel to Modern Judaism, Intellect in Quest of Understanding: Essays in Honor of Marvin Fox,* 3 vols. (Atlanta, 1989), 3:3–24.

were overwhelmed by the dazzling accumulation of new scientific data and the dizzying pace of scientific discovery. No educator and certainly no religious decisor could afford to be oblivious to this conspicuous promontory amid the intellectual expanse of early modern European culture.

A wonderful example of Lampronti's grappling with the challenge of contemporary science to traditional Jewish life involves a lively encounter with his former teacher, Judah Briel, over the issue of killing lice on the Sabbath.[14] Based on the common assumption that lice, unlike fleas, were not living creatures, the *halakha* had permitted the killing of lice on the Sabbath while prohibiting the killing of fleas.[15] The distinction between lice and fleas was clarified especially in Maimonides' code of Jewish law and by its commentators.[16] As Lampronti paraphrased it, the distinction Jewish law drew was "between creatures that reproduced themselves from a male and female or that come into existence from the earth as opposed to those creatures who come into existence from excrement or rotting fruit or the like."[17] Since it was commonly assumed that lice did not sexually reproduce themselves but emanated from moisture in the ground and were equivalent to worms that emanated from dung, it was permitted to kill them at any time.

Of course, by Lampronti's time the assumption of spontaneous generation of any creatures from moisture or dung had been increasingly challenged by contemporary science. Accordingly, he stated the obvious: "I would think that in our days when the naturalists *[ḥakhmei ha-toladot]* observed and witnessed, knew and wrote that every living thing originates from an egg—all this has

14. Lampronti, *Paḥad Yiẓḥak* (Lyck, 1874), "ẓidah," pp. 21a–22b. Boaz Cohen had already noticed this passage in his aforementioned essay and had quoted selections from it without extensive comment.

15. Lampronti refers to the following sources (I have added references to the editions I consulted): *Shulḥan Arukh,* Oraḥ Ḥayyim 316:9; Isaac Alfasi, *Hilkhot ha-Rif Shabbat* (Lemberg, 1868), chap. 14, p. 126; Joshua Boaz, *Shilte Gibborim,* 5, on the same page; and Jair Bacharach, *Ḥavvot Jair* (Frankfurt am Main, 1699), n. 164.

16. Maimonides, *Mishneh Torah,* Shabbat, end of c. 10 and 11:2, and esp. *Maggid Mishneh* in both places.

17. *Paḥad Yiẓḥak,* "ẓidah," p. 21b.

been proven in clear demonstrations—any careful person who fears for his life would avoid such creatures and would not kill either a flea or a louse and not place himself in a situation of possibly being obligated to make a sin offering. Regarding this, I would say that if the sages of Israel might have heard the proofs of the gentile sages, they might have reconsidered and acknowledged [the latter's] opinions."[18]

Yet Lampronti's seemingly self-evident conclusion was nevertheless questionable to him and required confirmation from an independent rabbinic authority in whose judgment he had confidence. Lampronti addressed his query to Briel, who replied fully and unambiguously. Abreast of contemporary scientific theories, Briel nevertheless reached the opposite conclusion from what Lampronti had expected and certainly wished to receive.

Briel's response to the challenge of contemporary scientific opinion was emphatic: "One should not change the rules based on the tradition of our forefathers on account of the research of Gentile scholars."[19] He offered two illustrations to substantiate his conclusion. He first cited the position of Jewish sources regarding the fascination of the evil eye. Like most medieval and early modern persons, Briel accepted the bewitching and harmful effects of the glance of the evil eye as fact.[20] Despite the many Gentile scholars who deny the occult power of the evil eye, he and Jewish law, so he maintained, knew better. Here was an obvious case where "the tradition of our rabbis is sufficient."[21]

His second illustration of the soundness of rabbinic opinion was the oft-quoted statement of the rabbis on whether the spheres were fixed and the stars moved or vice versa.[22] What perplexed numerous Jewish interpreters of this pas-

18. Ibid.
19. Ibid.
20. On the evil eye in Jewish sources, see the convenient summaries and lists of sources by D. Noy in *Encyclopedia Judaica*, 6: 977–1000, and by J. Tractenberg in *Jewish Magic and Superstition* (New York, 1970), pp. 54–56, 283, n. 26. Briel refers explicitly to Naḥmanides' discussion of the matter. Cf. Naḥmanides on Leviticus 18:19. For contemporary Christian sources, see the indices of vols. 6–8 of L. Thorndike, *A History of Magic and Experimental Science*, 8 vols. (New York, 1923–58), under "fascination."
21. *Paḥad Yiẓḥak,* "ẓidah," p. 21b.
22. B.T. Pesaḥim 94b. For a large selection of medieval discussions of the Talmudic passages, see I. Twersky, "Joseph Ibn Caspi: Portrait of a Medieval Jewish Intellectual," in *Studies*

sage was the startling admission by the Jewish sages that they were wrong and the Gentile scholars correct. Briel, like most previous Jewish exegetes, understood this passage as referring to whether the earth was immovable and at the center of the universe while the planets and the sun revolved around it, or whether the sun was immobile and at the center. The rabbis ostensibly had held the latter opinion, which had previously been considered wrong in light of Ptolemaic and Aristotelian science. In the post-Copernican age the rabbis finally had been vindicated: "But, in the end, after many hundred years had passed, all the Gentile astronomers with their investigations based on experience and demonstrations returned to the opinions of our sages and our ancient tradition. And, therefore, we should not budge from what was ruled by our *gemara,* even if all the winds of human sciences come and blow [against] it, for the wind of God speaks in us [compare 2 Samuel 23:2]."[23] Scientific opinion, Briel maintained, was deficient, since the Gentile scholars "knew and understood nature only in its superficialities regarding observable things and not in its internal nature as made known to the receivers of *ma'aseh bereshit* [literally, the act of creation: that is, the rabbis] who were enlightened."[24]

Before considering Lampronti's reaction to his teacher's responsum, we might review the larger context of Briel's defense of rabbinic naturalistic wisdom. By contrast, Maimonides' evaluation of the scientific knowledge of the rabbis had been resoundingly negative, as we have seen. Regarding natural matters, the rabbis never claimed to present the revealed truth, he argued, but only expressed their own fallible opinions.[25] Maimonides thus obviated the necessity of demonstrating the accuracy of all rabbinic statements about the natural world. His view was endorsed by a number of later Jewish thinkers[26] but was

---

in *Medieval Jewish History and Literature* (Cambridge, Mass., and London, 1979), p. 256, n. 52. The passage is also discussed at length with reference to the views of Moses Isserles, the Maharal of Prague, and David Gans in A. Neher, *Jewish Thought and the Scientific Revolution of the Sixteenth Century: David Gans (1541–1613) and His Times,* trans. D. Maisel (Oxford, 1986), pp. 205–218.

23. *Pahad Yizhak,* "zidah," pp. 21b.

24. Ibid.

25. Maimonides, *Moreh Nevukhim,* 2:8, 3:14, discussed in chap. 1 above.

26. See, for example, Isaac Arama, *Akedat Yizhak,* 5 vols. (Pressburg, 1849), sha'ar 36, siman 21.

either ignored or rejected by others. The Maharal of Prague recognized the truth of scientific claims but argued that the rabbis were not competitors with the naturalists. Their knowledge was of a different sort, the knowledge of the essence and not the appearance of things, as Briel later articulated. Rabbinic statements about the natural world represented a kind of metanaturalism, not a mere science of secondary physical causes.[27] Briel's younger contemporary David Gans referred to Brahe's reaction to the rabbinic passage on the spheres and stars. According to Gans, Brahe had insisted that the Jewish sages had been wrong to acknowledge the truth of the Ptolemaic position of the Gentile scholars. The truth—the heliocentric one—lay with them.[28] This passage was clearly the source of Briel's other response. Accordingly, Briel echoed Gans's argument that, in the long run, the accuracy of rabbinic science would prove to be true; he, like the Maharal of Prague, emphasized that the understanding of the rabbis was deeper than that of the naturalists.

Judah Briel's position was embellished by his student Solomon Aviad Sar Shalom Basilea (who was also Lampronti's close friend) in his *Emunat Ḥakhamim*. One of Basilea's major concerns was to exploit contemporary empirical knowledge to discredit the claims of Aristotelian science and to bolster those of the rabbis. He excoriated those who sought to discredit the scientific knowledge of the rabbis and enlisted the aid of his own scientific observations or those of others. When he was unable to reconcile what he knew of reality with the rabbinic view, he attributed the problem to his own finite human wisdom and not to that of the rabbis.[29] He openly declared: "We are unable to deny what the Torah has said and what the rabbis said in their tradition, even if our finite intelligence is unable to comprehend its reason."[30] He too was well aware of Brahe's confirmation of the position of the Jewish sages: "Experience has already shown us in these generations that the truth is that the spheres stand and the stars turn according to the view of the Jewish sages. However, human knowledge will never grasp even a part of the received knowledge of the rabbis until hundreds

27. See chap. 2 above.
28. This is also mentioned in chap. 2 above.
29. See chap. 7 above.
30. Basilea, *Sefer Emunat Ḥakhamim,* p. 7b.

and thousands of years have passed, as happened in the case of the stationary sphere and the moving stars, where all the Gentile scholars initially assumed that the opposite was the case. But afterwards, experience proved that the truth was with the rabbis."[31] In the new empiricism, Basilea had a formidable weapon to defend the rabbis' views on nature. But like Briel he maintained that Jewish tradition, especially the *kabbalah,* understands the essence of nature more profoundly and more fully than any naturalist utilizing the conventional tools of science.[32]

A similar strategy was adopted by David Nieto, an older contemporary of Lampronti and a fellow graduate of Padua, in his *Kuzari ha-Sheni.* In a large section of his defense of the Jewish faith, he reinterprets a number of rabbinic passages on nature to make them conform to contemporary scientific knowledge. At the same time, he underscores the hypothetical character of scientific propositions and the accidental nature of scientific discovery. All this he juxtaposes with the more substantial and reliable positions of the rabbis.[33]

Lampronti undoubtedly was familiar with the positions of Maimonides, the Maharal, and Gans on the credibility of rabbinic statements on nature. He was on intimate terms with Basilea and was probably familiar with his views, since he even praised the publication of his friend's book in the pages of *Pahad Yizhak.*[34] But apparently he had expected a different response from Judah Briel. Instead of endorsing his teacher's answer or at least acknowledging it in silence, he proceeds to praise it faintly and then openly challenges its assumptions: "I observed the decision of the distinguished master of Torah on lice and I declared: 'Very well done, although it goes against common sense completely, for in a confusing and doubtful situation among decisors . . . we should make the decision more severe rather than more lenient.'"[35] Having invited his teacher's answer and

31. *Sefer Emunat Ḥakhamim,* p. 9a.

32. Ibid., esp. chap. 15; cf. chap. 7 above.

33. His thought is fully discussed in chap. 11 below. Lampronti's close associate, Samson Morpurgo, also discussed the passage from B.T. Pesaḥim 94a in his sermons (in manuscript). See Hebrew University and National Library MS Heb 80 3609, fol. 33b. On Murpurgo, see chap. 7 above.

34. See *Pahad Yizhak,* ed. Ashkenazi, 3:5, and *Pahad Yizhak* (Reggio, 1813), letters 'yod-lamed," p. 26b.

35. *Pahad Yizhak,* "zidah," p. 21b.

examined the result, he had no recourse but to produce his own response and to challenge the views of Briel, which were obviously not to his liking.

Lampronti was not prepared to close his eyes to the simple fact that the law regarding lice was based on faulty assumptions, since "the scientists maintained with clear proofs that no species originates from mold, nor do eggs originate from moisture but from living creatures."[36] Lampronti's emphatic rejection of spontaneous generation was probably based on his reading of an important work on the subject that had first appeared in 1668 and was subsequently reprinted in a variety of editions: Francesco Redi's *Esperienze intorno alla generazione degli insetti*. Redi had observed under the microscope the morphological elements characteristic of eggs in various species of insects and concluded that the Aristotelian view of spontaneous generation was untenable. Even if it might appear that decaying animals or plants "give birth to an infinity of worms," the reality was quite different. The putrefying material had no other function than to provide "a suitable place or nest into which, at the time of procreation, the worms or eggs or other seed of worms are brought and hatched by the animals; and in this nest the worms, as soon as they are born, find sufficient food on which to nourish themselves excellently." Through experiments using wide-mouthed flasks containing meat or cheese, Redi confirmed his point.[37] His younger contemporary, Marcello Malpighi, widened Redi's experiments to include the insects of plant galls and reached the same conclusion.[38] For all intents and purposes, the idea of spontaneous generation had no credibility among scientific researchers by the end of the seventeenth century, and Lampronti knew it.

36. Ibid.

37. On Redi and his work, see L. Belloni in the *Dictionary of Scientific Biography* (New York, 1975), 11:341–42, who translates the lines quoted above. See also L. Belloni, "Francesco Redi, biologo," *Celebrazione dell'Accademia del Cimento nel tricentenario della fondazione* (Pisa, 1958), 53–70. I have consulted the modern French translation of Redi's work by A. Sempoux entitled *Expériences sur la génération des insectes et autres écrits de science et de littérature* (Louvain, 1970). A more extensive bibliography on Redi is on pp. xii–xiv. See, most recently, P. Findley, "Controlling the Experiment: Rhetoric, Court Patronage and the Experimental Method of Francesco Redi," *History of Science* 31 (1993): 35–64.

38. On Malpighi, see L. Belloni's essay in the *Dictionary of Scientific Biography* (New York, 1974), 9:62–66, and H. B. Adelmann, *Marcello Malpighi and the Evolution of Embryology* (Ithaca, 1966).

Lampronti consequently could not accept Briel's dismissal of the relevance of contemporary scientific opinion regarding the issue of lice. The *halakha* had to be reformulated in the light of this new understanding of natural processes. And he was unwilling to concede Briel's two other points either. For Lampronti, the lesson to be learned regarding the disagreement between the Jewish and Gentile sages over the mobility of the spheres or the stars was quite different from what Briel had claimed. The fact that the Jews had acknowledged the truth of the Gentile position indicates quite firmly "that not every statement made in the *gemara* derives from the [sanctified] tradition. Rather, the Jewish sages sometimes expressed themselves on the basis of their intelligence and human investigation [alone] and not according to the tradition. If this were not the case, why would they acknowledge [their mistake]?"[39] In maintaining that the views of the Jewish sages on such matters of astronomy were strictly personal opinions, he was following the position of Maimonides.

Lampronti continued: "And if in our own time there are Gentile sages like Copernicus who maintain that the spheres are stationary [as the Jewish sages had argued], the number who maintain and prove the opposite are also not insignificant. Such matters are not arithmetical sciences, that is, mathematics, whereby a person is able to present clear and accurate propositions and indubitable proof to which his opponent is unable to counter or respond. Rather [in this case], each party makes its separate claims and each presents its arguments in favor of its own opinions."[40]

Lampronti's uncertainty about the theory of heliocentricity is not unusual, even for the eighteenth century. A number of contemporary Jewish scientific writers, including Tobias Cohen and David Nieto, had voiced similar views.[41] Of greater interest is his argument regarding the theoretical nature of the sciences, that Copernicus need not be wrong since no one can offer certain proof, as in mathematics, to either affirm or deny his position. In upholding such a "mitigated skepticism,"[42] Lampronti not only aligned himself with such pious

39. *Paḥad Yiẓḥak,* "ẓidah," p. 21b.

40. Ibid., pp. 21b–22a.

41. See chap. 8 above and chap. 11 below.

42. See R. Popkin, *The History of Scepticism from Erasmus to Spinoza,* 2d ed. (Berkeley, 1979), chap. 7. I have already used the term in describing Figo's posture in chap. 6 above.

scientific enthusiasts as Gassendi and Mersenne, who viewed scientific theories as mere descriptions of appearances rather than of reality itself, but also shared a perception of several other Jewish thinkers. Both Nieto and Basilea had arrived at similar conclusions with respect to the scientific systems of Descartes, the atomists, the chemical philosophers, and the Aristotelians.[43] Each of these systems upheld rational and self-consistent understandings of the real world. But they were only hypothetical understandings; no position could make greater truth claims than the next. Rather, "each party makes its separate claims and brings its own arguments in favor of its opinions," as Lampronti had argued. Like his contemporaries, Lampronti understood precisely the theoretical nature of scientific claims. Briel might have countered by asking why Redi's understanding of generation was more valid than Aristotle's, if both were mere theories. And Lampronti's answer would probably have been that although both views ultimately rested on appearances, in the light of Redi's careful observations under the microscope, Redi's theory was more convincing and probably more correct than Aristotle's. The difference between the two, in this case, was attributable to the quality of the instruments of observation. Until Redi's theory was disproved with new and better evidence, his informed opinion would hold true. Although it was not identical with reality, it most closely approximated it.

Lampronti did agree with Briel in accepting the fascination of the evil eye.[44] Here too, he maintained, there were theoreticians in both camps—those who denied the notion of fascination and others, such as Pliny and Ovid, along with the rabbis, who affirmed its facticity.[45] That Lampronti could uphold a seemingly modernist anti-Aristotelian position in the case of Redi while simultaneously suspecting the Copernican view and displaying no discomfort at all with the notion of the evil eye reveals the confusing and often contradictory directions of religious thinkers shifting in the often murky and uncharted waters of the new sciences. And Briel, with all his conservatism regarding the unimpeachable authority of the rabbis and Aristotle alike, ironically wore the hat of the Coper-

43. See Basilea, *Sefer Emunat Ḥakhamim* (Mantua, 1730), pp. 4a–4b. Nieto is discussed in chap. 11 below.

44. *Paḥad Yizḥak,* "ẓidah," p. 22a.

45. See Pliny, *Natural History* 28, 6, and C. Thorndike, *A History of Magic and Experimental Science* (New York, 1958), 1:83, 217.

nican in the debate. Neither associate had yet worked out a clear and consistent strategy concerning the challenge of the new sciences to their faith; yet neither could afford to ignore it.

The case of lice was not the only instance of Lampronti's sensitivity to the intrusion of contemporary scientific opinion into the process of determining the *halakha*. Sometimes he willingly offers his medical and scientific knowledge, even citing known authorities, to affirm or deny a particular legal assumption.[46] At other times he is less tolerant, even belligerent about considering such "Gentile opinion," since the Jewish sages understand much more, "for God spoke truth through their mouths."[47] In one instance, he attempts to formulate a general strategy for dealing with the problem of the competing authorities of contemporary scientific opinion and rabbinic wisdom.

Lampronti offers this formulation when evaluating the credibility of a rabbinic passage that the kidneys in the human body are the seat of deliberation.[48] As the passage in the Talmud explains: "One kidney urges a person to do good and one to do bad, and it seems that the one to do good is on the right and the one to do evil is on the left." Here was as good a case as any for dismissing the scientific claims of rabbinic utterances. Lampronti's easiest tack would have been to invalidate this statement as part of the revealed tradition and to argue in a Maimonidean fashion that it was merely the opinion of an individual rabbi which could then be discounted. Instead, he proceeds to argue in a manner reminiscent of that of his teacher, Judah Briel, even to the extent of using the same language and references. He first declares that despite the seemingly impressive achievements of the natural philosophers, their knowledge remains superficial, since they do not possess a deep understanding of a thing, its constitution, manner of assembly, strength and vitality, its ultimate difference from other things, and the reason for a change in its form. In contrast, "the knowledge of our sages is deep, for they stood in the secret [that is, counsel] of God,

46. Consult the useful anthology of Margalit, but see esp. the following entries in the *Pahad Yizhak:* "oznayim la-kotel," "besar dagim," "nozot," "nital ha-lev," "ketoret," and "telata kevei havu."

47. See esp. his discussion of "nikkur."

48. *Pahad Yizhak,* "kelayot yo'azot," a discussion of a passage found in B.T. Berakhot 61a.

as it is written: 'The secret of the Lord is for those who fear Him [Psalm 25:14].'
This is the science of *ma'aseh bereshit* [literally, the act of creation], as R. Nissim
[Gerondi] explained in his sermons.[49] . . . One who knows and recognizes it can
do wonders much better than the naturalists who pride themselves in performing the science of alchemy and natural magic. In the final analysis, the human
eye cannot see what the [divine] eye that shines upon it observes, the light of
true knowledge."[50]

By quoting the same line in Psalms and the same reference to R. Nissim's
sermons, Lampronti was echoing the sentiments of his teacher in his aforementioned responsum that previously he had rejected.[51] Had he reversed himself
completely in now arguing that contemporary science as practiced in his day
was superficial and inferior in every respect to the deep insight and higher magic
of rabbinic sapience?

Perhaps sensing his own inconsistency, Lampronti attempts to explain his
overall exegetical strategy when interpreting rabbinic passages that purport to
offer information about the natural world:

When I come to [rabbinic] passages that deal with natural matters, I am accustomed to interpret them in either of two ways: First, according to a view
of the ancient philosophers [the ancient naturalists and their more recent
interpreters] even when they deviated from a view of one of our sages and
those who followed them. This is not a defect in the wisdom of our sages,
for many times they did not speak [with the authority] of the tradition in
such matters. In such a way, the author of the *Me'or Einayim* explained in
the name of Maimonides.[52] Or, second, by the truth which they [the rabbis]

49. See Nissim ben Reuben Gerondi, *Derashot ha-Ran,* ed. L. A. Feldman (Jerusalem, 1974),
sermon 1, 10–11.

50. Ibid.

51. Compare Briel's statement in his responsum *Paḥad Yiẓḥak,* "ẓidah," p. 21b: "So it is
written: 'He issues his commands to Jacob [Psalm 147:19] and 'the secret of the Lord is for
those who fear Him [Psalm 25:14].' The Gentile sages knew and understood nature only in
its superficialities regarding observable things and not in its internal nature as the receivers
of *ma'aseh bereshit* were enlightened, as R. Nissim explained in his sermons."

52. Azariah de' Rossi, *Me'or Einayim* (Vilna, 1866) quotes Maimonides *(Moreh Nebukhim*
3:14) in 1:156 and 2:269. Cf. L. Segal, *Religious Consciousness and Religious Tradition in Aẓariah*

knew by traditional knowledge even if it is hidden to the naturalists, even if it doesn't appear possible to reconcile the matter according to their [the naturalists'] way.

With respect to the passage on the kidneys, Lampronti adopts the second approach: "Although the doctors and naturalists didn't speak in such a way [about them], one should not bring a proof against their [the rabbis'] tradition, for Scripture speaks of God examining the hearts and kidneys . . . and the Torah associates them [the kidneys] with advice."[53]

Upon examining Lampronti's two approaches, one is struck by their sheer inconsistency. Lampronti had obviously hoped to dispel confusion by his clarification, yet he seems to have attained the opposite result. By stating clearly his first strategy, he reiterated the position of Maimonides that the rabbis were not transmitting the words of the prophets but only their individual opinions on matters of nature—the same approach he had taken in his responsum on not killing lice on the Sabbath. But there was a new twist in this formulation. He identified this position with that of Azariah de' Rossi, the sixteenth-century scholar of rabbinic and classical chronology and author of the highly acclaimed but controversial *Me'or Einayim*.[54] De' Rossi had indeed quoted the passage of Maimonides about rabbinic statements on astronomy, but on more than one occasion. Initially, he had cited the passage to refer specifically to matters of astronomy, but later he used the same passage to support a much broader and more audacious position.[55] De' Rossi argued that Maimonides' dictum could be understood to apply not only to astronomical matters but to all subjects un-

---

de' Rossi's *"Meor Einayim"* (Philadelphia, 1988), chap. 7; and see my remarks on de' Rossi in chaps. 1 and 2 above.

53. *Paḥad Yiẓḥak,* "kelayot yo'aẓot."

54. See R. Bonfil, "Some Reflections on the Place of Azariah de Rossi's *Me'or Enayim* in the Cultural Milieu of Italian Renaissance Jewry," in *Jewish Thought in the Sixteenth Century,* ed. B. Cooperman (Cambridge, Mass., and London, 1983), 23–48; Bonfil, ed., *Kitve Aẓariah min ha-Adumim* (Jerusalem, 1991). De' Rossi's views on the natural world are treated most recently by J. Weinberg, "The Voice of God: Jewish and Christian Responses to the Ferrara Earthquake of November 1570," *Italian Studies* 46 (1991): 69–81.

55. See the references in n. 52 above and Segal's discussion of them, which I have consulted.

SCIENCE AND JEWISH LAW

related to the incontestable matters of the Oral Law: "It is unnecessary to be particular where the sages' words do not conform to known truth since they had not spoken on the issue in the matter of a prophetic tradition but only as scholars of the time with respect to that matter, or because they heard it from scholars of those times."[56] Accordingly, de' Rossi argued, rabbinic opinion was not binding "in matters which by their very nature could not conceivably have been uttered at Sinai, as for example some historical account . . . or matters which you clearly know they stated as their own opinion, unobliged by Holy Scripture."[57]

Did Lampronti have in mind de' Rossi's first quotation of Maimonides or his second? In the second quotation de' Rossi had clearly stretched Maimonides' original intention to imply that any time the rabbis opined on speculative non-legal matters, they were not doing so in the name of a sacred tradition but were merely stating their own individual views. They were only reflecting the level of knowledge of their cultural surroundings, and therefore they could be wrong on any subject outside the narrow confines of the law. Any sensitive reader of *Me'or Einayim* would have noticed that this second reading of Maimonides was in fact the central and most provocative theme of de' Rossi's penetrating historicism. By going out of his way to quote Maimonides within the text of de' Rossi, instead of quoting Maimonides alone, Lampronti not only revealed his awareness of de' Rossi's daring position but seemed to concur with it. Accordingly, he felt fully justified in discounting the uninformed rabbinic view of spontaneous generation and adopting the more scientifically accurate contemporary opinion of Redi.

Yet Lampronti would not allow the first approach to stand without the second. When all is said and done, when no reconciliation between science and the rabbinic view seems possible, one is obligated to accept the rabbinic view, he contended. By appending his second approach, Lampronti again reversed himself completely, returning to the traditionalist camp of Nissim, Briel, Basilea, and others.

We are left in doubt as to the true position of Isaac Lampronti. In attempting

56. De' Rossi, *Me'or Einayim*, 2:269.
57. Ibid., 2:270.

to clarify his views, he had obfuscated them even more. Lampronti's equivocation regarding the authority of contemporary science, I contend, is more than an isolated example of a Jewish response to the new sciences of the early modern era. It is symptomatic of the formidable intellectual challenge science was mounting in a variety of guises and in multiple avenues of Jewish intellectual life, several of which we have already considered in this book. As it was for Christians, the process of rethinking privileged and cherished assumptions about the ultimate soundness and veracity of revealed traditions triggered by the scientific revolution constituted a Jewish intellectual endeavor of primary importance. And the sacred domain of the *halakha* was by no means immune from this new scrutiny.

Lampronti and his contemporaries, from Jonathan Eybeschutz to Ḥakham Ẓevi to Jacob Emden to other important rabbinic decisors, had more to worry about than the highly publicized heresy of the false messiah, Shabbatai Ẓevi, and his vociferous followers. They were involved to an unprecedented degree in the same process of evaluating and sifting contemporary scientific evidence in order to resolve issues of Jewish law.[58] That no consensus emerged, that they vacillated like Lampronti in both protesting and succumbing to the weight of the impressive, even dazzling findings of the new sciences, that they were becoming increasingly sensitive about seemingly outmoded and uninformed ancestral traditions, suggests above all how pervasive and significant a factor scientific culture had become in their mental universe. Their confusion and bewilderment no doubt reflect the same growing sense of insecurity and inferiority that we have seen in such writers as Tobias Cohen, Samson Morpurgo, and Solomon Basilea, engendered by the new intellectual vistas of their age. They no doubt had reason to believe that the religious and social foundations of Jewish communal life were beginning to erode.

58. A small sampling of representative texts on the problems raised by contemporary science would include Ḥakham Ẓevi Ashkenazi, *She'elot u-Teshuvot* (Jerusalem, 1970), nos. 64, 66, 74, 76, 77, 93; Jonathan Eybeschutz, *Kereti u-Feleti* (Warsaw, 1878; repr. Brooklyn, 1979), no. 40; idem, *Bene Ahuvah* (Prague, 1819; repr. Jerusalem, 1965), pt. 2, p. 47a; pt. 3, pp. 12a–15b; Jacob Emden, *Iggeret Bikkoret* (Zhitomir, 1868), pp. 3b–6b, 39b–43b; idem, *She'elat Yaveẓ* (Lemberg, 1884), pt. 1, nos. 41, 121; Samson Morpurgo, *Shemesh Ẓedakah* (Venice, 1743), no. 29; and Jacob Reischer, *Shevut Ya'akov* (Lemberg, 1860), pt. 1, no. 97. Other sources are collected by H. J. Zimmels in *Magicians, Theologians, and Doctors* (London, 1952).

The Community of Converso Physicians

RACE, MEDICINE, AND THE SHAPING OF A CULTURAL IDENTITY

Notwithstanding their large numbers and conspicuous presence in the Netherlands, Italy, southern France, Germany, and elsewhere from the late sixteenth century on, the converso émigrés who returned to Judaism, many of whom were university-trained physicians, have hardly been perceived as major contributors to the scientific revolution. Yosef Kaplan's recent assessment appears quite decisive: "Despite the relatively large number of Sephardic Jewish physicians in those generations, including prominent scientists (such as Amatus Lusitanus, Elijah Montalto, Abraham Zakut, known as Zacutus Lusitanus, and many others), they took no part in the scientific revolution in the field of medicine." Kaplan offers an explanation for this seeming anomaly: "This might derive from a certain paradox: In Spain and Portugal during the sixteenth and seventeenth centuries medicine had become 'a Jewish profession' because of the high percentage of 'New Christians' among the physicians in the Iberian peninsula. Many of them occupied prominent positions in this field and also taught in the most important universities: hence they were too closely involved in the classical medical establishment to be open to new initiatives and conceptual changes, which are known to have arisen outside the walls of the universities."[1]

1. I quote from a typescript version of an essay in the forthcoming proceedings of a conference devoted to Prof. Jacob Katz's *Tradition and Crisis,* held at Harvard University in 1988, entitled "An Alternative Path to Mod-

Kaplan's assessment of the scientific importance of this large professional community is generally confirmed by historians of Spanish medicine. In the second half of the sixteenth century, the innovations engendered by the Paracelsian revolution dramatically retreated, to be replaced by the study of the classic texts of Avicenna, Hippocrates, and Galen alone. The primary literary output of the medical establishment was commentaries on these texts, which were known primarily in their Latin translations. The commentaries were no more than scholastic glosses, containing little evidence of clinical observation and empirical verification of anatomical data.[2] Kaplan's sweeping conclusion regarding the converso community may be premature, however, in light of the fact that most of the medical writings of its distinguished membership have not yet been systematically studied. Moreover, it fails to factor in the intellectual stimulus many of these doctors received from medical environments outside of Spain, such as Germany and the Netherlands.[3] Perhaps the real contribution of this group lay in the practice rather than in the theory of medicine, as they themselves testify.[4]

---

ernity: The Portuguese Jews of Amsterdam in Early Modern Times," pp. 22–23. The article subsequently appeared in Hebrew as "The Path of Western Sephardi Jewry to Modernity," in *Pe'amim* 48 (1991): 85–103; the quotation appears on p. 92. See also Y. Kaplan, "Jewish Students at the University of Leiden in the Seventeenth Century" (in Hebrew), *Studies in the History of Dutch Jewry* 2 (1979): 65–76.

2. J. M. López Piñero and F. Bujoso Homan, "Tradición y renovación en la medicina española del siglo XVI," *Asclepio* 30–31 (1978–79): 285–306; Piñero, *La Introducción de la ciencia moderna en España* (Barcelona, 1968); idem, *Ciencia y técnica en la sociedad Española de los siglos XVI y XVII* (Barcelona, 1979), esp. pp. 73–77; G. Ballester, *Historia social de la medicina en la España de los siglos XIII al XVI* (Madrid, 1976); R. L. Kagan, "Universities in Castille, 1500–1700," *Past and Present* 49 (1970): 71; idem, *Students and Society in Early Modern Spain* (Baltimore, 1974).

3. See, for example, the up-to-date references to seventeenth-century medicine and chemistry in Rodrigo and Benedict de Castro's writing, discussed below in this chapter. One wonders whether it is possible to detect a shift in methodological perspective on the part of the transplanted converso physicians: from that of the classical medical establishment in Spain and Portugal to a more open and innovative one, the result of their new encounters with the northern European centers of medicine and science. The subject requires more careful investigation.

4. This is the claim made by Huarte de San Juan, as well as by Rodrigo and Benedict de Castro. See below.

Be that as it may, I would like to pose a different sort of question than the one Kaplan addresses: What contribution did the converso medical community make to shaping a Jewish cultural identity in the early modern period? Having examined the broader cultural import of eastern European and especially Italian Jewish encounters with medicine and scientific activity, we must now consider those of this new community as well. Surely the influx of hundreds of prominent doctors—many of them well known in their fields, carrying distinguished university degrees, often singled out and hounded by the Inquisition before gaining their freedom—could hardly go unnoticed by the Jewish communities they gradually infiltrated and in which they eventually set up medical practice. Their prominent positions in both Jewish and Christian society engendered a range of reactions regarding their professional competence, particularly in comparison with Christian physicians, their often affluent lifestyles, their sometimes tenuous loyalty to Jewish religious norms, and the nature of their affiliation with the organized Jewish community.[5] And their own adjustment to a new Jewish lifestyle, with its accompanying stresses and strains, as Jewish physicians now attending to Jewish as well as Christian patients, was bound to elicit from them an emerging sense of the Jewish nature of their medical enterprise.

The following observations about Sephardic physicians are necessarily preliminary both because of the vastness of the subject and because of my limited competency to evaluate properly the large corpus of medical writings these individuals left behind. Nevertheless, there is sufficient evidence to suggest that the intrusion of a relatively large community of medical professionals with a substantial education in medicine and the natural sciences did inject a new and important cultural element into the Jewish communities with which they affili-

5. I have not bothered to list the rich bibliography on the conversos and their western European diaspora of the seventeenth century. For additional references, see Y. Kaplan, "The Problem of the Anusim and New Christians in the Historical Research of the Last Generation" (in Hebrew), in M. Zimmerman, M. Stern, and Y. Salmon, eds., *Iyyunim Be-Historiografia* (Jerusalem, 1988), 117–44; Kaplan, "The Portuguese Community in Amsterdam in the Seventeenth Century: Between Tradition and Change" (in Hebrew), *Proceedings of the Israel Academy of Science and the Humanities* 7 (1988): 161–81; idem, *From Christianity to Judaism: The Story of Isaac Orobio de Castro* (Oxford, 1989); and his two synthetic essays on the western Sephardic diaspora in H. Beinart, ed., *Moreshet Sefarad* (Jerusalem, 1992), pp. 562–621 (translated into English as *The Sephardic Legacy* [Jerusalem, 1993]).

ated. Specifically, these physicians of Spanish and Portuguese origin found a common professional and cultural agenda with other Jewish graduates of medical schools in Italy and elsewhere in Europe, creating a kind of informal medical and scientific fellowship among Jews, and projecting themselves as a kind of intellectual and cultural elite within their own communities. They helped to define a Jewish cultural identity along strictly secular and professional lines. Several of them even contributed to discussions of the nature of religious belief and epistemological uncertainty, even applying their own rational and naturalistic sensibilities to a radical rereading of the biblical text and the Jewish religious tradition. But most significantly, despite their often limited exposure to Jewish learning and religious observance, their notions of the Jewish self in relation to the Christian other that most had repudiated were profoundly fused with their professional identities as medical writers and clinicians.

We might begin this discussion by recalling two areas alleged by others to constitute, in some respects, a specifically converso contribution to scientific discourse both within the Jewish community and beyond it: A strong skeptical posture undermining the shaky intellectual foundations of scholasticism and prescribing a probabilistic empiricism as a realistic basis for human knowledge, on the one hand; and on the other the application of scientific criteria to the study of sacred scripture, thereby unleashing a radical critique of the methods and assumptions of traditional biblical and religious study. The first area is primarily associated with the writing of Francisco Sanchez (1551–1623), the second with Isaac La Peyrère (1596–1676) and Benedict Spinoza (1632–1677).

Born and baptized in Tuy, in northwestern Spain, Sanchez studied medicine at the Collège de Guyenne in Bordeaux. After a long sojourn in Italy, where he was exposed to new approaches to medicine and scientific methodology, he returned to southern France, completing his doctorate at the University of Montpellier in 1574. He eventually taught philosophy and medicine at the University of Toulouse, an institution already renown for a Portuguese converso faculty that included Manuel Alvares, Pedro Vaz Castelo, and Baltazar Orobio de Castro, later called Isaac Orobio.[6]

6. For a succinct and up-to-date biography of Sanchez, see the introduction of E. Librick to Francisco Sanchez, *That Nothing Is Known (Quod nihil scitur)*, trans. D. F. S. Thomson

Sanchez's *Quod nihil scitur,* published in Lyons in 1581, is a lucid and pene-trating critique of Aristotelianism, laying the foundation for a new rationality resting on practical learning, empiricism, and experimentation. Sanchez's doubts about the scholastic system of knowledge and the syllogism led him to adopt a constructive skepticism that allowed for assent to probable testimonies based on the best and most consistently tested empirical data available.

Sanchez's skepticism has often been linked to that of Michel de Montaigne, although the former's work had a more circumscribed impact on a primarily philosophical and medical community. The evidence for a meaningful relation between the two is scanty, although Montaigne was distantly related to Sanchez through his mother. Both attended the Collège de Guyenne, although not at the same time, and both appear to have been affiliated with the Portuguese converso community of émigrés there and in Toulouse.[7]

Most recently, José Faur has attempted to read Sanchez's work with an eye to recapturing the faint Jewish identity of its author, thus reclaiming him for Jewish intellectual history and situating his new rationality within the context of the spiritual crisis precipitated in no small part by the converso situation. While admitting that Sanchez's innermost convictions about Judaism are never fully transparent, he adduces several tantalizing hints strewn throughout the book which suggest a positive feeling for Judaism, even a sense of pride and identifi-cation with the Jewish community. These include Sanchez's warm dedication to the converso doctor Jacob de Castro, his frequent use of Old Testament verses, especially from Ecclesiastes, and, most prominently, several unusual citations which, when decoded by Faur, reveal his indebtedness to Maimonides and even

---

(Cambridge, 1988). See A. Moreira de Sa, *Francisco Sanchez,* 2 vols. (Lisbon, 1947); Francisco Sanchez, *Opera philosophica,* ed. J. de Carvalho (Coimbra, 1955), Introduction. On the Collège de Guyenne, see E. Gaullieur, *Histoire du Collège de Guyenne* (Paris, 1874); R. Trinquet, *La Jeunesse de Montaigne* (Paris, 1972), pp. 409–507. On the Portuguese community at Toulouse, see J. Verissimo Serrão, *Les Portugais à l'Université de Toulouse, xiii–xvii siècles* (Paris, 1970); G. Nahon, *Les "Nations" juives portugaises du Sud-Ouest de la France (1684–1791)* (Paris, 1981); and Kaplan, *From Christianity to Judaism,* pp. 97–103.

7. See Limbrick, *That Nothing Is Known,* pp. 79–81. J. Faur, *In the Shadow of History: Jews and Conversos at the Dawn of Modernity* (Albany, 1992), pp.105–8.

to the rabbinic work *The Ethics of the Fathers [Avot]*.[8] Sanchez was clearly influenced by another thinker of converso background, Juan Luis Vives;[9] he also cites the converso doctor Amatus Lusitanus.[10] While the *Quid nihil scitur* can hardly be construed as a work of Jewish advocacy, Faur makes a plausible case that its author, at the very least, harbored a positive feeling toward Judaism and that his skeptical posture is somehow linked to the latter.

The problem with Faur's reading of Sanchez is obvious. As Faur admits, Sanchez's Jewish identity remains elusive, nor can it be shown that his constructive skepticism is ultimately attributable to his converso identity rather than to Galen, to his Italian university studies, or simply to his disillusionment with the scholastic curriculum of his day.[11] When one attempts to link his strivings to those of Montaigne or to an even larger group of converso thinkers, to propose a kind of converso mentality "rooted in the spiritual crisis of the Iberian peninsula,"[12] the evidence is slim indeed. No one would deny the existential challenges of the conversos, their sense of alienation and uprootedness, as factors in understanding the spiritual makeup of men like Sanchez and even Montaigne. The work of Americo Castro, Stephan Gilman, and others offers a persuasive argument for viewing the converso dilemma as a key to understanding a critical part of Spanish literary sensibility in the sixteenth century, and we shall have an opportunity to return to their work below. But can skepticism, as it emerged in the sixteenth century, be reduced o a converso mood or intellectual style? Is Sanchez's skepticism ultimately a Jewish or converso perspective on the reality of his day? Despite Sanchez's coded Jewish messages, such as citing Romans to disguise an authentic Maimonidean utterance,[13] he remained

8. Faur, *In the Shadow of History,* pp. 87–109.

9. On Vives, see R. Guerlac, *Jean Luis Vives against the Pseudodialecticians: A Humanist Critique on Medieval Logic* (Dordrecht, 1979); Limbrick, *That Nothing Is Known,* pp. 33–34; and C. G. Norena, *Juan Luis Vives* (The Hague, 1970).

10. Limbrick, *That Nothing Is Known,* p. 214.

11. Reading the editor's introduction to *That Nothing is Known,* for example, the reader is only faintly aware of the converso background as a relevant factor in understanding Sanchez's skepticism. For Limbrick, the medical background of Sanchez and its connection with philosophy are critical.

12. Faur, *In the Shadow of History,* p. 88.

13. Ibid., p. 95.

a Catholic in the heavily Catholic city of Toulouse. Although his impact on the medical and philosophical community of southern France is apparent, and he seems to have been known by Descartes and other Christian thinkers well into the seventeenth century,[14] there is virtually no evidence of his influence on Montaigne or, for that matter, on any other Jewish or converso thinker.

To what extent did a constructive skeptical position like that of Sanchez capture the mood of the larger community of conversos who had returned to Judaism in the late sixteenth and seventeenth centuries? The issue has not yet been fully addressed. We have observed the surprising skeptical tendencies of Simone Luzzatto, the Venetian rabbi,[15] but Luzzatto had no obvious links to the converso community; despite his direct access to the sources of Pyrrhonian skepticism in Italy, he reveals no awareness of Sanchez's book. In contrast to the depth and consistency of Luzzatto's skeptical ruminations, the single and isolated statements of other converso writers do not invite any general conclusions regarding an overall converso skeptical posture.

Yosef Yerushalmi has pointed to the following statement of Isaac Cardoso in his *Las Excelencias de los Hebreos:* "And, in truth, Israel does not cultivate human sciences, nor treat of uncertain philosophy nor of doubtful medicine, nor of false astrology, nor of fallacious chemistry, nor of secret magic. It does not care to know the histories of the nations, nor the chronologies of the times, nor the politics of the rulers. All of its intent and desire is to study the law, and to meditate on its precepts, in order to keep and do them."[16] Cardoso's position stands in sharp contrast to his general appreciation for the cultivation of the human sciences, articulated often in his *Philosophia libera.* Yerushalmi explains this apparent shift as part of a general cultural oscillation among contemporary Jews between attraction and resistance to "Gentile" wisdom. Yosef Kaplan, on the other hand, compares this passage of Cardoso with similar sentiments expressed by both Isaac Orobio de Castro and Antonio Enriques Gomez, and relates them all to the diffusion of skeptical currents in sixteenth- and seventeenth-century

14. Limbrick, *That Nothing Is Known,* pp. 79–86.

15. See chap. 5 above.

16. I. Cardoso, *Las Excelencias de los Hebreos* (Amsterdam, 1679), p. 135; Y. Yerushalmi, *From Spanish Court to Italian Ghetto: Isaac Cardoso: A Study in Seventeenth-Century Marranism and Jewish Apologetics* (New York, 1971), p. 371.

Europe. Kaplan judiciously balances such sentiments against the still powerful roots of Neoscholastic thought in each of these thinkers. Isaac Orobio's skeptical statements about the incapacity of human beings to comprehend supernatural matters emerge within his polemical writings against the Remonstrant theologian Philip van Limborch and the converso deist Juan de Prado.[17] His criticism of the study of chemistry is directed against hermeticism and Paracelsianism rather than against scientific inquiry in general.[18] In short, such utterances do not yield a systematic and comprehensive skeptical position but only a limited appreciation and flirtation with it. In his eclectic mind, Isaac Orobio could freely draw from the dominant streams of Neoscholastic thought while discovering a kind of "spiritual refuge" from its "conceptual constraints"[19] in skepticism. Whether or not he had access to Sanchez's or Montaigne's thinking from his own sojourn in Toulouse, skepticism only affected him lightly and selectively. In the absence of more compelling testimony, Kaplan seems correct to refrain from making far-reaching conclusions as to the links between the crypto-Jewish community and skeptical thought.[20] Sanchez's rigorous criticisms of scholastic reasoning and pedagogy apparently did not succeed in converting even the conversos who fully shared his background in medicine and philosophy.

Some twenty-five years ago, Richard Popkin cogently argued that the conflict between theology and science in the seventeenth century emerged neither from Copernican heliocentricism nor from the mechanistic philosophies but from the application of "scientific" techniques to the study of the Bible, ultimately undermining the miraculous and mysterious foundations of Judeo-Christianity. He singled out the radical theories of the alleged converso thinker Isaac La Peyrère (1596–1676) and his disciples (as Popkin called them) Benedict Spinoza and Richard Simon.[21] Assuming that La Peyrère's ancestry was converso, as Popkin maintains, the well-established fact that Spinoza was born to converso parents

17. Kaplan, *From Christianity to Judaism,* pp. 319–22.

18. See D. Ruderman, review of original Hebrew edition of Kaplan's *From Christianity to Judaism, Zion* 49 (1984): 306–13.

19. This is Kaplan's phrase, *From Christianity to Judaism,* p. 321.

20. Ibid., p. 321–22.

21. R. H. Popkin, "Scepticism, Theology, and the Scientific Revolution in the Seventeenth Century," in I. Lakatos and A. Musgrave, eds., *Problems in the Philosophy of Science* (Amster-

in Amsterdam tempt one to conclude that this new "scientific" assault on religion was propelled by forces stemming primarily from within the converso community. A closer look at Popkin's thesis is in order.

Popkin's initial observations on the significance of Isaac La Peyrère has led to several essays, a revised chapter in his classic account of European skepticism, and finally a complete monograph.[22] La Peyrère's significance for biblical criticism rests on his polygenetic account of the origins of humanity, commonly referred to as his pre-Adamite thesis: his denial that Moses was the author of the Torah and that various biblical accounts were accurate; and his attempt to separate human and Jewish history as depicted in the Bible by considering the physical, cultural, and geographical differences among various human groups. According to Popkin, La Peyrère's secularization of human history and its severance from biblical history launched major investigations in anthropology and biblical criticism in subsequent centuries. Although there is no evidence that La Peyrère and Spinoza knew each other, it seems clear that Spinoza was familiar with La Peyrère's ideas and that he was influenced by him without subscribing in the least to his bizarre messianic theories.[23]

Popkin admits that the circumstantial evidence for La Peyrère's converso background is not overwhelming and that all one can conclude is that he was most likely of Jewish origin.[24] On the basis of his unique messianic vision of a kind of fusion of Jewish and Christian theologies, Popkin maintains that La Peyrère held a distinctly "marrano" vision of the world, a "marrano" theology.[25]

---

dam, 1968), pp. 1–39. See also idem, "Biblical Criticism and Social Science," *Boston Studies in the Philosophy of Science* 14 (1974): 339–60.

22. R. H. Popkin, "The Marrano Theology of Isaac La Peyrère," *Studi internazionali di filosofia* 5 (1973): 97–126; idem, "The Development of Religious Scepticism and the Influence of Isaac La Peyrère: Pre-Adamism and Biblical Criticism," in R. R. Bolgar, ed., *Classical Influences on European Culture* (Cambridge, 1976), pp. 271–80; idem, "La Peyrère and Spinoza," in R. Shahan and J. Biro eds., *Spinoza: New Perspectives* (Norman, Okla., 1978), pp. 177–95; idem, "Menasseh Ben Israel and Isaac La Peyrère," *Studia Rosenthaliana* 8 (1974): 59–63; 18 (1984): 12–20; idem, *The History of Scepticism from Erasmus to Spinoza* (Berkeley, 1979), chap. 11; idem, *Isaac La Peyrère: His Life, Work, and Influence* (Leiden, 1987).

23. Popkin, "La Peyrère and Spinoza"; idem, *Isaac La Peyrère*, pp. 84–85.

24. See Popkin, *Isaac La Peyrère*, pp. 21–25, where he discusses the various scholarly views of La Peyrère's alleged converso background.

25. See esp. Popkin, "The Marrano Theology."

One might quibble about how typical a marrano theology this eccentric thinker was espousing or how serious his scientific commitments were, since they were so entangled in his religious and apocalyptic meditations. His pre-Adamite theory was certainly known to several of his contemporaries, including Menasseh ben Israel, Isaac Orobio de Castro, and the Italian Jewish physician Isaac Cantarini,[26] but its immediate impact on the converso community of the seventeenth century seems most circumscribed.

Given his seminal importance to Western thought, Spinoza might appear a more likely candidate in which to locate a specific converso attitude concerning the relations of science and religion. At first blush, this seems hardly the case, in view of Spinoza's very minor contribution to scientific writing. As Marjorie Grene remarks, Spinoza was "a stranger in an age of science" who displayed "no kinship whatsoever to a groping, experimental, cumulative, and critical approach from which modern science springs."[27] Spinoza was a rationalist who identified scientific knowledge with a comprehensive and deductive axiomatic system of thought, considered sensory perception as highly fallible, and interpreted nature by applying principles already known by the light of reason. Despite his expertise at lens grinding and optics, Spinoza's originality was neither in the natural sciences nor in mathematics but in political thinking and in biblical criticism.[28]

Spinoza stakes out his innovative approach to the latter at the opening of chapter 7 of the *Theologico-Political Treatise:* "I may sum up the matter by saying that the method of interpreting Scripture does not widely differ from the method of interpreting nature—in fact, it is almost the same. For as the interpretation of nature consists in the examination of the history of nature, and therefrom deducing definitions of natural phenomena on certain fixed axioms, so Scriptural interpretation proceeds by the examination of Scripture, and infer-

26. See R. H. Popkin, "Menasseh Ben Israël and Isaac La Peyrère"; *Isaac La Peyrère,* pp. 86–90.

27. M. Grene and D. Nails, eds., *Spinoza and the Sciences* (=*Boston Studies in the Philosophy of Science* 91) (Dordrecht, 1986), p. xii.

28. This is the consensus emerging from the aforementioned collection of Grene and Nails. Note esp. N. Maull, "Spinoza in the Century of Science," pp. 3–13; H. Siebrand, "Spinoza and the Rise of Modern Science in the Netherlands," pp. 61–91; and D. Savan, "Spinoza: Scientist and Theorist of Scientific Method," pp. 95–123.

ring the intention of its authors as a legitimate conclusion from its fundamental principles."[29]

He adds that just as knowledge of nature is sought from nature alone, the knowledge of scripture emerges directly from the text. And just as definitions of natural things are derived from observing "the diverse workings of nature," scriptural definitions emerge from investigating the various narratives about a given subject. Just as we do not manipulate our data to fix the appearance of nature, we also should not "wrest the meaning of texts to suit the dictates of our reason."[30] By extending a scientific outlook and methodology to the study of the biblical text, Spinoza was following the approach adopted by Azariah de' Rossi in the study of rabbinic homilies. As we have seen, de' Rossi applied scientific historical criteria to an evaluation of the authenticity of rabbinic dicta, justifying himself by citing Maimonides' statement that when the rabbis made statements about the heavens, they did so as finite individuals and not as spokesman of a revealed tradition, and thus they were liable to error. By enlarging Maimonides' strategy to include all rabbinic homilies, de' Rossi ignored the privileged status of rabbinic literature, treating it like any literary or historical document, and thus incurred the wrath of the Maharal of Prague.[31] Spinoza had merely taken the next logical step by extending the methods of historical scholarship to the biblical text as well. Despite Spinoza's strong objection to Maimonides' allegorical method of scriptural interpretation, he had merely followed a project begun by the sage of Fustat some five hundred years earlier.

Spinoza's argument against biblical miracles followed the same logical lines: they were not possible since they broke the knowable laws and limits of nature. The reports of their existence emerged from unscientific minds.[32] The science of the Bible, like natural science, was to be inductive, free of metaphysics, unprejudiced by prior assumptions, honestly attempting to approximate objective knowledge.

Spinoza's inductive methodology in reading the Bible was surely based on a scientific method of studying nature, but was it *his* method for studying nature?

29. Benedict Spinoza, *Theologico-Political Treatise,* trans. R. H. M. Elwes (New York, 1951), p. 99.

30. Ibid., pp. 100–103.

31. See chap. 1 and esp. chap. 9 above.

32. See Spinoza, *Theologico-Political Treatise,* chap. 6, pp. 81–97.

As Leo Strauss once argued, Spinoza could not think of "conquering" nature if it were the same as God.[33] And if he considered human intuition to be the highest form of knowledge and a deductive system to be the highest science, his method of studying scripture was not at all comparable to the way he studied the chemical and physical sciences. Thus his biblical analysis is more historical than "scientific" in his sense of the latter word.[34] Indeed, his biblical criticism appears unrelated, or only vaguely related, to the natural sciences as he perceived them.[35] Be that as it may, his naturalist method of studying the foundations of Judaism and Christianity, along with La Peyrère's widening of the anthropological horizons of ancient historical study, left a lasting impression on Simon, Bayle, and all future students of the biblical text.

Both La Peyrère and Spinoza thus adopted contemporary scholarly canons and applied them to the study of religion with devastating results. But are we entitled to see their scientific applications as stemming directly from their converso backgrounds? More significant, was their approach to the study of sacred scriptures at all characteristic of that of other members of the converso community? La Peyrère's messianic fantasies and Spinoza's general philosophical orientation are surely rooted in their converso backgrounds. But it is more difficult to claim that their specific appropriations of the methods of science for studying Judaism are directly related to this common background. If one examines the attitudes to Bible study on the part of fellow conversos such as Menasseh ben Israel,[36] Elijah Montalto,[37] Isaac Orobio de Castro,[38] and Isaac Cardoso,[39] the contrast is striking. All saw the biblical text as generally immune from such historical or

33. L. Strauss, *Spinoza's Critique of Religion* (New York, 1965), p. 15.

34. Cf. ibid., pp. 175, 251–63.

35. See A. Momigliano, "The Greater Danger: Science or Biblical Criticism? [Response to R. Popkin]" in Lakatos and Musgrave, *Problems in the Philosophy of Science*, p. 34.

36. Menasseh's *Consiliador* attempted to reconcile conflicting biblical passages while upholding the accuracy of the Bible.

37. On Montalto's view of the Bible as infallible, see B. Cooperman, "Eliahu Montalto's 'Suitable and Incontrovertible Propositions': A Seventeenth-Century Anti-Christian Polemic," in I. Twersky and B. Septimus, eds., *Jewish Thought in the Seventeenth Century* (Cambridge, Mass., 1987), pp. 488–92.

38. See Kaplan, *From Christianity to Judaism,* pp. 166–78.

39. See Yerushalmi, *From Spanish Court to Italian Ghetto,* pp. 242, 246, 422–32.

anthropological investigations. Despite their highly sophisticated medical and scientific backgrounds, they would not countenance "the student or physician", as Isaac Orobio De Castro remarked "whose own arrogance will not permit him to take the holy antidote of the doctrine of our sages and scholars."[40] They consistently displayed conservative and defensive temperaments regarding matters of the Jewish faith. Their science had nothing at all to do with the scholarly incursions into the sacred realm of faith launched by La Peyrère and Spinoza. Some of them could at least tolerate and even absorb a modest dosage of fideistic skepticism; they could do no more than condemn or consciously ignore the radical hermeneutical turn of the new biblical critics.

If neither the new skeptical mood nor the new biblical criticism adequately captures the contribution of the converso philosophical and medical community as a whole, but only that of a few exceptional members within it, we are forced to look elsewhere to grasp the significance of this group for Jewish history. As we stated at the outset of this chapter, the strictly scientific nature of their enterprise may not properly define their broader cultural role within the Jewish community. There remains a further and critical dimension to explore: the group's self-image and that which it projected to others, among both contemporary Jews and Christians.

Let us begin by closely examining one unusual chapter in the well-known pioneering study of national and cultural traits, the *Examen de ingenios para las sciencias* (Inquiry into the Nature and Kinds of Intelligence), written by the converso physician Juan Huarte de San Juan, first published in 1575 and then republished in 1594 and subsequently many times and in many translations.[41]

40. Quoted by Kaplan, *From Christianity to Judaism*, p. 151.

41. I have used the edition of the *Examen de Ingenios* edited by G. Serés (Madrid, 1989), cited below as Serés. On Huarte, see the classic study of M. De Iriarte, *El Doctor Huarte de San Juan y su Examen de Ingenios: Contribución a la historia del la psicología diferencial* (Madrid, 1948); G. A. Perouse, *L'Examen des esprits du Docteur Juan Huarte de San Juan: Sa Diffusion e son influence en France au XVIe et XVIIe siècles* (Paris, 1970); M. Read, *Juan Huarte de San Juan* (Boston, 1981); G. Carlos Noreña, "Huarte's Naturalistic Philosophy of Man," *Studies in Spanish Renaissance Thought* (The Hague, 1975), pp. 210–63. The English translations cited in the text are based on the *Examen de Ingenios or, the Tryal of Wits Discovering the Great Difference of Wits among Men,*

In this chapter Huarte considers at length the history of the Jews and the effect on them of social repression and persecution, and offers a kind of scientific explanation of why they possess a special talent for medical practice.

Huarte begins the chapter entitled "That the Theory of Physic Belongs Part to the Memory, and Part to the Understanding, and to the Practice, to the Imagination"[42] with the observation that great theoreticians do not necessarily make good physicians. He then poses the question the chapter will consider: "The difficulty, then, is to understand why the most learned doctors, though they employ all their lives in the working of cures, never become excellent in practice; whereas others who are but ignoramuses, with three or four rules of Physic, learnt in the schools, can do greater cures in less time."[43] The answer he offers is that imagination, not mere understanding, is a prerequisite to be a good diagnostician and that this character trait was developed not in Spain but first and foremost in the geographical area of Egypt.[44] He interrupts this discussion by relating the following anecdote:

> When Francis de Valois, king of France, was seized with a very tedious sickness, and that the physicians of his house and court could give him no ease, he said that every time the fever returned, that it was not possible for any Christian physician to cure him. . . . He ordered a courier to be dispatched to Spain, to desire the Emperor Charles the fifth, to send him a Jew doctor, the best of all the court. . . . There was no little laughing in Spain at his request, and all concluded that it was no other than the conceit of a man in fever. . . . They sent him a physician newly turned Christian, hoping thereby to comply with the king's curiosity. But the physician being arrived in France and

---

and What Sort of Learning Suits Best with Each Genius, English by Mr. Bellamy (London, 1698), cited below as Bellamy.

42. Serés, chap. 12, pp. 493–523, entitled "Donde se prueba que la teórica de la medicine, parte della pertenece a la memoria y parte al entendimiento, y la practica, a la imaginativa." Bellamy, pp. 279–313 (following the ordering of the 1594 edition as chap. 14).

43. Bellamy, p. 280; Serés, p. 494: "Y, asi, la dificultad no está sino en saber por qué razón los médicos muy letrados, aunque se ejerciten toda la vida en curar, jamás salen con la práctica; y otros, idiotas, con tres o cuatro reglas de medicina que aprendieron en las escuelas, en muy menos tiempo saben mejor curar."

44. Serés, pp. 503–504; Bellamy, p. 292.

286

brought to the king's presence, there past between them a most agreeable dialogue, wherein was discover'd, that the physician was a Christian, and therefore the king would take no physic at his hands. [Huarte relates the dialogue between the two about the nature of the messiah, whereby the doctor indicates his belief in Jesus Christ. The king is incensed by his response and orders him to leave.] . . . Then said the king, be gone to your own country in good time, for I have Christian physicians enough in my own court and house. I took you to be a Jew, who in my opinion are those that have a natural ability for cures. And so he took leave of him without allowing him to feel his pulse or examine his urine, or mingle the least word concerning his distemper, and forthwith sent to Constantinople for a Jew who recovered him only with Asses-milk.[45]

Huarte offers this remarkable story to illustrate that temperaments are shaped by differing geographical environments, and thus he proposes to prove "that the people of Israel, at their going from thence, eat and drank such fruits and waters, as are proper to make this difference of Imagination [thus confirming and justifying] the conceit of the king of France."[46] Upon recounting the an-

45. Bellamy, pp. 293–94; Serés, pp. 504–06: ". . . estando Francisco de Valois, rey de Francia, molestado de una prolija enfermedad, y viendo que los médicos du su casa y Corte no le daban remedio, decia todas las veces que le creciá la calentura que non era posible que los médicos cristianos supiesen curar . . . mandó despachar un correo a España, pidiendo al Emperador, nuestro señor, le enviase un médico judío, el mejor que hubiese en su corte. . . . La cual demanda fue harto reída en España, y todos concluyeron que era antojo de hombre que estaba con calentura . . . envió un médico cristiano nuevo, pareciéndole que con esto cumpliria con el antojo del rey. Pero puesto el médico en Francia y delante el rey, pasó un coloquio entre ambos muy gracioso, en el cual se descubrió que el médico era cristiano, y por tanto, no se quiso curar con él . . . Rey: Pues volveos en hora buena a vuestra tierra, porque médicos cristianos sobrados tengo en mi casa y corte. Por judío lo habia yo, los cuales en mi opinión son los que tienen habilidad natural para curar! Y, asi, lo despidió, sin quererle dar el pulso ni que viese la urina ni le hablase palabra tocante a su enfermedad. Y luego envió a Constantinopla por un judío, y con sola leche de borricas le curó."

46. Bellamy, p. 295; Serés, p. 507: "Luego si yo probare ahora que el pueblo de Israel estuvo de asiento muchos años en Egipto y que, saliendo de él, comió y bebió las aguas y manjares que son apropiados para hacer esta diferencia de imaginativa, habremos hecho demostración del la opinion del rey de Francia . . . ."

cient origins of the Hebrews, he offers a further insight, that because of the Jews' servitude and afflictions, they contracted "a good deal of adjust choler," the humor which is "the instrument of craft, of cunning, and of malice."[47] In such abysmal conditions, their imagination was "ever busied in contriving to do some damage to their master, and free themselves from slavery."[48] Their character was further enhanced by the climatic factors in Israel, which were virtually identical to those in Egypt. And during their sojourn in the desert, the Israelite nation fed on manna ("a delicate vapor raised by the force of the sun's heat from the earth,"[49] which turned into adjust choler), drank water from Moses's rod, and breathed desert air that was subtle and delicate, all of which sharpened their wit. Thus their sadness and toil combined with their climate and diet to shape their distinct character traits ("craft, cunning, intriguing, and malice" [as opposed to wisdom which is the moral kind]),[50] those particularly well suited for the proper diagnosis of the causes and cures of disease.

Huarte must then account for the retention of these same traits in Spanish doctors of Jewish origin far removed from their ancient captivity in the desert. He acknowledges a certain loss of vitality, but maintains that it would take four thousand years to eradicate these qualities altogether: "True it is, that they are not now so quick and sharp, as they were a thousand years ago . . . and also because they have mingled with women of the Gentile race, who wanted this difference of wit: But this is not to be denied them, that as yet they have not utterly lost it."[51]

47. Bellamy, p. 297; Serés, p. 508: ". . . engendran mucha cólera requemada por no tener libertad de hablar ni vengarse de sus injurias; y este humor, estando tostado, es el instrumento de la astucia, solercia y malicia."

48. Bellamy, p. 297; Serés, pp. 508–9: "Y, asi, se ve por experiencia que no hay peores costumbres ni condiciones, que las del señor esclavo, cuya imaginación esta siempre ocupada en cómo hará daño a su señor y se librará de la servidumbre."

49. Bellamy, p. 300; Serés, p. 512: "un vapor muy delicado que el sol levanta de la tierra."

50. Bellamy, p. 305; Serés, p. 517: "la solercia, astucia, versucia y malicia."

51. Bellamy, p. 313; Serés, p. 523: "Ello verdad es que no son ahora tan agudos y solertes como mil años atras . . . y por haberse mezclado con los que descienden de la gentilidad, los cuales carecen de esta diligencia de ingenio. Pero lo que no se les puede negar es que aún no lo han acabado de perder."

What is perplexing about Huarte's assigning the quality of craftiness to the Jewish doctor is the moral ambiguity of such an attribution. At one point he cites Plato, who defines craftiness as "that knowledge which is void of honesty," as distinct from wisdom "attended with honesty and simplicity, without double-dealing, or tricks."[52] Although the attribute has a negative connotation on the moral plane, it is positive when applied to the doctor's craft. The implication would seem to be that Jews are good doctors but dishonorable men!

To appreciate the significance of Huarte's excursus on the Jewish doctor, one needs to recall the social context of Jewish medicine in sixteenth-century Spain, particularly the predominance of doctors of Jewish origin in Spanish society and the widespread perception of the profession's Jewish character.[53] Despite the obvious need for well-trained doctors, the converso group, like Jewish doctors before them, incurred enormous resentment for their well-proven abilities and the power they held over their Christian patients. As Americo Castro put it: "Here it is useful in understanding the absurdity of the Spaniard's forbidding the Jews to serve as doctors to Christians at the same time that the legislators and the people who were themselves trying to exterminate the Jews, could not possibly do without the services of the Jewish physicians when they had so much as a stomach ache."[54]

The animosity toward the doctor of Jewish ancestry found full expression in the debates over *limpieza de sangre* (purity of blood) throughout the sixteenth and seventeenth centuries.[55] In 1594, for example, Alfonso Guerrero lamented the exalted position of the converso doctors, whom he regarded as Jewish. And in 1575 Simancas accused the Jews of criminal medicine, prescribing and preparing poisons for their patients, placing fatal venom under their fingertips and administering mortal drugs to their open wounds. Similarly, J. F. Ripa accused the Christian patient of the Jewish doctor of insulting Jesus and committing a

52. Bellamy, p. 299; Serés, p. 511: "scientia quae est remota a iusticia . . . Otro hay con rectitud y simplicidad, sin dobleces ni engaños."

53. See esp. J. Caro Baroja, *Los Judíos en la España moderna y contemporánea*, 3 vols. (Madrid, 1961), 2:162–94. Additional references follow.

54. A. Castro, *The Structure of Spanish History*, trans. E. L. King (Princeton, 1954), p. 494.

55. See generally A. A. Sicroff, *Les Controverses des statuts de pureté de sang en Espagne du XVe au XVIIe siècle* (Paris, 1960).

mortal sin. Jewish doctors were regularly accused of murdering their patients.[56]

Such slander against Jewish physicians was not new; only the intensity and regularity of the slander both in Spain and throughout Europe was exceptional. Most novel of all was the direct connection between racism and medicine. Thus Gerónimo de la Huarta, personal physician to Philip IV, proposed statutes of blood purity in the medical profession. To this he added his own brand of inflammatory rhetoric singling out the putrid odor of the Jewish physician caused by his murder of Christ, his permanent condition of hemorrhoids, and the flux of anal blood on his bare fingers. Dr. Juan de Quiñones even devoted an entire treatise to the menstruation of Jewish males, their hemorrhoidal condition, and the permanent odor that they supposedly endured.[57]

Such verbal abuse was still the least devastating part of the fate of these converso physicians. Hundreds of them were tried and convicted by the Inquisition, and many escaped the Iberian peninsula fearing for their lives. In an inventory of converso doctors tried by the Inquisitions in Spain and Portugal between 1550 and 1800, prepared for Dr. Harry Friedenwald by Yakov Malkiel in 1940 and now located in the National and University Library in Jerusalem, 239 names are listed.[58] This list complements earlier lists from other sources[59] and offers

56. All of these examples with full documentation are taken from H. Méchoulan, *Le Sang de l'autre ou l'honneur de Dieu: Indiens, Juifs, Morisques dans l'Espagne du siècle d'or* (Paris, 1979), pp. 153–61; see also Y. Kaplan, "Jews and Judaism in the Political and Social Thought of Spain in the Sixteenth and Seventeenth Centuries," in S. Almog, ed., *Anti-Semitism through the Ages* (Oxford and New York, 1988), pp. 153–60.

57. Méchoulan, *Sang*, p. 157; Yerushalmi, *From Spanish Court to Italian Ghetto*, pp. 122–36. See also the response of Isaac Cardoso to Quiñones' accusations in Yerushalmi, *From Spanish Court to Italian Ghetto*, pp. 435–37. On the connection between racism, Jewishness, and medicine in the nineteenth and twentieth centuries, see S. Gilman, *The Case of Sigmund Freud: Medicine and Identity at the Fin de Siècle* (Baltimore, 1993).

58. It is entitled "List of the Physicians Mentioned in the Rolls of the Spanish and Portuguese Inquisition, 1500–1800" and is taken from the *Collecção das Noticias dos Autos de fe que se tem celebrado nas' Inquisicoes deste Reyno de Portugal; e Listas das Pessoas que Nelles Sahirae Penitenciadas*, now in the possession of the Library of the Jewish Theological Seminary of America. It is listed in the catalogue of the Harry Friedenwald Library, published with *Jewish Luminaries in Medical History* (Baltimore, 1946), p. 162. It is compiled from testimonies in Coimbra, Evora, Lisbon, Granada, Majorca, Santiago, Cuenca, Valencia, Madrid, and Seville.

59. See, for example, P. A. d'Azevedo, "Médicos cristãos novos que se ausentaram de Portugal no principio do século XVII," *Arqivos de historia da medicina portuguesa*, n.s. 5 (1914):

telling testimony both to the large number of doctors among the victims of the Inquisition and to their high profile, university training, and professional success.

Huarte's chapter on the Jewish doctor is surely his personal response to the vilification and victimization of his professional group. In designating the diagnostic skills of the Jew as being acquired at birth and equating this medical talent with dishonor and cunning, he had clearly internalized the thinking of his accusers ("la mimesis de l'antagonisme").[60] Yet his transformation of a negative cultural trait into a positive medical one, his eloquent and passionate critique (in a later chapter of his book) of the false notion of honor based on birth and privilege, together with his audacious telling of the story of Francis's appreciation of a good Jewish doctor, evinces a distinctive pride and sense of self-respect in his Jewish ancestry. To the extent that it reflects the case of Huarte de San Juan, Americo Castro's sweeping and complex observation is worth citing: "These [Jewish] doctors were, beyond a shadow of a doubt, one of the channels through which flowed the didacticism, the sententious style, the integral expression of the person, the preoccupation with purity of blood, and many other phenomena (including the fierce passion of the Inquisition), which the converts were eventually to rivet into the Spanish consciousness."[61]

The penetrating observations of Castro's student Stephan Gilman on the

---

153–72; *Medicos perseguidos por la Inquisición Española* (Madrid, 1855). Friedenwald compiled his own list from these lists and other sources of information in "Spanish and Portuguese Physicians after the Expulsion at the End of the Fifteenth Century," in his *The Jews and Medicine,* 2 vols. (Baltimore, 1944), 2:701–72. For recent lists of Sephardic physicians in the Netherlands, see H. S. Hes, *Jewish Physicians in the Netherlands* (Assen, 1980); and Y. Emanuel, "New Information on the Portuguese Congregation of Amsterdam" (in Hebrew), *Oẓar Yehudai Sefarad* 6 (1963): 168–72.

60. The expression is that of René Girard in his *Deux choses cachées depuis la fondation du monde* (Paris, 1978), p. 35, cited by Y. Kaplan in "Political Concepts in the World of the Portuguese Jews of Amsterdam during the Seventeenth Century: The Problem of Exclusion and the Boundaries of Self-Identity," in Y. Kaplan, H. Méchoulan, and R. H. Popkin, eds., *Menasseh Ben Israel and His World* (Leiden, 1989), pp. 45–62; the reference is on p. 53. This essay is most suggestive to me for the subject of converso doctors and their identity formation, particularly their appropriation and internalization of racial notions of their oppressors.

61. Castro, *Structure of Spanish History,* p. 495.

converso dilemma are even more useful in understanding Huarte and other members of his professional group. Gilman, like Castro, viewed the conversos as members of a caste subject to intense scorn and suspicion, forced into a marginal position, and reacting to persecution in a number of characteristic ways, among them the cultivation of the intellect. For Gilman, such a condition is inherently paradoxical in that the member of this caste simultaneously sees himself both on the margin and at the center of society. Gilman's insight is particularly appropriate when viewing the converso physicians. Despite being told they were marginal, they knew all too well how essential their occupation was to the functioning of society. Thus they were both honored and suspected, trusted and resented at the same time, "at once wholly inside and wholly outside the society in which they lived . . . at once empowered to make the most crucial and delicate decisions and yet subject to the arbitrary power of Inquisitors and to the vilification of the masses."[62]

Gilman suggests a spectrum of converso responses to this predicament, ranging from aggressive resentment to ironical withdrawal and camouflage to acceptance, either partial or complete. In reality, these responses often converge in the same individual: "Resentful rejection and ironical devaluation of the surrounding society are inevitably accompanied by partial assimilation of the points of view of the dominant caste." However firmly the converso rejects the culture of his oppressor, he remains part of the same linguistic community, involving him constantly in dialogue—as a speaker or writer in Spanish and Portuguese—with much that he repudiates.[63]

Within the paradox of being both central and marginal, the converso unwittingly appropriated values relating to the confrontation of his self with others, particularly notions of nobility, rank, position, and honor. Thus Gilman concludes: "Against surrounding disesteem, in case after case, a facade of nobility was erected, defended, and after a while believed in."[64] The conversos represented themselves as *hidalgos* (noblemen), claiming the presumption of aristocracy.[65]

62. S. Gilman, *The Spain of Fernando de Rojas: The Intellectual and Social Landscape of "La Celestina"* (Princeton, 1972), pp. 117–24, 137–38.

63. Gilman, *Spain,* pp. 139–43.

64. Ibid., p. 144.

65. Ibid., p. 145.

The French king's humiliation of the Christian doctor who confessed to believing in Christ's redemption and his instant replacement by a Jew from Constantinople surely illustrate Huarte's devaluation of Christian practitioners of his craft, while empowering the lowly Jewish doctor who heals his patient with nothing more than asses' milk. Through his own definition of *hidalgua*, based on merit and achievement rather than birth or governmental privilege,[66] Huarte reverses the roles of oppressor and victim, of centrality and marginality, promoting the true *hidalgo* as the Turkish doctor with traces of manna still coursing through his veins. The reversal is not fully complete. He acknowledges that the downside of good medical instincts is a cunning and crafty character. Behind the facade of self-esteem Huarte had erected, remained the residue of a negative disesteem, an acceptance and acknowledgment of a deep-rooted stereotype of Jewish deviousness in the service of dishonorable ends.

In a recent essay, the Spanish historian of medicine Diego Gracia Guillén argues that medicine was not merely a victim of the Inquisition but was "also allied with the inquisitorial authorities in the task of corporally and morally disciplining Spanish society." Medicine in the sixteenth century became a judicial discipline, a normative science of social conduct, distinguishing normal from abnormal and pathological behavior. Not only did the Inquisition use medical arguments to justify its practices, Guillén maintains, but medicine itself also acquired "a certain inquisitorial nature," becoming "a collaborator with the Inquisition in the task of disciplining society."[67]

Guillén's observation parallels that of José Antonio Maravall in his well-known study of Baroque culture. Maravall sees the use of medicine for political ends as characteristic of the Baroque age in general. He notes that many seventeenth-century writers, including Descartes, believed in drawing upon medicine for ways to govern human conduct. Physicians considered themselves

---

66. See Huarte's discussion of nobility in Serés, pp. 550–56; Bellamy, pp. 344–48.

67. D. G. Guillén, "Judaism, Medicine, and the Inquisitorial Mind in Sixteenth-Century Spain," in A. Alcalá, ed., *The Spanish Inquisition and the Inquisitorial Mind*, translation of *Inquisición española y mentalidad inquisitorial* (Barcelona, 1984), Atlantic Studies on Society in Change no. 49 (New York, 1989), pp.375–400.

capable of speaking about politics, morality, and the economy.[68] Both Maravall and Guillén offer Huarte de San Juan as an example of a doctor whose discovery of a differential psychology among peoples and individuals empowered him with authority to address politicians, moralists, artists, and writers.[69]

Guillén singles out a new genre of literature that emerges in the late sixteenth century—written, not coincidentally, by converso physicians—demonstrating the link between medical and political authority. He analyzes two examples of this special medico-political literature: Henrique Jorge Enriquez's *Retrato del perfecto médico* and Rodrigo de Castro's *Medicus politicus*. For Guillén, this literature emerges as a by-product of the inquisitorial mentality, recognizing medicine's enormous power as a normalizing and controlling disciplinarian of both corporal and spiritual behavior. The physician conceives himself as "a governor, a politician who has the order of the microcosmos in his hands, just as the monarch governs the mezzocosmos—the republic—and God the world or macrocosmos." Guillén also points out that the intervention of the physician into the social sphere has its negative and insidious side. The doctor who saw himself capable of determining moral qualities on the basis of physical appearance could easily take the next step from a kind of moral biologism to racism, differentiating between noble and ignoble families on the basis of their blood type. Ironically, the converso physician of the Inquisition had unconsciously become a collaborator in a system of which he had been the most conspicuous victim.[70]

As we have see in the case of Huarte de San Juan, the converso physician was capable of sharing the values and mindset of his oppressors. Guillén and Maravall are no doubt correct in seeing the emergence of the new image of the *medicus politicus* as a product of both the Inquisition and Baroque culture. But, I suggest, the converso physician's attempt to stake out a political and moral role for the medical profession is not the result of these general forces alone. It is

68. J. A. Maravall, *Culture of the Baroque: Analysis of a Historical Structure,* trans. T. Cochran (Minneapolis, 1986), pp. 64–66. We might also note parenthetically the prominence of converso physicians in political roles in their newly established Jewish communities. Emanuel, "New Information," p. 168, for example, says that 18 out of a total of 60 doctors were serving as *parnasim* in Amsterdam in the seventeenth century.

69. Guillén, "Judaism," p. 386; Maravall, *Culture of the Baroque,* p. 66.

70. Guillén, "Judaism," pp. 384–95.

more directly linked to his quest for cultural identity, his attempt to define his Jewishness by integrating it with the most important factor that made him both unique and critical to Jewish and Christian society alike: his medical acumen.

In order to substantiate this observation, I propose to consider two works by converso physicians: the aforementioned treatise of Rodrigo de Castro of Hamburg and that of his son Benedict de Castro, the *Flagellum calumniantium sue apologia in qua anonymi cujusdam calumniae refutantur,* a defense of Jewish physicians. It is my contention that both compositions are closely linked as works of Jewish advocacy. When viewed together, they powerfully reveal an emerging sense of Jewish identification on the part of two members of a distinguished family of converso doctors, and to a great extent they articulate the shared convictions of many in their professional and ethnic community.

The full title of Rodrigo de Castro's work reads in translation: "The Political Physician, or Treatise of Medical Political Skills . . . in which not only are the mores and virtues of good doctors explained and the frauds and impostures of bad ones unveiled but also very many useful and joyful things about this new topic are proposed. A work very useful for doctors, patients, and nurses and for everyone interested in letters and politics."[71] Rodrigo de Castro (1550–1627) acquired considerable fame as a physician in Lisbon before settling in Hamburg in 1594 and eventually returning to the Jewish faith, at least officially, as late as 1612. Prior to that time, he lived as a Catholic and gave a Christian burial in 1603 to his first wife and a baptism to his two sons, Benedict and Andrea. His most famous medical work was his study of gynecology called *De universa mulierum morborum medicina,* published in Hamburg in 1603. He published the *Medicus politicus* eleven years later in the same city—perhaps not coincidentally after his public affiliation with the Jewish community.[72]

---

71. *Medicus politicus, sive de officiis medico-politicis tractatus . . . in quibus non solum bonorum medicorum mores ac virtutes exprimuntur, malorum vero fraudes et imposturae detegentur, verum etiam pleraque alia circa novum hoc argumentum utilia atque jucunda exactissime proponuntur. Opus admodum utile medicis, aegrotis, aegrotorum assistentibus, et cunctis aliis litterarum atque adeo politicae disciplinae cultoribus.*

72. On Rodrigo, see H. Kellenbenz, *Sephardim an der Unteren Elbe* (Wiesbaden, 1958), pp. 325–30; M. Kayserling in *Jewish Encyclopedia,* 3:609–11; Friedenwald, *Jews and Medicine,* 1:56–

Rodrigo's rise to prominence in Hamburg coincided with the growing domination of the city's Portuguese Jewish community. In 1612 the first official contract was negotiated with the city's officials, and soon after an "unofficial synagogue" was reported in use. By 1646 the prosperous community of Portuguese merchants, numbering as many as five hundred lived like ostentatious aristocrats, making no secret of their wealth and influence—in striking contrast to their Ashkenazic coreligionists in Hamburg. Rodrigo's reputation was so great that he was the only Jew allowed to own a comfortable house in the city.[73]

Some twenty years after Rodrigo's death but during the height of Benedict's career, the burgesses and clergy of the city under the leadership of Pastor Johannes Müller organized a protest against the conspicuous presence of the Sephardim in the city. In 1649 (the same year the Ashkenazim were expelled from Hamburg) Müller issued a series of public denunciations of the Jews, complaining of their noisy and extravagant religious ceremonies, their defilement of the Sabbath, their insults to Christian women, and their medical practice. He also called for new conversionary efforts against the Jews, including "a Christian rabbi" to teach them. Only in the 1650s did a structure of organized Jewish life with a professional rabbinate fully emerge.[74]

Rodrigo's *Medicus politicus,* we might infer, contains some of his first public utterances as a full-fledged member of the Jewish community, his "coming out of the closet," so to speak. Although the treatise may retain the residual mindset of the Inquisition, as Guillén has proposed, Rodrigo's embrace of Judaism and his

---

57, 60–61; 2:449–52; H. J. Schoeps, "Die Sephardische Artztfamilie de Castro: Ein Beitrag zur Medecin Geschichte des Barock," *Ein weites Feld: Gesamelte Aufsatz* (Berlin, 1980), pp. 137–62.

73. See J. Whaley, *Religious Toleration and Social Change in Hamburg, 1529–1819* (Cambridge, 1985), pp. 74–76; M. Isler, "Zur altesten Geschichte der Juden in Hamburg," *Zeitschrift der Vereins für Hamburgische Geschichte* 6 (1875): 467–76; A. Cassuto, *Gedenkschrift anläslich des 270 jährigen Bestenhens der portugiesische-jüdischen Gemeinde in Hamburg* (Amsterdam, 1927); idem, "Neue Funde zur ältesten Geschichte der Portugiesischen Juden in Hamburg," *Zeitschrift für die Geschichte der Juden in Deutschland* 3 (1931): 58–71; B. Z. Ornan Pinkus, "The Portuguese Community in Hamburg and Its Leadership in the Seventeenth Century" (in Hebrew), *Mi-Mizrah u-mi-Ma'arav* 5 (1986): 7–51; G. Bohn, "Die Sephardim in Hamburg," in A. Herzig, ed., *Die Juden in Hamburg 1590 bis 1900* (Hamburg, 1991), pp. 21–40.

74. Whaley, *Religious Toleration,* pp. 76–79, 82.

public identification with other Portuguese Jews resonate strongly throughout the text.

The centerpiece of his newly reclaimed identity is found in his eloquent commentary on Ben Sira 38 ("Show the physician due honor in view of your need of him, for the Lord has created him"), extolling the physician and his moral and religious role in society.[75] His text is studded with such biblical citations and examples establishing the connection between medicine, religion, and moral virtue.[76] Several times he returns to Ben Sira's notion of the divine origin of medicine;[77] adduces Solomon as an exemplar of his honored profession;[78] and, among the distinguished contemporary references he cites, includes a generous sampling of his own community of physicians—Amatus Lusitanus, Christophorus a Vega Hispanus, Ambrosius Nonius Lusitanus, Thomas Rodericus a Vega Lusitanus, and others.[79]

Most remarkable in Rodrigo's public testimonial to the Jewish "ministry" of the physician is his repudiation of Hermes and Paracelsus, on the one hand (the ideologue of an exclusive Christian ministry of medicine),[80] and his awareness and approbation of the kabbalah on the other. He is particularly fascinated by the

75. I have used the 1662 Hamburg edition of the *Medicus politicus* in the Friedenwald Collection, National and University Library, Jerusalem. See bk. 1, chap. 9, pp. 29–33.

76. *Medicus politicus,* pp. 30 (refers to Genesis 50, Exodus 21, and Ezekiel 47; 32 (Ezekiel 18); 51 (Isaiah 3); 117 (Psalms, Isaiah, etc.); 145 (Job 27, Psalm 5, Proverbs 12); 221 (Psalm 30); 228 (Exodus 15:26); 269 (Isaiah 5); 274 (Exodus 25, Numbers 10, Leviticus 23, Judges 5, 1 Kings 21, etc.).

77. Ibid., p. 34: "Sic quia Ecclesiasticus dixit, medici opera necessaria, & medicum honorandum propter necessitatem"; p. 75: "Quod consonat cum verbis Ecclesiastici dicentis: medicinam a Deo esse creatam, quam vir prudens non ab[h]orrebit"; p. 193: "A rege, inquit Ecclesiasticus, accipiet donationem, & disciplina medici exaltabit caput illi 9."

78. Ibid., p. 76: "Ita ferunt Salomonem e didisse naturalium disputationum opus ingens, admirabili rerum omnium sapientia refertum . . . ."

79. Ibid., pp. 88–90.

80. Ibid., p. 14: "Explicatur, atque rejicutur chymicorum secta! Theophrasto Paracelso, qui rejectis veterum rationibiis, principiis, & causis, nova principia & novas causas excogitavit, & ut in medicina monarchiam affectaret, novam sectam constituit, diversus per omnia ab Hippocratis & Galeni placitis." On the chemical philosophers, see chap. 8 above.

kabbalists' magical powers with words, their abilities to transform nature, and their skills in engendering sympathetic connections with the heavenly bodies.[81] He is credulous about the demonic origin of disease.[82] Where the pagan forms of magical healing defile the name of God, the kabbalist's are sanctified and efficacious.[83] He is intrigued by the analogies of the ten sefirot that prevail in the macrocosmos and microcosmos. He learns of the latter from his reading of Paulus Ricius's *De coelesti agricultura libri quattuor* (1541), as well as Joseph Gikatilla's *Sha'arai Orah (Portae lucis)*, part of which Ricius had translated into Latin in 1516.[84] He waxes eloquent about the Tabernacle, particularly its three parts representing the three worlds: earthly, heavenly, and divine.[85] He expounds upon the use of music in healing, which he attributes to David's psalms, offering ample biblical citations.[86] Finally, he offers his own exegesis on an obscure passage in Isaiah 3:7, where the word *keẓin* (chief of a people) is equated with *ḥovesh* (a dresser of wounds). The connection for him is emblematic of the thesis of his

---

81. Ibid., bk. 4, chap. 3, pp. 224–25: "De verbis & vocibus id confirmant ex fundamentis Cabalistarum, qui asservunt, litteris & syllabis quandam cum coelestibus corporibus & mentibus sympathiae connexionem: verba autem illa esse natura sua majoris efficaciae, quae sunt orta a lingua digniore, & a sanctiore dignitate instituta, quaeque sanctiores res significant."

82. Ibid., pp. 226–27

83. Ibid., p. 228.

84. Ibid., p. 229: "Non quod Cabalaeus ejusmodi interpretamenta ubique ad amussim prophetarum & sacri eloquii intellectum fuisse vel esse existimet: sed hoc unum intendit, ut concinna & reciproca hac phantasiae, rationis & mentis exercitatione denudentur animi vires a cogitatione terrena tollanturque ad superos, illisque adhaereant: tunc deinde totis viribus virtuti ad divinis oraculis studeat Cabalaeus, ut in iis decem sanctorum Dei nominum sensum dignoscat, sciatque & intelligat, singula praedictorum nominum clavis vicem genere, ad aliquod ex iis, quod seculi usus deposcit: ita ut analogia quadam eisdem decem nominibus sanctissimis, decem divina oracula correspondeant: decem item orbes coelestes, decem angelorum ordines, decem potissima membra hominis, ac rerum omnium ordines decem, quos praedicamenta vocamus. Ut eleganter ac fuse 4. Agricultura caelestis Rifius disputat, & Josephus Castiliensis in Porta lucis: quod si ita intellexerit Avicenna in eo, quem ex ipsius mente retulimus dogmate, non videtur omnino rejicienda Arabis sententia."

85. Ibid., pp. 235–37.

86. Ibid., pp. 265–74.

book—the political role of the physician—and the archetype of such a fusion of medicine and political role is none other than the Hebraic king Solomon.[87]

There can be little doubt to any reader of the *Medicus politicus* as to the book's Jewish provenance. Despite the poverty of rabbinic citations, Castro fortified his literacy of the Bible with kabbalistic references. He appears to have mastered them from Christian sources, especially Paulus Ricius. Despite the sober and rational tone of the treatise as a whole, he is enraptured by kabbalist sapience and embraces it as his own. In this he may have already planted the seeds for his son Benedict's infatuation with Jewish mystical fantasies, particularly his zealous and contentious endorsement of the false messiah Shabbatai Zevi. Whatever the case, Benedict surely endorsed his father's ideal of the Solomonic *ḥovesh* as *kaẕin* and, like him, promoted it as a thoroughly Jewish notion, underscoring both the unique contribution of Judaism to Western culture and the singular role of the contemporary Jewish physician within European society. What Rodrigo had implied through his plentiful citations from Hebraic wisdom, Benedict would make unambiguously explicit. There is no doubt that Benedict viewed his *Flagellum calumniantium* as a direct sequel to his father's *Medicus politicus*.

Benedict de Castro, known in Hebrew sources as Barukh Naḥmias, was born in Hamburg in 1597, attended the gymnasium of the city while receiving preparatory instruction from his father in medicine, and finally studied at several universities until he received a medical degree. In is not clear from what university he graduated, although Padua records the graduation of his brother Daniel

---

87. Ibid., bk. 1, chap. 12, p. 51: "Apprehendet, enim vir fratrem suum domesticum patris sui, & dicet, vestimentum tibi est, princeps *[keẕin]* esto noster, ruina autem haec sub manu tua. Respondebitque in die illa, dicens, non sum medicus *[ḥovesh]*, & in domo mea non est panis neque vestimentum, nolite me constituere principem populi: ubi in Ebraeo contextu pro voce medicus est *keẕin* quae vox curatorum significat, seu rei publicae gubernatorum, non autem medicum physicum quem Ebrei dicunt *rofeh* . . . & verbum *tehiyeh* [in Isaiah 3:6] ibi positum de futuro est, non de praesenti; atque ita totus sensus erit: non sum medicus sive curator, hoc est, non novi has calamitates curare, quia rem publicam gubernare non sum assuetus: & in domo mea non est panis, nec vestimentum, id est, non sum opulentus & potens, quae tria ad regiam dignitatem requiruntur . . . . Neque legimus populi Israelitici reges, praeter unum Salomonem medicos fuisse & plerique eorum admodum pueri sceptrum obtinuerunt."

(also known as Andrea) in 1633. In 1622 Benedict began to practice medicine in Hamburg and soon achieved considerable success, eventually assuming the position of physician-in-ordinary to Queen Christina of Sweden in 1645.[88] He devoted to her his only medical work, *Monamachia sive Certamen medicum quo verus in febre synocho putrida cum crucis inflammatione medendi usus per venae sectionem in brachio demonstratur,* published in Hamburg in 1647. He was apparently as well known as his illustrious father: Hugo Grotius called him "vir humanissimus" and he enlisted the most famous Portuguese physician of his day, Zacutus Lusitanus, to compose the preface for his book.[89]

After the appearance of Shabbatai Zevi, the board of elders of the Jewish community of Hamburg, with Benedict de Castro present, resolved to send a delegation to meet the alleged messiah. According to the testimony of Jacob Sasportas, who was in Hamburg at the time, a prayer for Shabbatai Zevi was introduced into the prayer service by March 1666. The retired rabbi, David Kohen de Lara, was contemptuous of this gesture and exited the synagogue every time the prayer was recited. On Yom Kippur eve, at the appointed time of the prayer, "this scholar walked out as was his custom, but then the *parnas* [a communal leader] Dr. Barukh Naḥmias got off his chair and grabbed him by his clothing and dishonored him, even lifting a hand to him, so that there was a great uproar in a place where they were obliged to scream and to ask forgiveness on all they had done."[90] Only three years later, Benedict was physically assaulted by a crowd enraged by the false charge that Jews had converted a Christian girl. Reduced to poverty in his old age, he died in 1684 in Hamburg but was buried in the cemetery of the Portuguese synagogue of Altona.[91]

88. See S. Akerman, *Queen Christina of Sweden and Her Circle: The Transformation of a Seventeenth-Century Philosophical Libertine* (Leiden, 1991), pp. 178–95, esp. 183.

89. On Benedict, see Kellenbenz, *Sephardim,* pp. 328–30; M. Kayserling in *Jewish Encyclopedia,* 3:609–11; Friedenwald, *Jews and Medicine,* 1:53–67, 292–93; 2:449–52; Schoeps, "Die Sephardische Artztfamilie." Daniel de Castro graduated from the University of Padua's medical school on June 19, 1633. See A. Modena and E. Morpurgo, *Medici e chirurghi ebrei dottorati e licenziati nell'Università di Padova dal 1616 al 1816,* ed. A. Luzzato, L. Münster, and V. Colorni (Bologna, 1967), p. 14, no. 30.

90. Jacob Sasportas, *Sefer Zizat Novel Zevi,* ed. I. Tishby (Jerusalem, 1954), pp. 132–33; G. Scholem, *Sabbatai Ṣevi: The Mystical Messiah* (Princeton, 1973), pp. 574–580.

91. Friedenwald, *Jews and Medicine,* 1:57.

Benedict's *Flagellum* was apparently first published at Antwerp in 1629 under the title *Trattado da Calumnia em o quel Brevemente se Mostram a Natureza, Causas e Effeitos deste Pernizioso Vicio,* and then published in its Latin edition in Amsterdam in 1631.[92] The full title in translation reads: "The Scourge of Calumniators, or Apology. In which the malicious charges of an anonymous author are refuted, the lust for lying of this person is disclosed, and the legitimate method of the most famous Portuguese physicians is commended, while the ignorance and temerity of empiric quacks are condemned as injurious to the commonwealth."[93]

Harry Friedenwald, the only previous scholar to study Benedict's apologia in any depth, offers a useful introduction to the context in which the book was written. It includes a long series of vilifications of Jewish doctors throughout the sixteenth century and well into the eighteenth.[94] In addition to the better-known statements of Luther, Reuchlin, and Paracelsus which Friedenwald quotes, one might add the longer vituperations of Margaritha, Wagenseil, Schudt, and Eisenmenger. As a whole, they constitute a long-standing tradition of incitement to physicians, primarily of Sephardic descent, who were practicing medicine throughout Germany.[95] Taken together with the hostile climate of Spain and Portugal from which the doctors had fled, and especially its racist overtones, this campaign of vilification allows us to appreciate fully the magnitude of the problem that these recent immigrants faced.

Friedenwald mentions one other volume, entitled *Medicaster Apella oder Juden Artzt* by a physician in Frankfurt named Ludovicus von Hoernigk, published in Strasbourg, also in 1631. This large work begins with a long genealogy of

92. According to M. Kayserling, *Jewish Encyclopedia,* 3:609.

93. *Flagellum calumniantium seu Apologia. In qua Anonymi cujusdam calumniae refutantur, ejusdem mentiendi libido detegitur: clarissimorum Lusitanorum Medicorum legitima methodus commendatur, empiricorum inscitia ac temeritas tamquam perniciosa republicae damnatur, auctore Philotheo Castello.* See Friedenwald, *Jews and Medicine,* 1:57–58.

94. Friedenwald, *Jews and Medicine,* 1:53–57

95. Antonio Margaritha, *Der gantze Juedische Glaube* (Leipzig, 1705), chap. 9, pp. 92–96; Johann Christoph Wagenseil, *Belehrung der juedisch-teutschen Red-und Schreibart* (Koeningsberg, 1699), preface; Johann Jacob Schudt, *Jüdische Merkwürdigkeiten* (Frankfurt, 1714–18), bk. 6, chap. 23, pp. 382–405; Johann Andreas Eisenmenger, *Endecktes Judenthum* (Berlin, 1711), pt. 2, chap. 3, pp. 227ff. See also generally S. Munter, *Alilot al Rofim Yehudiim be-Aspaklariah shel Toledot ha-Refu'ah* (Jerusalem, 1953)

Gentile doctors, those of Greek, Arabic, Italian, and German origin, but surprisingly mentions several Portuguese doctors, including Rodrigo de Castro, whom the author obviously considered a good Christian. The remainder of the book consists of a litany of charges against Jewish doctors, citing their medical incompetence, their misreading of Latin prescriptions, their inferiority in anatomy, and so on. A certain Isaac Schlam of Wertheimer is held up for special ridicule.[96]

Benedict de Castro wrote his *Scourge of Calumniators* under the pseudonym Philotheus Castellus. In the preface he describes a well-publicized booklet attacking Portuguese Jewish physicians, published anonymously that very year, to which his book was intended as a response. According to Friedenwald, following Gernet, the author of the booklet was Joachim Curtius (1585–1642), who published it anonymously under the title *Exhortatio celeberr. et excellentiss . . . dicata cur judei et agyptae a congressu et praxi medica arcendi sint et eliminandi* in Hamburg in 1631.[97] Friedenwald was not able to locate a copy, nor have I been. If this identification is correct, then the possibility of an earlier Portuguese edition of Benedict's apology published in Antwerp two years earlier has to be questioned. Be that as it may, it is Benedict's response as it appears in the extant Latin edition that is the focus of the discussion that follows.[98]

A stylized opening "to the benevolent reader," in which the circumstances of writing the book are set forth, is followed by a preface dedicated to the author by the famous Portuguese physician Zacutus Lusitanus of Amsterdam. As we shall see, Benedict returned the compliment in a letter of approbation printed in

96. Ludovicus von Hoernigk, *Medicaster Apella oder Juden Artzt* (Strassburg, 1631). Friedenwald mentions the work in a note in *Jews and Medicine*, 1:53–54. I inspected a copy in the Friedenwald Collection of the National and University Library, Jerusalem. The converso doctors are listed on p. 10. Isaac Schlam is discussed on pp. 138ff. and 166ff.

97. Friedenwald, *Jews and Medicine*, 1:56, citing Dr. Gernet, *Mittheilungen aus der aelteren Medicinal-Geschichte Hamburgs* (Hamburg, 1869), p. 176.

98. I have used the photographic copy of the *Flagellum* (Amsterdam, 1631) in the Friedenwald Collection. Yakov Malkiel's typescript of a partial English translation of the work (identified below as Malkiel) is also in the collection. Friedenwald relied on this work in publishing large selections in his essay in *Jews and Medicine*, 1:53–67. I have used his translations whenever possible.

Zacutus's major medical compendium. Zacutus launches an energetic defense of his Portuguese colleagues, who are "true, reliable, learned, delicate, charming, witty, urbane . . . and . . . exceedingly skillful and efficient in their medical practice."[99] They are also reverent and observant of God's precepts and generous to all humanity.

A second preface follows, composed by a graduate of the University of Alcala de Henares named Philaletes. He adopts a strategy which is not followed—indeed, is contradicted—by Benedict. He argues that religious faith is irrelevant in evaluating a physician. If it were relevant, Galen, Hippocrates, Avicenna, Rhazes, and others would be deemed unworthy of their profession—an obviously absurd conclusion. It therefore follows, Philaletes argues, that physicians do not involve themselves with matters of conscience affecting the soul but only with bodily problems. He concludes by extolling the background and university background of Jewish physicians all over Europe.[100]

Benedict's text then opens by comparing the bad writer to an abortive child, a beginning with no great significance except that the sources listed in the side margin include Rodrigo de Castro's *De universa mulierum morborum medicina,* an initial signal, perhaps, of a strong filial piety which he maintains throughout the book.[101] In the pages that follow, Benedict offers a general defense of the loyalty and piety of Jewish citizens, holding up the example of the Dutch and their support of the Jewish graduates of the University of Leiden.

He then turns to consider the attributes of Portuguese Jewish physicians. As in the case of Huarte de San Juan and his own father, Benedict emphasizes the diagnostic abilities of Jewish physicians. This leads him to consider the proper procedures of the doctor and to describe his role in society. Clearly echoing his father, Benedict declares that medical rules are unchangeable, flowing from the purest fountains of nature. Accordingly, the dispenser of such rules is deemed more influential than a king.[102]

99. *Flagellum,* praefatio, p. x (my pagination): "nonne hi sunt Medici maxime veri, fidi, docti, suaves, lepidi, gratiosi, urbani omni virtute decoranti, in facienda medicine dexterrimi."

100. Ibid., pp. xii–xv.

101. Ibid., p. 1.

102. Ibid., pp. 2–16. On p. 16: "Quum itaque sit tanta earum necessitas, tanta praestantia, enitendum omnino ut integrae purae & castae hauriantur, è saluberrimis, & purissimis naturae

After praising the talents of pagan physicians, he turns to the Jews. If pagans were great physicians, he contends, then "why should the Jews, inspired by the divinity, and guided by the stimulus of a noble disposition, to whom God has conceded the privilege of this art from the outset, so as to be their hereditary right, fail in achieving infinitely more?" He pauses to recount the achievements of Moses, who laid the foundations of medicine, and Solomon, who left an exhaustive history of plants. Then he proclaims: "But why should I dwell on the roots . . . when there is virtually no single part of medicine which cannot be traced to those old forefathers of the Hebrews, from whom, as if they were a fountain head, endless systems of streams flew aboard all over the world? Though they are separated by their actual location, all of them go back to one common source . . . and apart from the faculty of medicine, is it not true that in other sciences as well, many things due to this old Hebrew nation have been preserved for posterity?" To confirm this observation, he offers the following authorities: Hermes, Hippocrates, Plato, Josephus, Seneca, and Clearchus.[103]

Having established the priority of Jews in medicine, Benedict considers the qualities of the physician in general, emphasizing his ethical responsibility. Both the divine cosmos and the human body reveal a remarkable inner coherence of all things in nature that teaches humanity to offer friendship in its mutual relations. Referring to a most up-to-date list of contemporary practitioners—Fernelius, Dodeons, Sennert, and Sylvius—Benedict extols the divine function of the skilled physician, who holds power over life and death, who displays the ability to grasp nature's secrets and apply them practically, and who func-

fontibus . . . eos vero qui earum ope medicinam sint facturi magna dignitatis commendatione apud omnes extollant."

103. Ibid., pp. 22–25. On p. 22: "Quid ni Hebraei divino numine afflati, & sincerioris animi impulsi ducti, quibus Deus O. M. primo hanc artem gratis concessit, haereditario quodam iure, multo plura [23] or pulchriora praestare poterint? . . . [24] Sed quid ego stirpes memoro . . . cum nulla omnino medicinae nostrae pars sit, quae non ad antiquos illos Hebraeorum patres suos natales referat, a quibus tamquam a perenni fontis capite, infinita fluentorum diuortia per orbem terrarum dimanarunt: locis quidem disclusa, sed ex communi inter se principio confluentia. . . . neque in medica facultate solum, verum & in aliijs scientijs ex prima illa Hebraeorum gente quam plurima prodierunt in luminis auras [25] posteritati relicta."

tions as both a true philosopher and a practitioner.[104] Only men worthy of such a responsibility can be doctors: "Oh, immortal God, I invoke thy name, lest Thou sufferest that this holy gift [medicine] be dishonored by laymen and be polluted by enemies of nature."[105] Only the Portuguese physicians are capable of honoring this "holy gift": "Not for the sake of money, nor for the sake of honor, nor, finally, for the sake of ambition for their minds are only bent upon the expectation of better human health."[106]

It is Benedict's father, Rodrigo de Castro, who most embodies the divine mission of the Portuguese Jewish doctor:

... the splendor of the Commonwealth, the adornment of the Republic, who, by the monuments erected by his own spiritual work, has consecrated his immortal memory. His unique and everlasting fame, based on rare gifts of virtue and a manifold experience, has pervaded a great part of the universe. In addition to this, it is by his religious attitude, his search for truth and light which is so welcome to God, that he has proved so helpful to his state and to all human beings. . . . He cultivated the beautiful fields of that science [medicine], and its eternally flourishing gardens. . . . He wrote his *Medicus politicus,* full of sentences culled from all sciences, and in this book he propounded not only salutary precepts valuable for the future physician, but also imparted canons and rules that may be of some use for all adults.[107]

Benedict now offers his inventory of great Portuguese Jewish physicians, dividing them into two groups. The first he describes as "those who merely trace back their origin to the Hebrew race"; the second are "those who, essen-

104. Ibid., pp. 29–52; the list of doctors is on p. 47. It should be mentioned that Isaac Cardoso similarly underscored the divine function of the physician in his *Philosophia libera.* See Yerushalmi, *From Spanish Court to Jewish Ghetto,* pp. 231–32.

105. *Flagellum,* p. 53: "Proh Deum immortalem, tuum numen imploro, ne sanctum hoc donum (medicinam) à prophanis pollui, à naturae hostibus conspurcari patiare . . . ."

106. Ibid., p. 63: "Hoc faciunt medici Lusitani, non pecuniae, non honori, non [64] denique ambitioni adicti, sed tantum salutis humanae prospectui intenti ad poeoneas artes recurrunt . . . ."

107. Ibid., p. 66: "Rodericus à Castro medicorum splendor, & reipublicae ornamentum, qui se proprij ingenij monumentis immortali posteritatis memoriae consecravit, cuius prae-

tially and religiously, are still Hebrew." In the first group are such luminaries as Thomas Rodericus a Vega and Rodericus Fonseca; in the second are Elijah Montalto, Amatus Lusitanus, and Zacutus Lusitanus.[108] He closes with a moving eulogy on the Jewish martyrs Eleazar and Hannah and the latter's seven sons, based on the account in 2 Maccabees, praising their steadfastness of faith—a transparent analogue to the martyrs of the Inquisition.[109] He admonishes his calumniators to display Christian charity, even quoting Matthew and Paul.[110] Finally, he offers his work to all German doctors, those who follow classical procedures as well as proponents of the new chemical practices.[111]

Benedict, like his father, defined medicine as a profession having moral and spiritual dimensions. The good physician is empowered to treat the soul as well as the body, to affect the moral fiber of society, and to engender a social harmony that reflects the divine harmony of the cosmos. Benedict goes beyond his father in stipulating that the "holy task" of the physician is a specifically Jewish enterprise. To be a Jewish doctor is to assume the role traditionally assigned to the rabbi: to transform society through his healing powers, his assiduous learning, and his moral example. Benedict's text, like his father's, as Friedenwald points out, is deficient in its quotations of Jewish sources other than the Bible, Josephus, and the Book of Maccabees.[112] Nevertheless, it displays a powerful sense of Jewish pride and commitment. Its author had transformed the shame and racial stigma of the converso doctor into a badge of honor, and in so doing had defined medicine as the quintessentially Jewish task, linked to the mem-

---

clara aeterni, nominis fama raris virtutum dotibus, variaque rerum experientia & usu parta magnam universi orbis partem implevit, sic pietatis cultu, veritatis inquisitione & luce, grata Deo, utilia humano generi ac reipublicae praestitit . . . [67] amenissimos huius scientiae agros colere studuit, florida iugiter vireta excolere . . . . [68] Deinde in suo Medico Politico varijs omnium scientiarum hosculis referto, salutaria praecepta non tantum futuro medico necessaria proponit, vorum etiam & adultis canones & regulas utiles impartitur."

108. Ibid., pp. 70–77.

109. Ibid., pp. 84–90.

110. Ibid., p. 91.

111. Ibid., p. 99: "hujus civitatis tam in Hipp. & Galeni doctrina, quam in arte Chymica Celeberrimos compello."

112. Friedenwald, *Jews and Medicine,* 1:67.

ory of the holy martyrs of the past and to the divine commandments of Jewish survival and social responsibility of the present and future.

The two most illustrious members of the converso community of physicians in the sixteenth and seventeenth centuries were surely Amatus Lusitanus (1511–68) and Zacutus Lusitanus (1575–1642). Their lives and works have been studied by Lemos, Friedenwald, and others, and there is no need to review them here.[113] I wish only to underscore the aspect of their lives which they held in common with their colleagues treated above—namely, the organic linkage between their professional careers and their emerging senses of Jewish identity.

The most disquieting aspect of Amatus's career, after leaving Portugal, was the public scorn heaped upon him by the well-known commentator of Dioscorides, Pietro Andrea Mattioli (1500–1577).[114] Having established a successful medical career in Ferrara, while gaining the friendship of Brassavola, Canano, Falconer, and other distinguished scientists, Amatus must have felt confident enough in his own situation and abilities to offer some modest corrections of Mattioli's work in his own commentary on Dioscorides. He could not have been fully prepared for Mattioli's response:

> It seems truly wonderful that he [Amatus] should have sullied our religion and his own with every misdeed, dishonored it with shame and made himself guilty of crime towards it, and that only for that reason was he forced to live as an exile from his native Portugal. . . . I do not regard you as blind because of [your] ancient heathen superstition . . . but for the reason and conviction (to which you yourself have assuredly also come), that you have most perfidiously turned away from God, the Eternal. . . . For as you now present to adhere to our faith (so I learn), and then give yourself over to Jewish laws

113. See the numerous references to both in the index to Friedenwald, *Jews and Medicine.* The classic accounts of both are by Maximiano Lemos, *Amato Lusitano. A sua Vida e a sua obra* (Porto, 1907), and *Zacuto Lusitano. A sua Vida e a sua obra* (Porto, 1909). On Amatus, see also A. G. Keller's essay in *Dictionary of Scientific Bibliography,* 8:554–55.

114. On Mattioli, see J. Stannard, "P. A. Mattioli: Sixteenth-Century Commentators on Dioscorides," *University of Kansas Libraries, Bibliographical Contributions,* vol. 1 (Lawrence, Kan., 1969), pp. 59–81; G. Fabiani, *La Vita di Pietro Andrea Mattioli,* ed. L. Banchi (Siena, 1872).

and superstitions and thus insult not only your fellow beings, but also God, the Almighty, it is not to be wondered that you are false even to yourself and are losing your mind. Just as there is no faith and no religion within you, so in truth you are completely blind as to the medical art which you unworthily profess . . . and that driven by wild furies you have brought it about that you neither enlighten others nor yourself in medical practice, just as you are blind in your heresy to divine truth.[115]

Amatus reports that he had written a response and complains of censorship.[116] Lacking the response, we can only conjecture how Amatus might have viewed Mattioli's attack. Most likely he would have taken it as a telling indication of how a threatened Christian colleague perceived the clear nexus between this converso's professional and religious identities, and rather than deny the connection, he would have affirmed it unambiguously and wholeheartedly.

Zacutus Lusitanus's reflection on the connection between his medical and Jewish identities coincided with the culmination of his career: the publication of the first volume of his complete works during the year of his death in 1642. In the opening peroration he fully acknowledges his Jewish identity and merges it directly with his distinguished medical career and his devotion to study. Like his colleagues Rodrigo (he even quotes from the *Medicus politicus*) and Benedict de Castro, he views physicians "as the tutelaries of Divinity, sons of the gods."[117] But most telling of all are the approbatory letters and poems that celebrate the publication of the volume and the distinguished career of the author. They were written by a remarkable group of medical luminaries from all over Europe. Most conspicuous of all, and represented beyond their numbers in the medical community, are the converso physicians, Zacutus's professional and ethnic fraternity, who declare their solidarity and kinship with him. The list includes the two Castros (their letters were dated 1629) of Hamburg, Ludovico Nunez of Antwerp, Benjamin Mussafia of Hamburg, Moses de Luna of Cracow, Jacob Rosales of Hamburg, and many more. And as this proud and distin-

115. Quoted and translated in Friedenwald, *Jews and Medicine*, 2:349.

116. Ibid., p. 351.

117. Zacutus Lusitanus, *Opera omnia* (Amsterdam, 1642), 1:984, 904 (where he also quotes from the *Medicus politicus*).

guished group saluted their colleague in opening the volume, another, no less distinguished one symbolically closed it.

Conspicuously situated between the list of ancient and Arabic doctors in the "Elencus auctorum" at the end of the volume, a distinct inventory of Jewish medical authorities is offered the reader. This group includes Abraham ibn Ezra, David de Pomis, Benjamin Mussafia, Jacob Mantino, Elijah Montalto, Leone Ebreo, David Kimḥi, Isaac Abravanel, Menasseh ben Israel, Moses Maimonides, and several kings of ancient Israel, including, of course, Solomon Rex. The intermingling of traditional Jewish authorities with recent converso physicians seems innocuous enough. But perhaps we might view it as well as both a declaration of pride in Jewish ancestry and a bold assertion that Montalto and Mussafia, converso physicians of Zacutus's generation, personified and transmitted—like Kimḥi and ibn Ezra, and before them Solomon—the glorious traditions of Judaism to a new generation of Jews in seventeenth-century Europe.[118]

118. Another illustration of pride in Jewish ancestry is offered by Y. Kaplan in his study of Jewish medical students at Leiden (n. 1 above). He discusses in particular the dedications appended to the dissertations of Moses Orobio, the son of Isaac Orobio de Castro, and David Pina. Moses dedicates his composition to his father and to Benedict de Castro of Hamburg, along with two other rabbis of Amsterdam. Pina also singles out Isaac Orobio, among others. As Kaplan points out (p. 73), the dedications, particularly the one to Benedict, offer clear testimony of the students' perceptions that they were entering a profession ennobled by their Jewish forebears.

A Jewish Thinker in Newtonian England

DAVID NIETO AND HIS DEFENSE OF THE JEWISH FAITH

David Nieto (1654–1728), the first rabbi of the new Bevis Marks
Synagogue and the *ḥakham* of the Spanish and Portuguese congregation of London at the beginning of the eighteenth century,
is not an unstudied figure in recent Jewish historiography. From
the portrait of Moses Gaster to the later elaborations of Cecil
Roth and Moses Hyamson, and from the exhaustive bibliographical study of Israel Solomons to the pioneering study of Nieto's
thought by Jacob Petuchowski, Nieto's public career and theological writings have been examined as thoroughly as those of
any other Jewish intellectual figure of early modern Europe.[1] Yet
each of these studies was completed over thirty years ago. In
the interim, new scholarship in Jewish history, particularly in
the history of Marranism and Sabbatianism, has illumined the
broader cultural ambiance of Nieto's era.[2] Even more dramatic

---

1. M. Gaster, *History of the Ancient Synagogue of the Spanish and Portuguese
Jews* (London, 1901), pp. 101–16; C. Roth, *Essays and Portraits in Anglo-Jewish
History* (Philadelphia, 1962), pp. 113–29 (a Hebrew version of the same essay
is part of the introduction to *Ha-Kuzari ha-Sheni Hu Matteh Dan,* ed. J. L.
Maimon [Jerusalem, 1958]); A. Hyamson, *The Sephardim of England* (Lon-
don, 1951), index; I. Solomons, "David Nieto and Some of His Contempo-
raries," *Transactions of the Jewish Historical Society of England* 12 (1931): 1–101;
J. J. Petuchowski, *The Theology of Haham David Nieto: An Eighteenth-Century
Defense of the Jewish Tradition* (New York, 1954, 1970).

2. I refer especially to G. Scholem's many studies, first and foremost
Sabbatai Ṣevi: The Mystical Messiah (Princeton, 1973). See also the work of

has been the plethora of scholarship on English political and cultural history, and especially the history of scientific thought.[3] In the light of new insights offered by both scholarly literatures, Nieto's career and intellectual achievements require a fresh look, particularly because Nieto's "Jewish" preoccupations were so closely intertwined with the larger cultural—especially scientific—concerns of his newly adopted country.

David Nieto came to England in 1701 to assume the chief rabbinic post of the fledgling community of Jews of Sephardic descent, primarily former conversos. Since his contract stipulated that he could not practice medicine, despite the prestigious medical degree he held from the University of Padua,[4] he fully understood his new calling as that of a public figure, the chief representative of his coreligionists in England, and their primary spokesman and religious leader. His primary concern was to be the welfare of his community, its legal status, its economic and social condition, as well as its spiritual well-being. At the same time, Nieto was more than a public official and religious functionary. In inviting him to England, the Sephardim had engaged one of the most original minds of eighteenth-century Jewry, a prolific writer in Hebrew and Spanish, well edu-

---

Y. Liebes mentioned in the Introduction, n. 21, above; E. Carlebach, *In Pursuit of Heresy* (New York, 1990), Y. Kaplan, *From Christianity to Judaism* (Oxford, 1989), N. Yosha, "The Philosophic Background of Sabbatian Theology: Guidelines towards an Understanding of Abraham Michael Cardoso's Theory of the Divine," in A. Mirsky, A. Grossman, and Y. Kaplan, eds., *Galut Aḥar Golah* (Jerusalem, 1988), pp. 541–72; idem, "Ha-Parshanut ha-Pilosofit shel R. Avraham Cohen Herrera le-Kabbalat ha-Ari," unpublished Ph.D. diss., Hebrew University, 1991; Y. Yerushalmi, *From Spanish Court to Italian Ghetto* (New York, 1991); the many essays and books of M. Benayahu and I. Tishby on Sabbatianism; D. Katz's *Philosemitism and the Readmission of the Jews into England, 1603–1655* (Oxford and New York, 1982); and J. Israel's *European Jewry in the Age of Mercantilism, 1550–1750* (Oxford, 1985).

3. The literature is too vast to list here. A recent overview which stresses the connection between political and scientific culture in early modern Europe is M. Jacob, *The Cultural Meaning of the Scientific Revolution* (Philadelphia, 1988), including a useful bibliographical essay. This should be compared with C. Russell, *Science and Social Change in Britain and Europe, 1700–1900* (New York, 1983), and M. Hunter, *Science and Society in Restoration England* (Cambridge, 1981), with its useful bibliographical essay, recently updated in his *Establishing the New Science: The Experience of the Early Royal Society* (Woodbridge, England, 1989), pp. 356–68.

4. See Solomons, "David Nieto," p. 8

cated in Jewish and secular subjects. Like many of the other figures we have examined above, especially those of Italian provenance, he had studied medicine and rabbinics and had pursued simultaneously a rabbinic and medical career while in Italy. Upon his arrival in England, he already held a reputation as a serious scholar of Judaism and was well versed in the sciences and in several European languages, as his correspondence with Theopold Unger and other Christian intellectuals indicates.[5] Although he was apparently insecure about his inability to speak and write fluent English,[6] he was certainly able to hold his own among his new countrymen as an expositor of Judaism in an era of formidable intellectual challenges. To appreciate fully Nieto's place in the history of Jewish civilization, we must consider both of his faces—the political as well as the intellectual—and particularly how they intersected throughout his distinguished career on English soil.

As Nieto's writings testify, he considered the profound impact of the sciences on European culture and society a supreme intellectual challenge to the viability of Judaism at the turn of the century. In England, especially, Nieto encountered a highly sophisticated society of scientists and churchmen who had creatively wedded the new advances in science to their own political and religious aspirations. These "virtuosi," first prominently Puritan and later Anglican, had found in the new scientific discoveries a potent vehicle by which to enhance their understanding of the Christian faith.[7] In early modern Europe, and particularly in England, as Margaret Jacob has argued, ideas about the natural world often

5. Cf. ibid., pp. 21–24, 38–44.

6. In a letter to Dr. John Covel, the Master of Christ's Church, Cambridge, written in 1705–6, Nieto claimed he could not write English. See ibid., p. 22.

7. See esp. R. Merton, *Science, Technology and Society in Seventeenth-Century England* (New York, 1970); C. Webster, *The Great Instauration: Science, Medicine, and Reform* (London, 1975); Webster, ed., *The Intellectual Revolution of the Seventeenth Century* (London, 1974); C. Hill, *The Intellectual Origins of the English Revolution* (Oxford, 1965); J. Jacob, "Restoration, Reformation, and the Origins of the Royal Society," *History of Science* 13 (1975): 155–76; R. S. Westfall, *Science and Religion in Seventeenth-Century England* (New Haven, 1958); J. Jacob and M. Jacob, "The Anglican Origins of Modern Science," *Isis* 71 (1980): 251–67; and M. Jacob, *The Newtonians and the English Revolution* (Ithaca, 1976). Compare, however, the works by Russell and Hunter mentioned in n. 3 above; L. Mulligan, "Puritans and English Science: A Critique of Webster," *Isis* 71 (1980): 456–69; and the references in the following footnote.

bore a direct relation to the way people understood the social and moral order.[8] In the seventeenth century, such thinkers as Hobbes, Descartes, and Spinoza had articulated mechanical philosophies of nature which assumed that nature, not God, was a sufficient explanation for the cause and workings of the material environment. Among such "heretics," a philosophy of pantheistic materialism, claiming that God could be located only within natural objects, readily served as a philosophical justification for democratic belief. Since all things in nature shared a sense of divinity, all were ostensibly equal. The ways of nature militated against all social and political hierarchies and called for a total social leveling and a radical dismemberment of political power and privilege. Such philosophies of nature were accordingly deemed dangerous to those responsible for perpetuating the social order. They not only undermined traditional Christian orthodoxies, they also challenged the self-interest and stable polity of governments, which fostered religious ideologies and behavior that might buttress the political foundations of their Protestant kingdoms.[9]

8. This is a central point of Jacob's *Newtonians,* whose influence on the writing of this chapter is apparent. See also her essay "Christianity and the Newtonian World View" in *God and Nature: Historical Essays on the Encounter between Christianity and Science* (Berkeley, 1986), pp. 238–255; *Cultural Meaning of the Scientific Revolution,* pp. 73–135; and P. M. Heimann, "Science and the English Enlightenment," *History of Science* 16 (1978): 143–51. Jacob's work, nevertheless, has evoked a considerable degree of criticism regarding her oversimplification of Newtonianism and her neglect of orthodox hostility to it. See, for example, the works of Hunter and Russell, esp. chap. 4; J. Force, *William Whiston, Honest Newtonian* (Cambridge, 1985); G. Holmes, "Science, Reason, and Religion in the Age of Newton," *British Journal for the History of Science* 12 (1979): 164–71; C. B. Wilde, "Hutchinsonian Natural Philosophy and Religious Controversy in Eighteenth-Century Britain," *History of Science* 18 (1980): 1–24; and A. Guerrini, "The Tory Newtonians: Gregory Pitcaire and Their Circle," *Journal of British Studies* 15 (1986): 288–311.

9. See esp. P. Hazard, *The European Mind* (New Haven, 1953); C. Hill, *The World Turned Upside Down* (New York, 1972); M. Jacob, *The Radical Enlightenment: Pantheists, Freemasons, and Republicans* (London and Boston, 1981); C. Giuntini, *Panteismo e ideologia republicana: John Toland (1670–1722)* (Bologna, 1979); R. Kargon, *Atomism in England from Harriot to Newton* (Oxford, 1966); R. Colie, "Spinoza in England, 1665–1730," *Proceedings of the American Philosophical Society* 107 (1963): 183–219; S. I. Mintz, *The Hunting of Leviathan* (Cambridge, 1962); Hunter, *Science and Society,* chap. 7; idem, "Science and Heterodoxy," in R. S. Westman and

In opposition to these heretics stood the Christian Anglican proponents of the new science. They became especially prominent in England after the revolution of 1688–89 and were at the height of their power and influence during Nieto's career in London in the first decades of the eighteenth century. Their heroes were Boyle and Newton, whom they lionized as the architects of a new Christian vision of the universe stamped with the seal of the Divinity. They defined their Christian faith as a natural religion or natural theology that glorified the new science while repudiating the outmoded Aristotelianism of the universities and the mechanical philosophies of Hobbes and Descartes, with their materialistic and potentially atheistic implications. They were equally disdainful of the newest version of pantheism made prominent by the political radical John Toland. In their place, they proposed a mechanical philosophy requiring God's active engagement in the workings of nature. The new discoveries revealed more distinctly than ever the manifold glimpses of the divine presence in everything. Science insured a faith in traditional Christian truths, so they argued, and also provided the most effective underpinning for their vision of a stable and prosperous social order ruled by human self-interest but controlled and directed by religious moderation and good taste. If the scientists had unveiled a blueprint of the harmony and stability operating in nature, it could and should be correlated with the proper workings of the social and economic order. Order in nature prescribed social and political stability in the world of government, church hierarchies, and capitalist markets.[10]

This new vision of Anglican Latitudinarian religiosity that nurtured stability and harmony in the natural and social realms, balancing the pursuit of self-interest with religious and political duty, was ultimately bound to clash with all forms of radicalism—religious, political, and economic. The spokesmen of this new orthodoxy saw as their primary purpose the defeat of all atheists, deists, freethinkers, and enthusiasts, who were often lumped together as the primary

---

D. C. Lindberg, eds., *Reappraisals of the Scientific Revolution* (Cambridge, 1990); and R. E. Sullivan, *John Toland and the Deist Controversy: A Study in Adaptations* (Cambridge, Mass., and London, 1982).

10. These themes are fully developed by M. Jacob in *Newtonians*. See as well the other works cited in nn. 7 and 8.

enemies of religion and the state. Uncontrolled extremism in the religious realm, pejoratively called religious "enthusiasm," was viewed as a critical threat to ecclesiastical power and as an illegitimate religious sensibility that might undermine the carefully calibrated sense of balance and order within the church, the political realm, and the marketplace.[11]

The most prominent platform for disseminating this new vision of Anglican Christianity confirmed by science was the prestigious Boyle lectures, established with income from the estate of Robert Boyle and held annually from 1692 to 1714. The lectures offer an extraordinary index of official Anglican theology bearing the scientific and political establishment's seal of approval. Among the most prominent of the Boyle lecturers was Samuel Clarke, whose erudite addresses on the being and attributes of God of 1704 and the obligations of the natural religion and the certainty of the Christian revelation of 1705 encapsulate as well as any of the lectures the essence of the new theological fusion between Christianity and Newtonian science. These lectures in particular bear an uncanny resemblance to Nieto's own theological writings, as we shall soon observe.[12]

Nieto's intellectual and political consciousness was undoubtedly shaped by

11. On the attacks against enthusiasm, see G. Williamson, "The Restoration Revolt against Enthusiasm," *Studies in Philology* 30 (1935): 571–604 (repr. in his *Seventeenth-Century Contexts* [London, 1960], pp. 202–39); P. B. Wood, "Methodology and Apologetics: Thomas Sprat's *History of the Royal Society," The British Journal for the History of Science* 13 (1980): 1–26; M. Heyd, "The Reaction to Enthusiasm in the Seventeenth Century: Towards an Integrative Approach," *Journal of Modern History* 53 (1981): 258–80; idem, "The New Experimental Philosophy: A Manifestation of 'Enthusiasm' or an Anidote to It?" *Minerva* 25 (1987): 423–40; and idem, *"Be Sober and Reasonable": Science, Medicine, and the Critique of Enthusiasm in the Seventeenth and Early Eighteenth Centuries* (forthcoming).

12. The Boyle lectures are treated in Jacob, *Newtonians,* chaps. 4 and 5. See also J. Dahm, "Science and Apologetics in the Early Boyle Lectures," *Church History* 39 (1970): 172–86. Hunter's argument that the lectures were neither homogeneous nor focused exclusively on Newtonian science is an important corrective to Jacob's treatment. See his works cited in nn. 3 and 8, esp. James Force's study of Clarke's colleague Whiston. On Clarke, compare J. P. Ferguson, *An Eighteenth-Century Heretic: Dr. Samuel Clarke* (Kineton, England, 1976), and L. Stewart, "Samuel Clarke, Newtonianism, and the Factions of Post-Revolutionary England," *Journal of the History of Ideas* 42 (1981): 53–72. I have read Clarke's two sermons in Samuel Clarke, *The Works, 1738, in Four Volumes* (New York and London, 1978), 2: 513–733.

the dominant ideology so forcefully articulated by the Anglican religious establishment. Nieto's vision of traditional Judaism as formulated in his highly polemical writings can be fully appreciated only by comparing it with that of his Anglican colleagues. From the time of his first publication in London until his death, he creatively adopted positions and theological solutions paralleling their own in the cause of traditional Judaism. Having only stepped off the boat as a new immigrant several months earlier, he composed in Spanish in December 1701 a prayer which begins: "A fervid and humble prayer addressed to the Great and Omnipotent God of Israel by the Congregation of Jews in London, in which they implore the assistance and help of Heaven at the Deliberations of His Majesty the Invincible King William III, their sovereign, of his Supreme Council, and of both the Chambers of his August Parliament."[13] An encomium to the political establishment was certainly consistent with other forms of political flattery in which Jewish leaders had indulged for centuries. But Nieto's prayer, when viewed together with his elaborate discussion of Judaism and the sciences, his ruminations on God and nature, his polemics with the Sabbatian enthusiast Nehemiah Ḥiyya Ḥayon, and the general direction of his public and literary career, suggest a consistent and distinctive ideological position unmistakably reminiscent of the image of his Anglican counterparts. Nieto quickly learned that Judaism could survive within English society only by both demonstrating the constant political loyalty of Jewish immigrants to the Crown and to the leadership elite and by appropriating the conceptual language and ideological underpinnings of its religious establishment. English Jews would remain Jews, so Nieto believed, if their religious aspirations and sensibilities were in tune both with their own economic and social aspirations and with those of their Christian neighbors. To these objectives he devoted his most creative energies.

It is difficult to point to any single inspiration for Nieto. The fonts of his literary imagination were still located in traditional Jewish sources; he was especially indebted to Judah ha-Levi's great classic and its dialogical form in the writing of his largest work, the *Mateh Dan*. But surely Jewish texts alone could not account for the strategies he now employed in defense of his ancestral faith. If any contemporary source expresses Nieto's most characteristic lines of argu-

13. See Solomons, "David Nieto," p. 8.

ment, it is Samuel Clarke's Boyle lectures of 1704–5. We shall examine the possibility of a relationship between the two authors below. In any event, it is clear that Nieto's positions paralleled those of Clarke and his Newtonian circle and that all of Nieto's major writings reveal a conscious and creative response to his cultural environment. All of his three works unambiguously display the ability of a Jewish thinker to absorb the dominant theological positions of his Christian contemporaries and to reformulate them as Jewish theology before a recently constituted congregation of assimilated, secularized, highly ambitious but politically and culturally insecure Jewish merchants.

Nieto's first major work was his *De la Divina Providencia,* published in London in 1704. Written in his preferred dialogical form in the wake of a controversy which had seriously threatened his good name and his brief tenure as religious leader, it was meant to clarify Nieto's position on divine providence and its relation to nature. In a sermon on the same topic delivered on November 20, 1703, some of his listeners were alarmed to hear the *ḥakham* identify nature with God. One member of the congregation, Joshua Ẓarfatti, petitioned the congregation to condemn their religious leader as a heretic. A long controversy ensued involving several members of the London congregation, the attorney general, and eventually Ḥakham Ẓevi Ashkenazi of Amsterdam.[14] Although the details have been discussed before, the precise context of the debate and Nieto's published work have yet to be clarified. Most interpreters have understood the alarm of Nieto's detractors as merely stemming from their belief that he was a Spinozist. Although Spinoza is nowhere mentioned explicitly either in Nieto's summary of the sermon or in his lengthier dialogue, scholars assumed that the allegations of heresy were Spinozist even though Nieto's thoughts were obviously misconstrued. In fact, Spinoza's pantheistic ideas were well known in

14. The work and the controversy are discussed in ibid., pp. 10–17, as well as in the other works mentioned in n. 1 above. See also A. Barzel, "General Nature and Particular Nature" (in Hebrew), *Da'at* 17 (1986): 67–80. I have used the original Spanish edition published by James Dover, as well as the English translation by E. H. Lindo of 1853, listed as Codex Adler (6c), in Solomons, "David Nieto," p. 66, and now located in the library of the Hebrew Union College–Jewish Institute of Religion in Cincinnati. My thanks to the library for providing me with a copy of this manuscript.

England by the early eighteenth century and were certainly familiar to some of Nieto's accusers.[15] But pantheism as a religious philosophy was certainly a broader phenomenon than Spinoza's ideas and clearly could have suggested wider associations for Nieto's listeners.

To fully appreciate Nieto's reflections on divine providence and the acrimony they elicited, we should mention not one but three distinct views. First was the view which Nieto's enemies thought they heard their ḥakham express, namely, his alleged pantheism. The first stirrings of pantheism, also known as materialism, in England were among sectarian radicals in the 1650s and later among Whig circles after the revolution of 1688. The most prominent pantheist in Nieto's day was John Toland, who had proclaimed nature, not God, to be the sole object of worship and study. The origins of this ideology could be traced to certain magical and naturalistic views of the Renaissance, and only later was it merged with Hobbesian materialism and Spinozist tendencies. In fact, Toland himself was the first to equate pantheism with Spinozism as late as 1709. As a challenge to the dualist nature of Christian metaphysics, and specifically the transcendent nature of God, pantheism was troublesome enough as a religious philosophy. As the foundation for a political philosophy that preached social equality for all, since God is in all nature and all natural things are equal, it clearly resonated with dangerous social implications for those who staked their own existence on the preservation of the existing social order.[16]

But Nieto had no sympathy for pantheism, nor did he intend to discuss it in his sermon. Rather, he presented another view which he found most objectionable. At the opening of the first dialogue of *De la Divina Providencia,* Nieto spells out this position through the mouthpiece of Simon. Simon claims that God gave nature the faculty and power to govern the world, arranging the whole in so fixed and inalterable a manner while reserving the intervention of occasional miracles for himself.[17] Simon marshals a number of biblical and rabbinic quotations to confirm this idea, including the rabbinic statement "The world follows its course."[18] When Reuven, Simon's interlocutor, presents Nieto's position that

15. See R. Colie, "Spinoza in England."
16. For references, see n. 9 above.
17. *De la Divina Providencia,* pp. 2–3; *On Divine Providence,* pp. 9–11.
18. B.T. Avodah Zarah 54b and elsewhere.

God and nature are the same, Simon parries with two primary objections. He claims that if God and nature are one, all creatures are then identical with God. Moreover, if God performs all that nature does, there is no place for the miraculous. Accordingly, the natural should come from nature, the miraculous from God.[19]

What follows is a sustained critique of Simon's position by Reuven. At one point, Reuven even identifies Simon's position with that of the deists, "who believed that there was only one God but He didn't trouble himself in the government of the world. They say that nature directs [this machine] and governs everything in its way . . . that God left the power of governing the world to a supposed universal nature as a prince who leaves the government to his minister."[20] Reuven concludes that this is enormous heresy and blasphemy; instead, only God governs the world.

To whom was Nieto referring when presenting Simon's view? He might have had in mind the views of Henry More and Ralph Cudworth, the two most prominent Cambridge Platonists, as well as those of John Ray, the famous "virtuoso," regarding the idea known as "plastic nature." Clearly opposed to the mechanistic and pantheistic views of nature which denied God any will at all, they settled instead for likening nature to a kind of semidiety, lieutenant, or viceregent of God, providing Him an instrument through which He could govern the universe and intervene when necessary to perform miracles. By assigning general nature the responsibility for regularly governing the world, they absolved God of the responsibility of evil.[21] Robert Boyle objected strenuously to this notion

19. *De la Divina Providencia,* pp. 4–5; *On Divine Providence,* pp. 11–12.

20. *De la Divina Providencia,* p. 9; *On Divine Providence,* p. 17. Compare Russell, *Science and Social Change,* pp. 45–46.

21. On the notion of plastic nature, see, for example, the following statement of Ralph Cudworth: "Since neither all things are produced fortuitously, or by the unguided mechanism of matter, nor God himself may reasonably be thought to do all things immediately and miraculously; it may well be concluded, that there is a plastic nature under him, as an inferior and subordinate instrument, which doth drudgingly execute that part of his providence, which consists in the regular and orderly motion of matter." *The True Intellectual System of the Universe,* ed. J. L. Mosheim, trans. J. Harrison (1678; repr. London, 1845), 1: 223–24 (quoted in Hunter, *Science and Society,* pp. 181–82). See also Westfall, *Science and Religion,* pp. 84–85, 94–95; Colie,

of plastic nature and consistently maintained that the universal and benevolent order of nature was identical with divine providence.[22] Samuel Clarke, his disciple and later disseminator of his views, identified this notion with a kind of deism and maintained that it unavoidably led to absolute atheism.[23]

It is the third view, the view of Reuven, with which Nieto identifies and which is brought by him to counter the allegedly pernicious view of Simon, which Nieto, like Clarke, understands as deism, heresy, blasphemy, and "absolute atheism." It is this third view which is the centerpiece of his sermon and treatise and to which all his energy is directed, and it is this view which is badly misinterpreted as pantheism by his detractors, when in reality he meant something else entirely. A close reading of Samuel Clarke's sermon on the obligations of the natural religion, published at almost the same time as Nieto's treatise, makes the rabbi's position unambiguous.[24]

Clarke's long discourse had carefully delineated the various kinds of deism that undermined the true Christian faith. The view Nieto had identified with that of Simon was the first Clarke discussed.[25] Upon declaring this position to be atheistic, Clarke maintained that creation depended on God's continual power over it, (quoting Matthew) "with whom not a sparrow falls to the ground and with whom the very hairs of our head are all numbered." A world left to its own resources to form "a world of adventures" is nothing more than a philosophical vanity for Clarke. On the contrary, everything in the universe displays the marks of the Creator—"that from the brightest star in the firmament of heaven, to the meanest pebble on the face of the earth, there is no one piece of matter

---

"Spinoza in England," p. 197; and idem, *Light and Enlightenment: A Study of the Cambridge Platonists and the Dutch Arminians* (Cambridge, 1957), chap. 7; Mintz, *Hunting of Leviathan,* chap. 5; and R. A. Green, "Henry Moore and Robert Boyle on the Spirit of Nature," *Journal of the History of Ideas* 23 (1962): 451–74.

22. Colie, "Spinoza in England," p. 197; J. E. McGuire, "Boyle's Conception of Nature," *Journal of the History of Ideas* 33 (1972): 523–42; Heimann, "Science and the English Enlightenment," pp. 145–46.

23. Clarke, *Works,* pp. 600–602.

24. Ibid., 581–733.

25. Ibid., pp. 600–607, esp. pp. 600–602.

which does not afford such instances of admirable artifice and exact proportion and contrivance, as exceeds all the wit of man."[26]

Such pious sentiments about divine providence were a commonplace among English "virtuosi" of the seventeenth century, but Clarke's sermon makes them of particular importance to Nieto. In response to the argument that reserves the ordinary for nature and the miraculous for God, Clarke emphatically denies that the distinction between the natural and the miraculous is meaningful. It is in God's power to do everything equally well. Thus either nothing should be considered a miracle or everything should be; in either case, they are all the effects of God's acting upon matter continually. And thus Clarke concludes: "There is no such thing, as what men commonly call the course of nature, or the power of nature. The course of nature, truly and properly speaking, is nothing else but the will of God producing certain effects in a continued, regular, constant, and uniform manner: which course of manner or acting, being in every moment, perfectly arbitrary, is as easy to be altered at any time, as to be preserved."[27]

Nieto did not require Clarke's felicitous phrasing to frame his own argument. He could and did enlist the authority of Jewish luminaries from Judah Ha-Levi to Judah Moscato to Jacob Abendana.[28] Nevertheless, Nieto's text is strewn with tantalizing hints that its author may have had Clarke's arguments or similar ones in mind when composing his own work. In the second dialogue, Nieto allows Reuven to respond to Simon concerning the need for divine miracles. Reuven's first strategy is to downplay the importance of miracles in establishing truths "rooted in the inmost recesses of our hearts." But he then argues, like Clarke, that there is no difference between the natural and the miraculous, since all are engendered by the divine will. He insists that he can prove his case by not making use "of modern authorities who have power but to opine, but only of acknowledged ancients who founded dogmas and established doctrines."[29] But the mere mention of "modern authorities" suggests that he is familiar with their opinions. Moreover, the examples that follow appear to indicate that those modern opinions were simply too appealing to be ignored.

26. Ibid., pp. 601–602, 647.
27. Ibid., pp. 696–98.
28. *De la Divina Providencia*, pp. 12–14; *On Divine Providence*, pp. 21–23.
29. *De la Divine Providencia*, pp. 35–37; *On Divine Providence*, pp. 42–44.

Curiously, Nieto offers the example of wheat in arguing that divine providence is the sole cause of nature. Naturalists, he says, assume "that God put
into the earth invisible corpuscules, divided and spread in a manner that they
unite to the sown grain as modern atomists contend. Or it must be believed
that the wheat comes invisibly from the ambient air where it is supposed to
be divided into corpuscules. . . . This formulation be conceived how it may, no
understanding will be induced to believe . . . that an inanimate thing like the
earth can form another object superior to itself."[30] He next turns to the analogy
of clocks to prove his case: "Suppose a rustic who never saw clocks were to see
the hands of a clock without knowing the art of the wheel of the pendulum.
He will consider and declare that those metal hands have an inward virtue." He
clearly confuses the effect with the cause, as do those who argue that nature
and not God is the cause.[31]

The language of corpuscules and clocks under the aegis of God's protecting
hand is unmistakably the language of Robert Boyle, a language so commonly
evoked by Newtonians and other admirers of Boyle in the early eighteenth century.[32] In these latter examples, Nieto was not borrowing directly from Clarke
to argue his case for the misuse of the term *universal nature* and for impiously
attributing "power and strength to secondary causes" rather than to God. Nevertheless, Nieto and Clarke obviously shared an intellectual agenda and a kinship
of spirit. Both admirers of Boyle, they were in essential agreement about the
need to defend a traditional view of divine providence against the dangerous
implications of the notion that God and his creation were virtually separate.
Nieto had protested too loudly about his lack of reliance on modern authorities.
Boyle was his hero too, whether he admitted it or not!

Mateh Dan, Nieto's magnum opus, was published in London in 1714 and
represented his most comprehensive defense of traditional Jewish faith and practice. His wide-ranging arguments in support of the Oral Law, their traditional

30. *De la Divina Providencia,* p. 53; *On Divine Providence,* p. 55a.

31. *De la Divine Providencia,* pp. 54–55; *On Divine Providence,* p. 60.

32. See M. Boaz, *Robert Boyle and Seventeenth-Century Chemistry* (Cambridge, 1958);
McGuire, "Boyle's Conception of Nature."

Jewish sources, and the audience of ex-conversos to whom they were appropriately addressed have been noted by Jacob Petuchowski and need not detain us here. What is critical for our discussion is Nieto's extensive use of science to bolster the authority of the rabbis and to present effectively the virtues of the Jewish faith. Even a superficial reading of *Mateh Dan* displays how seriously Nieto took the scientific context of his contemporaries. Like his Christian colleagues, the followers of Boyle and Newton, he acknowledged that an argument for the viability of his faith would be credible only if couched in the language of science. Judaism had to be shown to be open and willing to embrace science. Furthermore, it had to be demonstrated how the Jewish faith might complement and enhance the moral and spiritual life of the individual, particularly in areas where science might prove insufficient and incapable of penetrating. Nieto would have to preserve a precarious balance between praising science and pointing out its limitations and inadequacies as gently as possible.

Nieto devotes the fourth book of *Mateh Dan* to these two objectives. Aligning himself with a sizable number of earlier Jewish thinkers who had argued for the legitimacy of scientific pursuit in Judaism, Nieto eloquently presents the case that the rabbis had not only permitted scientific studies but had excelled in them. He even points out that kabbalists like Cordovero and Herrera were not adverse to employing natural arguments to explicate their theosophies.[33] Nieto notes with pride how rabbinic literature is replete with learning in a variety of disciplines, from rhetoric to geography, surgery, engineering, and astronomy.[34] Although he admits that the rabbis were interested in the sciences only to the extent that they helped to clarify problems of Jewish law, he stresses in strong Baconian language that their considerable knowledge was based not on speculation but on experience.[35]

Having identified his empiricist leanings, Nieto is ready to evaluate the epistemological basis of the the new mechanical philosophies of his day as potentially competing with the veracity of his own religious faith. What follows is a fully informed and accurate summary of the four primary theories of the origin

33. *Mateh Dan* (Jerusalem, 1958), p. 93.
34. Ibid., pp. 100–123.
35. Ibid., pp. 107, 123.

of matter: those of Aristotle, Gassendi, Descartes, and the chemical philosophers. He discusses the virtues and limitations of each theory and then concludes
that despite their obvious rationality and consistency, they are all hypothetical.
Since there are four and not one, and since each claims to be the truth, he cannot view any of them as certain but only as possible, plausible explanations of
reality.[36] Nieto is also conversant with the claims of Copernican astronomy and
of those who argue for the plurality of worlds beyond the known universe. He
admits the reasonableness of both theories and is willing to accept them as long
as they do not contradict accepted positions of traditional faith. On the basis of
the latter criterion, he approves of the second theory but rejects the first, since
it contradicts an explicit biblical statement.[37]

The speculative nature of the regnant theories of matter is not the only limitation of seventeenth-century science. Despite the dramatic impact of recent
discoveries, especially in his own day—Nieto explicitly mentions the barometer, the thermometer, and the telescope—scientific discovery in his estimation
is accidental and incomplete.[38] It can never claim to understand reality in its
totality. Nieto's enthusiastic endorsement of empiricism is thus tempered by
a skepticism that acknowledges science as a partial but never complete truth.
In light of the incompleteness of scientific achievement, there remains a place
for the rabbis and the divine origin of their sacred revelation. In arguing for
the compatibility of science and Judaism, and simultaneously against the claims
of the self-sufficiency of science devoid of religiosity, Nieto followed the well-
trodden path of Christian scientific practitioners like Mersenne and Gassendi,
as well as that of a recent group of Jewish enthusiasts located especially in
Italy.[39] His defense also mirrored that of Samuel Clarke, who had argued quite
forcefully at the end of his lecture on the truth and certainty of the Christian
religion that mankind required the saving truth of Christian revelation, since a
mechanical understanding of the world alone was insufficient.[40]

36. Ibid., pp. 141–47. For the precise background for this section, see M. Boaz, "The
Establishment of the Mechanical Philosophy," *Osiris* 10 (1952): 412–541.

37. Ibid., pp. 126–31.

38. Ibid., pp. 148–55.

39. On this, see esp. chaps. 6 and 7 above.

40. Clarke, *Works,* pp. 702–28.

Nieto, in *Mateh Dan,* had squarely faced the challenge the new sciences presented to Judaism and had devised the most effective strategies he could muster. Nevertheless, his full justification and rationale for Judaism and the oral law remained somewhat less than convincing and even a bit untidy. Faced with the formidable challenge of explaining the seemingly fantastic *midrashim* of the rabbis before a "sober and reasonable" audience, he could do more than admit his inability to fathom their meaning. So he argued that although we do not yet understand the meaning of many rabbinic homilies, we continue to learn more each day about the facts of nature, which will eventually confirm what presently remains unconfirmed.[41] His one attempt to explain the rabbinic *bat kol* (a kind of heavenly communication) as an illusion of auditory perception seems forced and specious.[42] Even more problematic is his notion of the commandments. Despite a long and revered tradition of exploring the rational reasons for the divine commandments, Nieto will have no part of it. The *mizvot* of Judaism function like sacraments in Christianity. They are deemed holy and require no rational justification.[43] Perhaps his effort to remove the commandments from the realm of rational speculation is his way of acknowledging that any such reflections are inadequate before the critical inquiry of the new empiricism. His other arguments in support of the oral law are neither original nor fully persuasive, as Petuchowski has pointed out.[44] Nieto had accepted the formidable challenge of articulating a Jewish theology in consonance with the highest standards of rationality of his day. His new defense of faith had addressed directly and passionately the intellectual demands of the new sciences. The results were mixed and less than conclusive. In the highly secularized and intense intellectual climate of Newtonian England, any rational defense of traditional Jewish faith, even as engaging and as novel as Nieto's, was to prove vulnerable and implausible even to some of his own students.

A year later, in 1715, Nieto published *Esh ha-Dat,* a critique of Nehemiah Ḥiyya Ḥayon. He was probably urged to do so by his colleagues Moses Ḥagiz

41. See Petuchowski's summary *The Theology,* pp. 99–105.
42. *Mateh Dan,* pp. 161–64.
43. See Petuchowski, *Theology,* pp. 64–68.
44. Ibid., pp. 69–98.

and Zevi Ashkenazi, who had hounded the notorious heresiarch since the beginning of his public career in Europe.[45] It is unclear to what degree Nieto had his heart in this project of heresy hunting. He must have felt obliged to respond to Ashkenazi, who had come to his support during the controversy over the sermon on divine providence. Hagiz had been in London and was certainly a persuasive crusader in his own right. No doubt Nieto found the public teachings of Hayon obnoxious, even though it remains unclear to what degree he had systematically studied the latter's writings. He knew enough to make the ideological connection between Hayon and Abraham Cardoso, the disciple of the messianic pretender Shabbatai Zevi and the architect of his own version of Zevi's ideology.[46] Although Nieto challenges several of Hayon's alleged pronouncements in the first part of the work, again using his familiar dialogical form, by the second part he seems to ignore Hayon entirely to pursue other related issues of faith. As a critique of Hayon's theology, *Esh ha-Dat* is weak and insubstantial; as a portrait of Nieto's ultimate concerns, it is even more revealing than his other writings.

Recent scholarship on Hayon has clarified beyond a doubt that the commotion over his public appearances and writings had little to do with messianism or Shabbatai Zevi.[47] He was certainly associated with the apostate messiah, but the issues his detractors raised were of a different sort. Hayon was Cardoso's faithful disciple, and he worked to disseminate his master's teachings throughout Europe. These teachings were antiphilosophical at their core, although they were informed by philosophical knowledge. Cardoso had taught that a dualistic separation existed between the immanent first cause of the philosophers and a totally hidden and transcendent God of Israel. Hayon preached this dualism while questioning the possibility of the simple, pure, immanent diety known to men; instead he suggested a trinitarian notion of the godhead, obviously conjuring up Christian associations in the minds of some of his critics. Hayon also advocated free inquiry and public disclosure of the most esoteric teachings of

45. The latest reconstruction of the Hayon controversy, from the perspective of Moses Hagiz, is Carlebach, *Pursuit of Heresy,* pp. 75–159; on Nieto, see esp. pp. 144–48.

46. See ibid., p. 98.

47. I refer specifically to Liebes's essays (mentioned in the Introduction, n. 21) and Carlebach's *Pursuit of Heresy.*

Judaism, implying that submission to rabbinic authority was unnecessary and even undesirable.[48]

In his critique of Ḥayon, Nieto ignores Ḥayon's trinitarian concept, perhaps in deference to the Christian readers of his work, or perhaps because it simply did not offend him as much as another concept Ḥayon had championed. He faults Ḥayon primarily for his dualistic notion of a Jewish God who has no relation to the world and to those smaller "gods" who direct and govern the created world.[49] To the readers of Nieto's treatise on divine providence, the issue was a familiar one. Ḥayon's dualism was no more than a variation of the notion of plastic nature, and such a position for Nieto was deistic. To posit a distinctly Jewish God as unconcerned and unrelated to his creation was to portray Judaism as a religion closer to paganism than to Islam and Christianity. For Nieto, a Judaism which failed to acknowledge that one God created the heaven and earth, and that there were an ongoing divine providence and a system of rewards and punishments, was not Judaism at all. Not only the two other major Western religions but most of the civilized world shared such essential notions of faith. And why, Nieto asked, would Ḥayon prescribe a unique Jewish faith unrelated to Christianity, Islam, or philosophical inquiry? Surely the power of Judaism was to be located in the truths it shared with the other religions, not in positions that contradicted those truths.[50] Finally, if doctrines of faith could be proven rationally, even one like transubstantiation, why was this to be considered a disgrace to the Jewish people rather than a distinct virtue and advantage?[51]

Nieto's formulations of Ḥayon's faults transparently reveal the rabbi's primary motivation in attacking Ḥayon. For Nieto, Ḥayon was a deist because he understood the Jewish God to be unconcerned with and unrelated to his creation. And such deism, as Samuel Clarke had indicated, would lead ultimately to "absolute atheism." Furthermore, Ḥayon was a dangerous enthusiast who claimed direct inspiration from God and who sought to undermine the existing

48. See the summaries of Ḥayon's theosophy by G. Scholem in *Encyclopedia Judaica,* 7:1500–03, and by Carlebach in *Pursuit of Heresy,* pp. 86–104.

49. *Esh ha-Dat* (London, 1715), p. 9a.

50. Ibid., pp. 15b–16b.

51. Ibid., pp. 16b–17a.

hierarchy of rabbinic authority.[52] Nieto firmly believed that the rabbinate, particularly the educated rabbinate armed with the tools of modern science, was
solely responsible for determining the boundaries of normal behavior. These
norms, as Nieto understood them, required Jews to be sober and reasonable and
self-restrained, to live within the limits imposed by both rabbinic and secular authorities. By labeling Hayon a pagan idol worshiper, Nieto placed him squarely
beyond the limits of normal propriety. Nieto, the rabbi, doctor, educated in the
ways of philosophy and science, had come to judge the unstable enthusiast and
found his behavior dangerously unacceptable.[53]

If there remains any doubt about Nieto's basic fears regarding Hayon, his
additional comments in the Spanish supplement to *Esh ha-Dat* are even clearer.[54]
In this writing, Nieto unambiguously expresses his credo as a public religious
leader. His major objective is to gain civic acceptability for the Jewish minority
living in a Christian environment.[55] Jewish religious institutions can be legitimated only on the assumption that Jews conduct themselves by the same norms
the Christians do. Hayon's irresponsible pronouncements undermine the public
credibility of the Anglo-Jewish community. By differentiating between a transcendent Jewish God and an immanent first cause of the philosophers, Hayon
had severed the Jewish faith from a universal notion of monotheism shared by
the two faiths. If God was not the first cause, He could not be unique, eternal, or
omnipotent, as Western monotheistic faiths grounded in reason had portrayed
him. By undermining the common foundation of the two faiths, Hayon had
done an injustice not only to Jewish theology but to Jewish civic acceptance,
and this was, in Nieto's eyes, "heregia, libertinage, atheismo."[56] By contrast,
Nieto required a Jewish faith fully displaying its common principles with the

52. Note Carlebach's designation of Hayon as an enthusiast (*Pursuit of Heresy*, p. 89), and
see the literature on enthusiasm in n. 11 above.

53. My formulation here is influenced by Michael Heyd's essays on enthusiasm listed in
n. 11 above.

54. See R. Loewe, "The Spanish Supplement to Nieto's '*Esh Dath*,'" *Proceedings of the
American Academy for Jewish Research* 48 (1981): 167–96.

55. Ibid., p. 282.

56. Ibid., pp. 286–89. On the term *libertinage*, see Jacob, *Cultural Meaning of the Scientific
Revolution*, p. 45.

dominant Christian one and validated by rational, scientific arguments. Such a faith, like that of the Boyle lecturers, affirmed the stability and harmony of the social order against all radical sectarians, deists, atheists, and enthusiasts like Nehemiah Ḥayon.

In the second part of *Esh ha-Dat,* Nieto conveniently forgets the embarrassing Ḥayon to underscore the aspects of Judaism that Jews hold in common with the rest of civilized humanity. His points again sound like a Jewish version of Samuel Clarke's discourse, this time resembling Clarke's discourse of 1704 concerning the being and attributes of God.[57] Like Clarke, Nieto offers his proofs of God's existence based on teleological and cosmological arguments that were standard for the early eighteenth century.[58] We might see such parallel lines of thought between the Jewish and Christian clergyman as a mere coincidence if not for the fact that Nieto adds a seemingly innocent anecdote regarding an alleged conversation with a disbeliever who lacked a rational foundation for affirming an eternal God. Nieto prefaces this account by distinguishing between two kinds of heretics: the first, ignorant barbarians who are incapable of knowing better; the second, those who are intelligent but simply cannot comprehend God's existence without positing his beginning. The second group mistakenly attribute eternity to creation instead of to the creator.[59]

We might not pause to summarize such a relatively insignificant conversation were it not that Clarke had deliberated on the same problem in a remarkably similar way. He begins his address by reflecting on three types of atheists. The first are wholly ignorant or stupid, while the second "through habitual debauchery have brought themselves to a custom of mocking and scoffing at all religion, and will not hearken to any fair reasoning." Only the third type use speculative reasoning and can be influenced by rational argument; they alone are the subject of his remarks.[60] Nieto had collapsed the first two categories into one, but clearly he preserved the distinction between atheists who

57. Clark, *Works,* pp. 511–77.

58. They are summarized by Petuchowski in *Theology,* pp. 107–14. See *Esh ha-Dat,* 29a–31a, and Clarke, *Works,* pp. 542–70.

59. *Esh ha-Dat,* p. 31b.

60. Clarke, *Works,* pp. 521–23.

were helplessly lost in their perversity and those who could be cured by the charm of persuasive logic. Having located the atheist he hoped to engage in discussion, Clarke immediately turned to the challenge of conceiving an eternal God, as opposed to an eternal matter or motion proposed by such atheists as Toland.[61] Nieto's response to his heretic who struggles with the difficulty of comprehending the eternity of God is strikingly similar to Clarke's discussion. Might Nieto have consulted Clarke's address of 1704 when composing the second half of *Esh ha-Dat,* and could he even have been aware of Clarke's second address, published the following year, in constructing his earlier argument on divine providence? Such circumstantial evidence is enticing if not compelling. Whatever the case, the parallels between Nieto's and Clarke's lines of argumentation in each of their compositions strongly recommend a universe of discourse shared by religious thinkers and communal leaders.

Seen as a whole, Nieto's major writings suggest a consistent and well-conceived educational strategy for presenting the Jewish faith in a social environment that was isolated from the mainstream of Jewish culture, highly secularized, and only tenuously attached to traditional Jewish norms. By choosing to construct his own public image of Judaism along lines similar to the Anglican social and intellectual elite, he hoped to make the most effective case for Jewish faith and to insure the civic welfare of the Jewish community. An examination of Nieto's theology thus offers a remarkable test case of adaptation and reformulation of Judaism in light of the formidable challenge scientific advances had posed to traditional faith.

Nieto's intellectual efforts surely left a positive impression on members of his congregation, especially on a small coterie of disciples, most of them physicians, who maintained affectionate ties with their master until his death in 1728. Yet Nieto's example of enlightened Jewish faith and civic virtue proved insufficient to secure the Jewish loyalty of one of his most brilliant students and colleagues. Some thirty years after Nieto died, Dr. Jacob de Castro Sarmento wrote to the elders of the Spanish and Portuguese congregation announcing his intention to withdraw from the community on the grounds that "the different opinion and

61. Ibid., pp. 524–31.

sentiments I have entertained long ago . . . entirely dissenting from those of the Synagogue . . . do not permit me any longer to keep up the appearance of a membership in your body. I therefore now take my leave of you, hereby renouncing expressly that communion in which I have been considered with yourselves."[62] Sarmento's break with his ancestral heritage as embodied in the legacy of David Nieto dramatically adumbrated the wave of defections from traditional Judaism in years to come. In the long run, even Nieto's elaborate reconstruction of Judaism, like Mendelssohn's after him, could not withstand the mighty forces of Jewish social disintegration unleashed by the rapidly changing political and cultural ambiance of Enlightenment and revolutionary Europe.

62. The passage is quoted in R. Barnett, "Dr. Jacob de Castro Sarmento and Sephardim in Medical Practice in Eighteenth-Century London," *Transactions of the Jewish Historical Society of England* 27 (1978–80): 94.

Physico-Theology and Jewish Thought at the End of the Eighteenth Century

MORDECHAI SCHNABER LEVISON AND SOME

OF HIS CONTEMPORARIES

In 1744 Israel ben Moses Ha-Levi of Zamosc (1710–1772) published a seemingly traditional Hebrew commentary on *Ru'ah Hen,*
a medieval philosophical dictionary commonly attributed to the
Maimonidean Jacob Anatoli.[1] Zamosc is known primarily as a
Talmudic scholar with interests in mathematics and the sciences
who, during his sojourn in Berlin, became an early teacher of
Moses Mendelssohn.[2] In electing to explicate a medieval classic,
as he had also done in the cases of Judah Ha-Levi's *Sefer ha-
Kuzari* and Bahya ibn Pakuda's *Hovot ha-Levavot,* he was seem-

1. *Sefer Ru'ah Hen* (Warsaw, 1826; repr. Jerusalem, 1970, ed. W. J. Lebens-
sohn).

2. On Israel Zamosc, see A. Altmann, *Moses Mendelssohn: A Biographical
Study* (University, Ala., 1973), pp. 21–22; E. Shveid, *Toledot ha-Hagut ha-
Yehudit be-Et hahadasha: Ha-Me'ah ha-Teshah Esreh* (Jerusalem, 1977), pp.
111–12; and H. M. Graupe, *The Rise of Modern Judaism: An Intellectual History
of German Jewry, 1650–1943,* trans. J. Robinson (Huntington, N.Y., 1978),
p. 66. More generally, see I. Eisenstein-Barzilay, "The Background of the
Berlin Haskalah," *Essays on Jewish Life and Thought Presented in Honor of Salo
Wittmayer Baron,* ed. J. L. Blau, A. Hertzberg, P. Freidman, and I. Mendelssohn (New York, 1959), pp. 183–97; J. Eschelbacher, "Die Anfange all-
gemeiner Bildung unter den deutschen Juden vor Mendelssohn," *Festschrift
zum siebzigsten Gerburtstage Martin Philippsons* (Leipzig, 1916), pp. 168–77; and
the additional references in the *Encyclopaedia Judaica,* 16:929.

ingly revealing once again his strong allegiance to the past and to the traditional roots of medieval Jewish thought. Thus it is surprising to discover the following description in his discussion of the element of air according to Aristotle:

> Know that according to what the moderns have discovered by their experiments, this air is sponge-like, that is, compressed or diffused when a force acts upon it, but then returns to its place when the force is released. This and other precious discoveries have been known through this wonderful instrument invented some ninety years ago, the mother of the new inventions, called in German *luftpumpe*. It is constructed with wisdom and intelligence in order to remove air from any desired container. . . . This convinced many scholars of our time to believe that a vacuum can exist in a narrow space as a result of experiments and clever devices as one famous scholar of our time presented in his book of natural experiments. One takes a sac (*blase* in German) that is not inflated but whose mouth is well clamped down so that no external air can get inside and puts it within a glass container with a narrow mouth attached to a brass valve . . . in order to enable the opening and closing of the mouth as needed with this valve. When we erect this glass container so that its mouth is open to this pump, our eyes will then behold that when the air begins to leave the glass container, the sac will then raise itself and begin to inflate until it is entirely inflated as all the air has been removed from the container. And again if we open a place so that the external air enters the container, it will deflate to the point it had been from the beginning. And this is a wonderful thing. . . . Thus it [air] is sponge-like without a doubt.[3]

Zamosc referred either to the air-pump of Otto von Guericke described by Caspar Schott in his *Mechanica hydraulico-pneumatica* of 1657, or more likely to the improved version described by Robert Boyle in his *New Experiments Physico-Mechanical*, published in 1660.[4] Although this device had been available for

3. *Sefer Ru'aḥ Ḥen*, p. 18b.

4. On the background of the air-pump, especially that of Boyle, see S. Shapin and S. Schaffer, *Leviathan and the Air-Pump: Hobbes, Boyle, and the Experimental Life* (Princeton, 1985), esp. chap. 2; A. Rupert Hall, *The Revolution in Science, 1500–1750* (London and New York, 1983), pp.

almost a century, as Zamosc pointed out, it apparently had been unknown to his Hebrew readership and thus he presented it to them as a novelty. Notwithstanding Tobias Cohen's and David Nieto's interest in new scientific instruments such as the telescope, microscope, and thermometer, neither mentions the air-pump in his writing at the beginning of the eighteenth century, nor do they elicit any serious interest in pneumatics in general. Whether or not Zamosc's enthusiastic description was the first in Hebrew literature, several of his Jewish contemporaries soon displayed similar excitement with the new experiments concerning the character of air.

Aaron Solomon Gumpertz, also called Aaron ben Zalman Emmerich (1723–1769), a medical graduate of the University of Frankfurt, also a teacher of Mendelssohn and apparently a student of Zamosc,[5] published a small essay on the value of science called *Ma'amar ha-Maddah* in 1765 in Hamburg.[6] Gumpertz's main point was to argue that the study of the sciences had no relation to the divine sciences and was therefore not injurious to Jewish faith. His prime example also focuses on the vacuum and the weight of air. This time he does not mention the air-pump per se but does recall the pneumatic devices of the seventeenth century, including those of Galileo and Gaspero Berti and especially the famous experiment of Evangelista Torricelli, later publicized and refined by Mersenne and Pascal in France.[7]

Gumpertz begins with the example of water being raised in a well or in a long vertical pipe. When pumped upward, the water will not rise beyond a certain level, leaving what appears to be a vacuous space from the top to the water level in the tube. In Gumpertz's words, the ancients "were astonished by this phenomenon and sought an explanation for this sign. They decreed a general

---

260–62; M. Daumas, *Les Instruments scientifiques aux XVIIe et XVIIIe siècles* (Paris, 1953); and R. Westfall, *The Construction of Modern Science: Mechanisms and Mechanics* (Cambridge, 1977).

5. On Gumpertz, see Altmann, *Moses Mendelssohn,* pp. 23–25; Barzilay-Eisenstein, "Background of the Berlin Haskalah"; D. Kaufmann and M. Freudenthal, *Die Familie Gomperz* (Frankfurt am Main, 1907); and Eschelbacher, "Anfange."

6. Published as an appendix to his *Sefer Megillat Sod,* a commentary on Abraham ibn Ezra's commentary to the five *megillot* in the edition of Vilna, 1836, which I have consulted.

7. For further information on these experiments, see the works cited in n. 4 above, esp. those by Hall, Daumas, and Westfall.

rule that there is no vacuum in nature and whenever there is a vacuum in nature, it strives to fill itself so that there will no longer be a vacuum there." The moderns recognized the weakness of this explanation and replicated the experiment in their long tubes, first with water and then with mercury and alcohol. They concluded that the column of water always rose to about thirty-two feet and that when mercury was used, since it is about fourteen times as dense as water, the column was only about two feet high, leaving in both cases a "Toricellian space" at the top. The moderns thus "abandoned the method of the ancients and sought another explanation . . . for this phenomenon which they discovered from their assumptions about the nature of air. These were investigated by way of experiments that concluded that air has a perceived weight like the weight of water." They thus determined the weight of air in relation to water, as well as that of mercury to water. Gumpertz concludes: "And from now on, they accepted this hypothesis as the correct truth established in nature. They likewise proceeded with all their investigations of nature . . . so they will not decree or decide on any hypothesis or idea in nature until they examine it with many experiments like these. So how can any person imagine that such methods will harm, God forbid, the opinions and beliefs [of the Jewish faith]? On the contrary, they do not rest at all on their own opinions but only on experiment and experience."[8]

One reader of Gumpertz's scientific manifesto who "borrowed" freely from it in his own scientific work was Mordechai Gumpel Schnaber (1741–97), known as George Levison in the English works he wrote. Since he is the primary subject of this chapter, I shall have occasion to return to several salient features of his biography below.[9] At this stage, let us briefly consider his remarks on the air-pump in his *Ma'amar ha-Torah ve-ha-Ḥokhmah*, published in London in 1771.

Levison discusses the pump on two separate occasions. He first inserts several comments in challenging the ancient view that everything desires to return to its natural place and that air and fire lack weight. "However, the moderns demonstrated with the instrument of the air-pump *[keli ha-meraken ha-avir]* the negation of [these] two assumptions. The first was negated when they observed in the glass container from which air had been removed that heavy and light

8. *Sefer Megillat Sod,* pp. 25b–26a.
9. For further references to him, see n. 39 below.

things fell equally at the same time. They negated the second assumption after noticing the decrease in weight of an object measured in air and then measured when the air was removed, a reduction attributable to the absence of air which had initially enhanced its weight."[10]

Later, in a separate chapter on air, Levison returns to the air-pump, this time identifying its inventor as Otto von Guericke, "a citizen of Magdenberg," and adding that "the scholar [Robert] Boyle" had improved it. Von Guericke's motivation, according to Levison, was to disprove the assumption of the ancients that no vacuum was possible in nature. Before proceeding to explain the construction of the pump, he adds the following reservation: "Although I am unable to explain well its activity without an illustration and even with an illustration one cannot understand the construction of the air-pump *without seeing it with your own eyes* [my emphasis], nevertheless, I will explain its operation as well as I possibly can."[11]

His description of the pump is more detailed than that of Zamosc and is too long to quote extensively here. He accurately describes the pumping apparatus and the receiver, the hollow brass cylinder, its internal piston covered with leather, the opening with a stopcock connecting the receiver to the pumping device, the valve allowing air to enter or be evacuated, and so forth. He also supplies a description of the "Torricelli tube," or barometer, for measuring "the weight of the air."[12]

Three Hebrew descriptions of pneumatic devices, including two of the air-pump, written in 1744, 1765, and 1771—more than a century after the devices initially appeared in Europe—suggest a belated awareness of discoveries in the physical sciences among Jewish writers, at least in comparison to the more up-to-date information they appear to have obtained in medicine and the life sciences.[13] Despite the notable contributions of the Italians Galileo and Torricelli, the fact that most seventeenth-century experiments in pneumatics were

10. *Ma'amar ha-Torah ve-ha-Ḥokhmah* (London, 1771), p. 27.

11. Ibid., p. 70.

12. Ibid., pp. 70–72. For background, see the references in n. 4 above, esp. Shapin and Schaffer, *Leviathan.*

13. Compare, for example, Tobias Cohen's up-to-date knowledge of medicine and the life sciences discussed in chap. 8 above.

carried out in Germany, France, and England, and thus were relatively inaccessible to Italian Jewish students of the sciences, might explain such belatedness. Nevertheless, by the end of the eighteenth century, Jewish authors writing in Hebrew were finally struck by pneumatical experiments, as this sampling amply suggests.

To appreciate why each of the three writers chose to highlight the Torricelli experiment or the air-pump of von Guericke and Boyle, one needs to consider the function of these devices as emblems of the new scientific culture of the seventeenth century. As Steven Shapin and Simon Schaffer have shown, the air-pump symbolized the new experimental philosophy of Robert Boyle and his colleagues.[14] A. Rupert Hall observed that it "was the unfailing pièce de résistance of the incipient scientific laboratory."[15] It was featured in all public displays of scientific achievement as both a source of entertainment and an object of public worship. Boyle even suggested that experiments using the instrument might best be performed on Sundays as part of the celebration of God's glories.[16] Accompanying the textbooks explicating the new experiments for a lay audience was an elaborate iconography of the air-pump and similar devices, ornately illustrated in all their glory.

The project of Boyle and his contemporaries rested on a set of social conventions for generating and explaining what they considered matters of fact. As Shapin and Schaffer explain, the new scientists insisted that their experiments be witnessed and not taken on faith. The experimental laboratory thus became a kind of social space for them, although restricted to witnesses with the appropriate intellectual and moral qualifications. Given the limitations on the number of witnesses observing the experiment or its replications, the proponents of the new experimental philosophy insisted on a framework of "virtual witnessing" whereby the text and the iconography documenting the experiment could replicate to some extent the image of the experimental scene in the reader's mind. Through the creation of a simple, modest scientific prose accompanying the visual images, faithfully presenting both successful and failed experiments,

14. Shapin and Schaffer, *Leviathan,* esp. pp. 30–35.

15. Hall, *Revolution in Science,* p. 262; also quoted in Shapin and Schaffer, *Leviathan,* p. 30.

16. Shapin and Schaffer, *Leviathan,* p. 319. See also H. Fisch, "The Scientist as Priest: A Note on Robert Boyle's Natural Theology," *Isis* 44 (1953): 252–65.

Boyle and his colleagues hoped to validate and publicize their knowledge claims within the larger political and religious communities of Europe.[17] Thus, one should not miss the import of Levison's remark that his description of the air-pump should be witnessed with one's eyes and, at the very least, observed through an illustration in a book (an obvious limitation of Levison's own work). In other words, Levison, as we shall soon observe, fully imbibed the pedagogic and political objectives of the new experimentalists and attempted to inculcate these same ideals within a community of Jewish readers through his enthusiastic endorsement of the air-pump and similar achievements of the new science. For him, as well as for Zamosc and Gumpertz, there was no better example than "the mother of the new inventions," as Zamosc had called it, to dramatize the enormous impact the new scientific discoveries held for Jews and other citizens of eighteenth-century Europe.

Previous discussions of Jewish intellectual life in the second half of the eighteenth century have focused on the impact of the cultural and political movement known as the *Haskalah,* or Jewish Enlightenment, either within its initial ambiance of Berlin or in its other cultural and social guises in eastern Europe well into the nineteenth century. Jacob Katz's understanding of the phenomenon of Haskalah as a conscious shift from "tradition" to "crisis" has been particularly influential in recent historiography:

> The social turning point to which we have alluded is revealed in the emergence of a new type, the *maskil,* who added to his knowledge of the Torah a command of foreign languages, general erudition, and an interest in what was happening in the non-Jewish world. This type became increasingly numerous beginning with the 1760s, and it soon constituted a subgroup in Jewish society. It demanded for itself not only the right of existence but also the privilege of leadership.
>
> After the emergence of the *maskilim,* new ideals pertaining to daily living, the organization and leadership of society, and the methods of education came to be formulated in a programmatic manner. When the maskilim began to gather strength, a feeling of crisis arose in the consciousness even of those

17. Shapin and Schaffer, *Leviathan,* pp. 36–79.

who continued to adhere to the values of the tradition in which they were reared.[18]

Katz's sociological model of what he came to call a semineutral society,[19] as found especially in Mendelssohn's Berlin, auguring a new structural relation between Jews and non-Jews in Western Europe, has dominated all subsequent discussions of this cultural period. In identifying intellectual figures who appear to exhibit certain "maskilic" tendencies prior to Mendelssohn, some historians have labeled such types as precursors or forerunners of the Haskalah. The discussion among Katz, his critics, and his students has continued to focus on the precise criteria of defining the Haskalah as a meaningful watershed in viewing Jewish cultural and social history in both western and eastern Europe.[20]

Zamosc, Gumpertz, and Levison all lived within the period known as the Haskalah and would appear to qualify as maskilim by Katz's criteria. Indeed, Zamosc and Gumpertz, both teachers and older associates of Mendelssohn, have also been labeled precursors of the Berlin Haskalah who paved the way for Mendelssohn's cultural and political aspirations.[21] Levison is harder to categorize. While apparently sympathetic to many of the ideals of the Berlin Haskalah— he even published an essay advocating the revival of Hebrew in the journal of

18. J. Katz, *Tradition and Crisis: Jewish Society at the End of the Middle Ages* (New York, 1961), p. 246.

19. See J. Katz, *Out of the Ghetto: The Social Background of Jewish Emancipation, 1770–1870* (Cambridge, Mass., 1973), chap. 4.

20. The bibliography is too vast to cite here. See esp. J. Katz, *Emancipation and Assimilation: Studies in Modern Jewish History* (Westmead, 1972); Katz, ed., *Toward Modernity: The European Jewish Model* (New Brunswick, 1987), esp. the article by E. Etkes; A. Shohat, *Im Ḥilufei Tekufot* (Jerusalem, 1960) and the review by B. Mevorah in *Kiryat Sefer* 37 (1961–62):154–55; Katz, *Out of the Ghetto*, pp. 34–37; Eisenstein-Barzilay, "Background of the Berlin Haskalah"; M. Eliav, *Ha-Ḥinukh ha-Yehudi be-Germania Bi-Tekufat ha-Haskalah ve-ha-Imanzipazia* (Jerusalem, 1960); T. Tsmariyon, *Moshe Mendelssohn ve-ha-Idi'ologia shel ha-Haskalah* (Tel Aviv, 1984); M. Pelli, *The Age of Haskalah: Studies in Hebrew Literature of the Enlightenment in Germany* (Leiden, 1979); and I. Bartal, " 'Ost' and 'West': Varieties of Jewish Enlightenment," to be published in the proceedings of a conference in honor of Katz's *Tradition and Crisis* sponsored by the Center of Jewish Studies of Harvard University.

21. See the references in nn. 2 and 5 above.

Mendelssohn's disciples, *Me'asef*[22]—he had little contact with Mendelssohn and his circle, and even criticized Mendelssohn in print.[23] His professional concerns as an active medical practitioner and writer appear to have taken priority over any strong political allegiance to the Haskalah movement.

In selecting these three thinkers, primarily the last, as the subject of the final chapter of this book, I do not intend to explore their relationship to the Haskalah either as full-fledged participants or as precursors. My objective is not to contextualize their thought as either pre- or post-maskilic, or as illustrating the break between medieval and modern mentalities, or even as a kind of transitional combination of old and new. This has been suggested by previous scholars. Rather, I would like to view it simply as a product of the continuous encounter of Jews with the scientific culture of Europe that had emerged with particular intensity from the late sixteenth century on and, at the same time, as a unique and novel expression of and response to particular developments within the scientific culture of the eighteenth century. As a preliminary excursion into the scientific thinking of Jewish thinkers in this later period, this chapter does not attempt to survey what remains a vast and unexplored terrain.[24] In focusing on the unusual figure of Levison, I wish only to exemplify the richness of the dialogue between Judaism and science in this period while eschewing the larger and more complex story of the place of medicine and science within the social and political contexts of Jewish life in the last two centuries. In closing this work with Levison, I view his interaction with scientific culture as an integral part of a broader process that had emerged some two centuries earlier

22. *Ha-Me'asef* (Königsberg, 1784), 4:184; and see T. Tsmariyon, *Ha-Me'asef: Ketav ha-Et ha-Moderni ha-Rishon be-Ivrit* (Tel Aviv, 1988), pp. 72–73.

23. In his commentary on Ecclesiastes, *Tokhahat Megillah* (Hamburg, 1784); and see below.

24. I have not bothered to list here the vast bibliography dealing with the Enlightenment and scientific developments during this era. A cursory but useful survey of scholarship is R. Porter, *The Enlightenment* (Hampshire and London, 1990), with an up-to-date list of older and recent interpretations from Cassirer, Becker, and Gay to Darnton, Chartier, and M. Jacob. A good survey of the sciences during the Enlightenment is T. L. Hankins, *Science and the Enlightenment* (Cambridge, 1985). Also useful is G. S. Rousseau and R. Porter, *The Ferment of Knowledge: Studies in the Historiography of Eighteenth-Century Science* (Cambridge, 1980).

in Italy, in eastern Europe, and in the western Sephardic diaspora, and in some respects as representing a culmination of that process. The subsequent story of Judaism's encounters with science, still essentially untold, displays certain continuities with this earlier period, but at the same time it reveals a substantial break with the past, accelerated by the dynamics of political emancipation, cultural and religious assimilation, new and violent forms of anti-Semitism, and the economic, social, and religious restructuring of Jewish life that marked the modern period. This is a subject for another book.

Both Zamosc and Gumpertz, in their works cited above, generally adopt positions vis-à-vis science that echo those of Jewish writers of the previous two centuries. Zamosc, in his comments on *Ru'aḥ Ḥen,* ultimately subverts the positions taken in this medieval philosophical text, consistently juxtaposing those of the past with those of his own age. In a manner reminiscent of Basilea or Nieto, he sees the invalidation of the Aristotelian cosmology as a vindication of the rabbis and their once discredited positions. He thus interprets the dispute between the sages and the Gentile scholars in the Talmud [B.T. Pesaḥim 94] much as Moses Isserles, David Gans, and Isaac Lampronti did.[25] He is emphatic in rejecting Aristotle's notion of the fifth essence of the heavenly spheres but is unwilling to decide conclusively whether the earth is a planet that revolves around the sun, as Copernicus claimed, or whether the earth is stationary while the rest of the planets revolve around the sun, the view of Tycho Brahe. Although the former position is "closer to the ways of astronomy" and is accepted by the majority of scholars of his day, it "has a bad odor of heresy in it." Therefore Zamosc is more comfortable with Brahe's view, despite the overwhelming evidence in favor of Copernicus.[26]

Like Tobias Cohen, he is familiar with the views of the chemical philosophers and their notion of five elements.[27] As with heliocentricity, he is still reluctant to abandon the notion of four elements since it is mentioned both in the *Sefer*

25. *Sefer Ru'aḥ Ḥen,* p. 2a. See chap. 9 above.
26. Ibid., p. 2b.
27. Ibid., pp. 2b–3a.

Yeẓirah and in the *Zohar*.[28] Like Nieto, he accurately portrays the views of the atomists and the Cartesians on the composition of matter.[29]

Zamosc ultimately diverges from earlier thinkers in two ways: first, in his constant emphasis on the novelty of scientific discovery and method of his day, and second, in his special interest in the new botanical and biological discoveries and their importance in confirming traditional views of divine providence and divine creation. By pitting modern theories against those stated in his medieval text, he consistently underscores the scientific ignorance of Maimonidean learning. At one point, perhaps aware how repetitive he has been in this regard, he admits that he sees no value in belaboring this obvious point.[30]

Besides his notice of the air-pump, Zamosc is equally impressed by the microscope and the visual advantage it offers contemporary naturalists. He points out that with the microscope the moderns have disproved the medieval view of spontaneous generation, an issue we have already observed in Lampronti's writing. Moreover, he maintains that by witnessing the origin of life in small seeds under the microscope, the actual blueprint of the full-blown creature, whether plant or animal, is discernible.[31] Zamosc alludes to the notion of preformation, a popular theory of his time which held that the adult existed "preformed" in the embryo. Both the rejection of spontaneous generation and the acceptance of preformation forcefully confirm for Zamosc God's power to create something out of nothing:[32]

> Thus from now on, the moderns among the Gentile scholars deny the power of creation to inanimate creatures and rather state that from the day God made the earth and all its host, and every plant and its seed within it, He commanded that the blueprint of the plant be created in each seed—with its fruit and seed and the seed of its seed—everything in its complete and

28. Ibid., p. 3a.
29. Ibid., p. 17b.
30. Ibid., p. 20a.
31. Ibid., pp. 3a–4a.
32. On the debates over spontaneous generation and preformation, see J. Farley, *The Spontaneous Generation Controversy from Descartes to Oparin* (Baltimore and London, 1977), esp. pp. 1–30; and see below.

correct form laid out and folded in the first seed from the days of creation until the end of the duration of the world determined by blessed God. . . . How excellent is this report which proves [the doctrine of] creation out of nothing, for it would be necessary to assume an infinite being in the seed for those who believed in the eternity of the world, and this is disgraceful.[33]

Zamosc also mentions Galileo's observations of tiny creatures under the microscope, further testifying to the fecundity and brilliance of God's creation.[34] Levison, as we shall soon see, pursued these themes even more elaborately in his writing.

The importance of Gumpertz's comparatively modest work lies in articulating the boundaries separating physics from metaphysics, allowing the faithful to feel secure in investigating nature in its own right. The argument, as we have seen, is not new and simply follows the well-trodden path laid out by the Maharal.[35] Nevertheless, several nuances in Gumpertz's formulation are worthy of closer attention, reflecting more specifically the cultural ambiance in which he wrote.

After an eloquent encomium on the inspiring delights of discovering the natural world and a strong denunciation of pernicious atheistic notions, Gumpertz reaches his major theme: "Everyone universally acknowledges that the ways of human investigation and the ways of the true *kabbalah* are distinct, for a person is incapable of comprehending absolute truth with the devices of his own intellect without divine assistance and emanation." Since mathematics and the natural sciences "have no business with the divine religion," and since anyone who studies these fields acknowledges "his deficiency from the beginning of his investigation," the religious person should never be threatened by the study

33. *Sefer Ru'aḥ Ḥen,* p. 3b.

34. Ibid., p. 4a. Zamosc also composed an entire work on the sciences that he called *Arubot ha-Shamayim,* which was never printed. I briefly inspected Jewish Theological Seminary MS mic. 2612, apparently a fragment of a larger work. The preserved section generally follows a Ptolemaic view of astronomy, although Copernicus and Brahe are quoted. Zamosc appears more daring and critical of medieval science in *Sefer Ru'aḥ Ḥen,* but his thought in general requires further study.

35. See chap. 2 above.

of nature. The general principle to be followed, according to Gumpertz, is that "investigation based on human intelligence in lofty matters like these [divine knowledge above nature] is never certain or absolute. However, it serves as a basis and a [helping] hand for understanding the Torah."[36]

The problem arose in earlier times, when it was "the custom of the ancients to mix and confuse natural science with what is beyond nature, which in our generation is no longer the case." The advantage of this age is its recognition of the limits of human knowledge, where scholars treat every subject in its own right, "particularly with respect to natural science, where they have chosen a new methodology, namely, experimentation, observation, examination, and cunning, performing many experiments with different instruments with the special purpose of testing their theories regarding the powers of nature."[37] Gumpertz's example of the Torricellian experiment follows, with his vigorous denial, quoted above, that information about such an experiment could be perilous to one's faith. He adds finally that the devices of the experimentalist are inappropriate to the study of the divine, since "the separate intelligences [of the divine realm] do not fall within the realm of the senses; no eye has seen them except the intelligence given from the Heavens alone."[38]

The emphasis on experimentation, on knowledge based on sensory perception, on its contingency and fallibility, unintrusive with respect to matters of faith and revelation, bears the distinctive coloring of sensationalist approaches to natural study associated with the philosophies of Locke and Boyle. This impression is reinforced when Gumpertz uses his description of pneumatic experiments to illustrate and confirm his epistemological discussion. The emphasis on experimentation also appears to be what impressed Levison, to the extent that he incorporated parts of *Ma'amar ha-Maddah* into the introduction of his own compendium of the sciences. It offers an excellent opening into Levison's more learned and sophisticated writing on science and religion. Levison, however, would eventually puncture the seemingly well-protected barriers between natural science and divine faith which Gumpertz overconfidently deemed impenetrable.

36. *Sefer Megillat Sod,* pp. 25a–b.
37. Ibid., p. 25b.
38. Ibid., p. 26a.

Mordechai Gumpel Schnaber Levison was perhaps the most colorful Jewish intellectual of his times. His concept of the relationship of science and religion represents a most original contribution to eighteenth-century Jewish thought. Despite the important studies of his biography and writings by Hans Joachim Schoeps and Heinz Mosche Graupe, and despite the fact that two Swedish novels have been devoted to his life, Levison deserves fuller and more systematic study.[39] While Levison's primary writings in Jewish thought were in Hebrew, he also produced a large number of works in English, German, and French. Most have barely been noticed at all, and several appear to have been lost.[40] The following analysis represents a modest attempt to situate his thought

39. H. J. Schoeps, "Gumpertz Levison-Leben und Werk: Eines Gelehrten Abenteurers des 18. Jahrhunderts," *Zeitschrift für Religions- und Geistesgeschichte* 4 (1952): 150–61, repr. in his *Studien zur unbekannten Religions- und Geistesgeschichte* (Berlin, 1963), pp. 216–27, and translated as "La Vie et l'oeuvre de Gumpertz Levison," *Revue d'histoire de la médicine hébraïque* 27 (1955): 133–43 (my references are to the French translation); H. M. Graupe, "Mordechai Gumpel (Levison)," *Bulletin des Leo Baeck Instituts* 5 (1962): 1–12; C. Roth, "The Haskalah in England," *Essays Presented to . . . Isaac Brodie* (London, 1967), pp. 367–68; Pelli, *Age of the Haskalah,* pp. 131–50 (with additional bibliography in n. 1); and Shveid, *Toledot,* pp. 113–16.

40. The following list of Levison's works is based on Schoeps, "Vie et l'oeuvre" and Graupe, "Mordechai Gumpel" together with my own additions; I suspect other works by this prolific author may yet be located: *Ma'amar ha-Torah ve-ha-Ḥokhmah* (London, 1771); *Tokhaḥat Megillah* (Hamburg, 1784); *Solet Minḥah Belulah* (Altona, 1797); *Shelosh Esrei Yesodei ha-Torah* (Altona?, 1792); *An Account of the Epidemical Sore Throat with the Method of Treatment, Illustrated by Cases and Observations* (London, 1778); *Beschreibung der Londonshen medicinishchen Praxis den deutschen Artzen vorgelegt* (Berlin and Stettin, 1782), with a preface by J. Cre. A. Theden, dedicated to Gustave III (Levison describes himself as professor named by the king of Sweden); *An Essay on the Blood, in Which the Objections to Mr. Hunter's Opinion Concerning the Blood Are Examined and Removed* (London, 1776); *Tokhaḥat Megulah* (a response to his detractors in London: see C. Roth, *Magna Bibliothceca Anglo-Judaica* [London, 1937], p. 271); his translation of *A Plain System of Alchymy* for Auguste Nordenskjold in 1779 (see Schoeps, "Vie et l'oeuvre," p. 135); *Eine leichte und fassliche Heilmethode für deijenigen von beyden Geschlechtern, so an einer Schwache der Gerbursglieder und Nerven nebst deren traurigen Folgen, so aus Onanie oder sonst einer Ursach entstanden, heimlich leiden. Von den Verfassern der Deutschen Gesunheitszeitung,* apparently based on his journal essays originally published in *Die Arzte* (Hamburg, 1787; repr. Breslau, 1789); *Der Mensch moralisch und physisch Dargestelt* (1797 and 1800) (see Schoeps, "Vie et l'oeuvre," p. 142, n. 35); *The Spirit and Union of the Natural, Moral, and Divine Law* (mentioned as published in

within the context of the themes of this book. It is based primarily on two of his Hebrew works: the aforementioned *Ma'amar ha-Torah,* published in London in 1771, and his *Shelosh-Esre Yesodei ha-Torah,* a commentary on Maimonides' thirteen principles of faith, probably published in Altona in 1792.

Schoeps has unearthed considerable documentation to sketch the outlines of Levison's life and professional career as a doctor. Born in Berlin to a distinguished rabbinic family, he studied with the distinguished Talmudist David Fraenkel before making his way to London sometime before 1771. There he became a student in the famous medical school of the surgeon and physiologist John Hunter. Upon completion of his medical studies, he was appointed a physician at the General Medical Asylum of the duke of Portland, probably sometime after 1776.[41] Throughout the 1770s he published several works, including *Ma'amar ha-Torah ve-ha-Ḥokhmah,* which he referred to in English as "A Dissertation on the Law and Science," and two medical works in English: *An Essay on the Blood, in which the Objections to Mr. Hunter's Opinion Concerning the Blood Are Examined and Removed* (London, 1776), dedicated to John Hunter's equally famous brother, William; and *An Account of the Epidemical Sore Throat with the Method of Treatment, Illustrated by Cases and Observations* (London, 1778). In the latter work he mentions another composition already published with the intriguing title *The Spirit and Union of the Natural, Moral, and Divine Law.* In *Ma'amar* he again refers to the work as *Sefer Ru'aḥ ha-Dat,* but I have found no trace of it in either English or Hebrew.

Before concluding this summary of the English phase of his life, it is worth pausing to consider the significance of Levison's apprenticeship under Hunter,

---

his work on the sore throat and in the *Ma'amar* as *Sefer Ru'aḥ ha-Dat,* but not located); *A Dissertation on Law and Science* (mentioned in his work on the sore throat, probably the same as *Ma'amar*); *Abhandlung über das Blut* (1782), translation of *An Essay on the Blood; Beschreibung der epidemischen Braune* (1783); *Sefer ha-Shorashim,* mentioned in *Tokhaḥat Megillah;* and a manuscript fragment of a larger philosophical work in Hebrew, including a letter to Emden, Jewish Theological Seminary MS 2481, entitled *Ma'amar Mahazeh Shaddai.*

41. Schoeps, "Vie et l'oeuvre," p. 134, dates his appointment around 1700, but the Asylum was not founded until 1776. See W. H. Bynum, "Physicians, Hospitals, and Career Structures in Eighteenth-Century London," in W. F. Bynum and R. Porter, eds., *William Hunter and the Eighteenth-Century Medical World* (Cambridge, 1985), p. 126.

both professionally and intellectually. The Hunters were not merely good physicians but two of the most influential medical men in England and Europe. Through their medical schools, museum, and roster of well-connected patients, they exerted enormous influence within the medical community and beyond it. And their entrepreneurial skills brought them much personal wealth and prestige.[42] That a German-speaking rabbinical student could gain entrance to John Hunter's private school, then employment in a Christian hospital upon completion of his studies, and openly publish medical works in English identifying himself as John Hunter's disciple represents no small feat. Beyond the professional competence Levison gained, one might surmise that he also grew intellectually under Hunter's tutelage. Traces of Hunter's general medical and scientific assumptions are discernible in Levison's thought, specifically the notion of plenitude and continuity in nature; the idea of a descending scale of perfection of animals; the absence of mechanical or chemical explanations of physiological processes (Levison discusses Hunter's ideas about both blood and the process of digestion); a general delight in the wonders of nature; and a strong commitment to a sensationalist epistemology. On the other hand, one should not overestimate Hunter's influence on his bright pupil. Levison says little about Hunter's passionate interest in comparative anatomy. He ignores Hunter's critique of Linnaeus's system of classification and Hunter's vitalistic theories, and his deep religious concerns find no counterpart in Hunter's general disinterest in spiritual matters. Nevertheless, Hunter's impact on Levison is undeniable and can probably be documented more extensively through a systematic reading of all of Levison's medical writings.[43]

42. On the Hunter brothers, see Bynum and Porter, *William Hunter,* esp. the essays by Porter, Bynum, Rolfe, and Gelfand; S. Cross, "John Hunter, The Animal Oeconomy, and Late Eighteenth-Century Physiological Discourse," in *Studies in the History of Biology,* ed. W. Coleman and C. Limoges (Baltimore, 1981), pp. 1–110; E. Finch, "The Influence of the Hunters on Medical Education," *Annals of the Royal College of Surgeons of England* 20 (1957): 205–48; G. Qvist, *John Hunter, 1728–1793* (London, 1981); and J. Kobler, *The Reluctant Surgeon: A Biography of John Hunter, Medical Genius and Great Inquirer of Johnson's England* (Garden City, N.Y., 1962).

43. On John Hunter's medical philosophy and methodology, see the sophisticated treatment by Cross mentioned in the previous note.

The next phase of Levison's life is well documented thanks to Schoeps' fascinating archival discoveries. In London, Levison became acquainted with Auguste Nordeskjold, a young medical student from Sweden who was soon to become a well-known doctor in his own right. The two shared an interest in alchemy. Levison even assisted his young friend in translating the latter's *A Plain System of Alchymy* into English. Nordeskjold facilitated Levison's contact with the royal court of Sweden. Remarkably, the Swedish king Gustave III invited Levison to Stockholm, where he received the prestigious title of professor of medicine. Upon his arrival in 1780 he was involved first in plans to establish an alchemical laboratory and later in setting up an entire institute for medicine, described in detail in a document Schoeps discovered.

Levison's power and prestige were short-lived. Negotiations with the Swedish court soon broke down. He was forced to return to London, found himself embroiled in a personal dispute resulting in a duel, and eventually took up residence in Hamburg, where he practiced medicine until his death in 1797. During this later period he continued to publish medical works, notably an account of the London medical scene for German doctors, a work on human passions and their impact on health, another work on epidemics, and even a sexual manual. For several years he edited a medical journal. His conspicuous presence in Hamburg inevitably incurred the wrath of the local physicians, who criticized him publicly. In the last period of his life, Levison also published several Hebrew works, including a commentary on Ecclesiastes written as a critique of a similar project by Moses Mendelssohn, the aforementioned commentary on Maimonides' thirteen principles of faith, a compendium of rabbinic homilies, a collection of Hebrew notes on various topics partially extant in manuscript, and a work on Hebrew grammar.[44]

In view of his remarkable career as a physician and prolific writer, Levison invites comparison with Moses Mendelssohn, Solomon Maimon, and other exceptional Jewish figures. As with Mendelssohn in Berlin, Levison's Jewishness appears not to have hampered him in forging social and professional relations with elite social circles in London and Stockholm, at least not initially. These

44. This is based primarily on Graupe, "Mordechai Gumpel," Schoeps, "Vie et l'oeuvre," and the list of works in n. 40 above.

contacts not only afforded him educational and professional opportunities and access to the latest medical information, they also catapulted him to the top of his profession, allowing him to publish widely, earning him a reputation as a master doctor, and enabling him to disseminate his sophisticated knowledge in books written in Western languages. In this latter accomplishment, he had few precursors in the Jewish community of early modern Europe, with the notable exception of a handful of famous converso physicians in the seventeenth century.[45] Like them, and like Mendelssohn, he ultimately became ensnared in public conflict and humiliation where his Jewish identity was at issue.

Unlike Mendelssohn's writings, however, Levison's barely address the issues of Jewish-Christian relations or the defense of Jewish particularity within a seemingly universalized culture. On the contrary, the title of Levison's composition on "the spirit and union of the natural, moral and divine law" appears to suggest an ecumenical posture whereby the issue of science and religion is addressed abstractly in broad human terms. Levison's Hebrew works, although obviously written for Jewish readers, embrace themes that could be fully appreciated by any enlightened Christian. Levison's interest in Mendelssohn's philosophy rested exclusively on his "universalist" themes: his commentary on the meaning of human existence according to Ecclesiastes and on the Socratic quest for immortality as discussed in the *Phaedon*.[46] About *Jerusalem*, Mendelssohn's belated effort to define his Jewish identity against the other, Levison apparently was silent. The primary theological concern so evident in his two principal Hebrew works is the relationship between science and religion. Levison creatively wedded the philosophical and cultural environments of London and Stockholm to biblical, rabbinic, and kabbalistic sources in order to construct a Jewish theology of nature appropriate to his times. He believed that this theology would be palatable to all intelligent Jews, allowing them to engage in scientific study while maintaining a spiritual link with their ancestral heritage. That Levison's effort could ultimately undermine the singularity of Jewish faith and its traditional understanding of revelation appears to have been missed by this author, who approached his task with a clear sense of Jewish commitment

45. See chap. 10 above.

46. He discusses the latter work in his *Shelosh Esrei Yesodei ha-Torah*, pp. 79b–80b.

and naive faithfulness in his educational mission. As we shall soon see, Levison's project illustrates the obstacles and tensions of conjoining Judaism with a sensationalist epistemology based on Locke and a physico-theology based on Linnaeus.

Of Levison's two Hebrew works—the treatise on law and science and the commentary on Maimonides' articles of faith—the second, written some twenty years after the first, is by far the more significant as a statement of religious philosophy and reflects a greater degree of sophistication and maturity. Levison's first work is not without interest, however. The introduction closely replicates the argument of Gumpertz, extolling the majesty of nature study in revering God and proclaiming that the sciences are unrelated to matters of faith. Levison even reproduces Gumpertz's list of Jewish luminaries involved in the sciences, ranging from Saadia and Baḥya ibn Pakuda to Mordechai Yaffe and Joseph Delmedigo.[47]

The remainder of the book represents a survey of the sciences of his day, intended as an introduction for the Hebrew reader. Levison intended to cover all the physical and life sciences in a conventional order, from the macrocosm to the microcosm, but he succeeded in completing only half the task in the single book he published; the mineral, plant, and animal worlds and the study of the human body were left out entirely. He begins with a description of the Copernican universe, advocating a nonliteralist reading of the Bible and arguing, as Zamosc had done through a citation of Joseph Delmedigo, that the rabbis were vindicated by the new cosmology.[48] A discussion of the sun and moon follow, with ample references to seventeenth-century scholars. Levison refers, for example, to the *Selenagraphia* of Johannes Hevelius (1611–87) and his mapping of lunar topography.[49]

Levison's most extensive discussion concerns Newtonian physics, including the three laws of motion, which he explains clearly and succinctly.[50] His nar-

47. *Ma'amar,* pp. 6–9
48. Ibid., pp. 18–20.
49. Ibid., pp. 21–22.
50. Ibid., pp. 28–30.

rative is filled with faithful descriptions of mechanical experiments referring to a wide array of seventeenth-century (but not eighteenth-century) researchers, including Boyle, Descartes, Borelli, Huygens, von Guericke, and Torrecelli.[51] He refers to Musschenbroeck's experiments on cohesion and the pyrometer and presents the aforementioned delineation of the air-pump.[52] His review of new findings related to the four elements ends with a discussion of water vapors and ice.[53] He closes with a brief peroration on how these new discoveries never imagined by the ancients reveal God's glory and demonstrate the wisdom of the rabbis. How the rabbis' sapience is confirmed by such a textbook of the "Gentile" sciences is never seriously explained. Levison promises more in a second volume that was apparently never published.[54]

Schoeps and Graupe describe a great commotion within the Jewish community of London over Levison's heretical views and indecent behavior. Levison was apparently barred from the synagogue, forced to defend himself from public ridicule in a pamphlet printed by his detractors. It is hard to understand how *Ma'amar ha-Torah ve-ha-Ḥokhmah* might have been connected to such hostility. Levison's dry, matter-of-fact presentation of some of the sciences was hardly the kind of work capable of eliciting any strong emotion from his readers. Levison lacked the eloquence and persuasive powers of Gumpertz. His long descriptions could have been read in full only by the most persistent of readers. He was surely not the first Hebrew writer to advocate a Copernican cosmology, and even if he was the first to present Newton's laws of motion to a Hebrew readership, such an effort was neither daring nor controversial in 1771. Levison's first Hebrew work seems to have had little impact, despite the excerpts he published in *Ha-Me'asef* some thirteen years later.[55] How many serious readers of Hebrew books existed in London of 1771 and how well the book circulated on the Continent are questions that require more study. Whatever the case,

51. Ibid., pp. 31–47

52. Ibid., pp. 55–62, 70–72. On Levison's reliance on Musschenbroek, see S. Bolag, "A Selection of Scientific Sources in the Hebrew Writings of the Seventeenth and Eighteenth Centuries" (in Hebrew), *Koroth* 9 (1989): 141–45.

53. *Ma'amar*, pp. 82–84.

54. Ibid., p. 85.

55. See n. 22 above.

Levison's controversy with the established Jewish community seems to have little to do with his unfinished scientific textbook.

When Levison decided to publish a commentary on Maimonides' thirteen principles some twenty years later, his agenda was quite different. Instead of a mere digest of scientific information, he now elected to reflect on the essence of the Jewish faith from the perspective of his own epistemological assumptions shaped within the medical and scientific community. Appearing some five years before his death, the *Shelosh-Esre Yesodei ha-Torah* represents his fullest and most thoughtful statement about the relationship between his scientific and Jewish identities. Following a convention adopted by several of his Jewish contemporaries in presenting their own reflections in the form of a commentary on a medieval philosophical text,[56] Levison hardly addresses Maimonides at all but merely utilizes the basic framework of thirteen principles to tackle each issue in his own way.

Levison begins his work like a good Maimonidean in defining man's highest ideal as knowledge of truth and in setting limits to human understanding in relation to divine knowledge revealed in the Torah.[57] But Levison soon reveals his independence from the medieval philosopher. He quickly mentions Joseph Albo's attempt to limit Maimonides' principles of faith to three and then suggests that one principle, not three or thirteen—that of knowing God—constitutes the only essential foundation of Judaism, while all the rest are derivative from it. He clarifies the unique status of this principle in relation to the other commandments in the following way: "For all the other commandments are capable of changing over time, since they only fall in the category of faith, but this foundational principle [the knowledge of one God] never changes even for an hour, since it is truth."[58] Within a Maimonidean context, indeed within

56. On the maskilic interest in Maimonides, see J. Lehmann, "Maimonides, Mendelssohn and the *Me'asfim:* Philosophy and the Biographical Imagination in the Early Haskalah," *Leo Baeck Institute Yearbook* 20 (1975): 87–108; and J. Harris, "The Image of Maimonides in Nineteenth-Century Jewish Historiography," *Proceedings of the American Academy for Jewish Research* 54 (1987): 117–39.

57. *Shelosh Esre Yesodei ha-Torah* [= *Yesodei ha-Torah*], pp. 1a–1b.

58. Ibid., p. 2a.

a traditional Jewish context, the formulation is strange. How can all the other commandments of Judaism be subject to change? What does Levison mean that they are "only faith" as opposed to knowledge of God, which is considered "truth"? Levison's usage of the terms *faith* and *truth* is not haphazard, as a full explication of them soon follows.

Levison defines "truth" as follows: "We know all those things that exist outside of ourselves and their essences through our senses and through all the experiments done with them through various instruments which enlarge or diminish, distance or bring closer; and all of them [the instruments] offer testimony together to all possessors of the senses and experience that their subject is what it is. This is truth which is an image of a thing and its appearance (for the essence and substance of things we do not know, but only their image and appearance)."[59]

Such a perception of the truth is surely liable to error, Levison admits, but the error is generated not by the senses per se but through our faulty judgment in interpreting them. On the other hand, "when all our senses together examine an object and collectively testify to its essence, then this object is truthful, since we have no recourse for knowing the truth other than the discernment of the senses together."[60] Levison elaborates on a procedure for determining truth claims: "We shall perform an experiment on them [specific objects] with all our senses and with various instruments, and we will also ask other people if they likewise acknowledge their reality and think the way we think. Thus, through many experiments and through many witnesses, an object can be verified to exist." Levison illustrates this method with a botanical example, that of determining that the seed of a date plant actually produces the date.[61]

Having defined "truth," Levison turns to the concept of "faith." He first explains that it is subject to time: "Sometimes we believe in something today that we didn't believe in yesterday and that we shall not believe in tomorrow, since only a fool believes in everything." Faith is a kind of trust not contradicted by

59. Ibid., p. 11a.
60. Ibid., p. 11b.
61. Ibid., pp. 12a–b.

reason. Something that reason proves to be false cannot be accepted on faith alone: "We do not believe that the sun is greater than the earth simply on the testimony of our forefathers, but only because we are incapable of imagining that it is smaller than the earth."[62]

Faith appropriately emerges within the human condition, where knowledge of the entire truth is unattainable: "It is a sign of deficiency in the strength of believers" who can never know all that God has created before or after their existence on earth. But there must be limits to what we believe. We should investigate what is within our capacity to know and "believe only what is beyond our intelligence and what the angels of God and his prophets have related." And we should be careful in believing in the words of a truthful prophet "who will offer a proof of his words."[63]

Finally, Levison offers the following clarification and illustration regarding the reciprocal relationship between truth and faith. No person can know anything without first accepting on faith the instruction of his master, relying on the latter's knowledge to acquire one's own knowledge firsthand. Levison's example is also taken from the natural world: "If the first person who told us of the magnet or about electricity was righteous and reliable, it is appropriate that we accept what he said on faith so long as there is no proof that contradicts it . . . and in this manner reason itself offers testimony on the virtue of faith."[64]

Levison's indebtedness to Locke's *Essay Concerning Human Understanding* in the above formulation is obvious. Locke's sensationalist epistemology emphatically rejected innate ideas and assumed that all human knowledge rested on probabilities. Probable propositions were of two kinds: those dealing with matters of fact and observation that human testimony can confirm, and those "which being beyond the discovery of our Senses, are not capable of any such Testimony."[65] The first kind is based on our constant observation, from which we draw a reasonable conjecture. When we encounter conflicting testimonies,

62. Ibid., p. 13a.

63. Ibid., p. 13b.

64. Ibid., p. 15a.

65. J. Locke, *An Essay Concerning Human Understanding*, 4.16.5, discussed in J. W. Yolton, *Locke: An Introduction* (Oxford and New York, 1985), p. 83.

we can only weigh all sides, arriving at the most plausible but not conclusive opinion.[66]

Faith for Locke was defined as "the assent to any proposition, not thus made by the deductions of reason; but upon the credit of the proposer, as coming from God, in some extraordinary way of communication." When our natural faculties are able to ascertain a probable fact, revelation is unnecessary. A revealed truth based on faith can never contradict the evidence of our understanding: "Faith can never convince us of anything that contradicts our knowledge. Because though Faith be founded on the testimony of God . . . yet we cannot have an assurance of the truth of its being a divine revelation, greater than our knowledge."[67]

As John Yolton points out, although Locke assigned reason the task of discerning a true revelation from a false one, he never clarified the criteria for making such a judgment. He strongly condemned mindless enthusiasts who suffered from "the conceits of a warmed or over-weening brain" but never provided an unambiguous answer as to how reason can distinguish between heavenly messages and the utterances of insanity.[68] His well-publicized debate with Bishop Edward Stillingfleet underscored the problematics of his position and his difficulty in accepting unquestioningly the tenets of the Christian faith. When the bishop pressed him on the absolute nature of Christian faith, he replied: "The Bible speaks of the assurance of faith, but nowhere that I can remember of the certainty of faith. Believing is not knowing."[69] As John Biddle puts it, Locke apparently believed that faith in God's revelation could somehow offer an assurance beyond all doubt, even though the divine authority of revelation was only a matter of probability.[70]

66. *Essay*, 4.16.6, 4.16.9.; and Yolton, *Locke*, p. 84.

67. *Essay*, 4.16.14, 4.18.5; and Yolton, *Locke*, pp. 85–86.

68. Yolton, *Locke*, pp. 88–90.

69. Ibid., pp. 92–94; the citation is on p. 94.

70. J. C. Biddle, "Locke's Critique of Innate Principles and Toland's Deism," in J. W. Yolton, ed., *Philosophy, Religion, and Science in the Seventeenth and Eighteenth Centuries* (Rochester, N.Y., 1990), pp. 140–51 (the reference is on p. 145); originally published in *Journal of the History of Ideas* 37 (1976): 411–22. See also, in the same volume, G. A. J. Rodgers, "Locke's *Essay* and Newton's *Principia*," pp. 366–81 (originally published in *Journal of the History of Ideas* 39 [1978]:

It appears that Levison not only followed Locke in distinguishing truth from faith; he also shared the same lack of clarity and consistency in establishing the criteria by which good faith is distinguished from bad. For Levison, as for Locke, Boyle, and their followers, knowledge is based exclusively on what the eye observes; it is probabilistic and fallibilistic. Probability is enhanced by the uniformity and regularity of our findings and by the number and reliability of our witnesses. But certainty of knowledge is unattainable by any means, and faith cannot offer us more than our human capacity allows.[71]

What alarmed Stillingfleet about Locke's position would certainly have alarmed the rabbis about Levison's book, including those who wrote endorsements of the book in its opening pages, if they had actually understood the full implications of his position. Like Locke, Levison backed away from a fideistic position. He would not take comfort in the security and certitude of faith that offered human beings solace from their contingent experience and finite knowledge. Faith, instead, is not only uncertain; it is less certain than the tentative knowledge human beings possess. It is neither timeless nor stable but fleetingly shifts from day to day, a position that goes beyond that of Locke.[72] When it contradicts empiricist reason, even though reason can never be absolute but only tentative, faith should be discarded.

What remains of Judaism, then, is its one foundational principle, the knowledge of God, which is grounded in reason—that is, in sensation and reflection. Any other principles derive from this one truth and all the remaining commandments of Judaism "are capable of changing over time," since they are grounded in faith, not truth. If one is to take Levison at his word, he has not only "reformed" Judaism with this epistemology;[73] he has undermined its very foundation. Knowing God is analogous to knowing that a seed produces a date or that the forces of gravitation or electricity are real. As Shapin and Schaffer have argued with respect to Boyle, the scientist's laboratory ultimately produced a

---

217–32); and idem, "The Empiricism of Locke and Newton," in S. C. Brown, ed., *Philosophers of the Enlightenment* (Sussex, 1979), 1–33.

71. Cf. Shapin and Schaffer, *Leviathan,* esp. pp. 21–25, and *Essay,* 4.14.1–2.

72. *Yesodei ha-Torah,* p. 13a.

73. I refer to the rather imprecise formulation of Pelli (see n. 39 above), who calls Levison in the title of his article the "first religious reform theoretician."

theology where empirical facts and schemata were deployed to convince men of the existence and attributes of God.[74] In Levison's radical formulation, he had suddenly overturned the uneasy alliance between natural philosophy and Jewish thought that had functioned at least since the time of the Maharal and the decline of medieval scholasticism. Basilea, we recall, had typified the Jewish thinkers through the early eighteenth century who had integrated contemporary physics with traditional, even kabbalistic metaphysics.[75] Levison's faithful adoption of Lockean epistemology with his enthusiastic endorsement of the Boylean program of experimentalism would no longer allow for such a merger. Jewish faith as understood by Saadia, Ha-Levi, and Nieto was seemingly devalued and demoralized.

If the Jewish faith rested only on the principle of knowing God and this knowledge rested entirely on human sensation and reflection as practiced in the scientific laboratory, then it was incumbent upon Levison to demonstrate how science as practiced in his day could reveal God's existence, his creation of the world, and his providence over all his creatures. This indeed becomes the primary task of the book. While previous Jewish thinkers had regularly employed the evidence of the splendorous design of creation to substantiate the Jewish faith, as we often have seen, Levison's effort in this regard surpasses them all in its comprehensiveness and in its profound understanding of natural processes. In this he reveals his indebtedness to a towering figure of eighteenth-century science, Carl Linnaeus, and to a theological system commonly known as physico-theology. If Locke and, to a lesser extent, Hunter constituted the primary English sources of Levison's religious philosophy, Linnaeus may be said to have represented his primary Swedish one.

The physico-theological tradition became prominent in the late sixteenth and early seventeenth centuries through the writing of such well-known figures as Pieter van Musschenbroeck and J. Albert Favbricus in Holland, and John Ray and William Derham in England. Physico-theology was based on the assumption of a remarkable system of balance and compensation that functioned

74. Shapin and Schaffer, *Leviathan*, p. 340.
75. See chap. 7 above.

throughout the universe. God had provided just the right number for everything on earth, "enough to keep up the species, but not to overcharge the world," as Derham put it. Thus, he adds, "the balance of the animal world is throughout all ages kept even, and by a curious harmony, and just proportion between the increase of all animals, and the length of their lives, the world is through all ages well, but not overstored."[76]

Linnaeus, a Swedish professor of natural history, had read Derham and the other physico-theologians and found their understanding of nature well suited to his deep sense of Christian piety. In his *Oeconomia naturae* of 1749, he sketched an elaborate science of ecology, followed by several other highly popular, accessible, and homiletical treatises, quickly translated into English and several other languages, including *De curiositate, Nemesis divina,* and *Politia naturae.* Linnaeus succinctly defined the theme of the economy of nature: "In order, therefore, to perpetuate the established course of nature in a continued series, the divine wisdom has thought fit, that all living creatures should constantly be employed in producing individuals; that all natural things should contribute and lend a helping hand to preserve every species; and lastly, that the death and destruction of one thing should always be subservient to the restitution of another." For Linnaeus, the most remarkable example of the world's ecological system was the propagation of plant seeds, which he maintained was effected "by an intercourse between different sexes, as experience testifies."[77] As Sten Lindroth

76. W. Derham, *Physico-Theology: Or, A Demonstration of the Being and Attributes of God, from his Works on Creation,* 3d ed. (London, 1714), p. 171; cited and discussed in W. Lepenies, "Linnaeus's *Nemesis Divina* and the Idea of Retaliation in the Eighteenth Century," in J. Weinstock, ed., *Contemporary Perspectives on Linnaeus* (Lanham, N.Y., 1985), pp. 94–95 (originally published in *Isis* 73 [1982]: 11–27). On physico-theology, see W. Philipp, "Physicotheology in the age of Enlightenment, Appearance and History," *Studies on Voltaire and the Eighteenth Century* 57 (1967): 1233–67.

77. C. Linneaus, "The Oeconomy of Nature," in *Miscellaneous Tracts Relating to Natural History, Husbandry and Physick,* trans. B. Stillingfleet (London, 1791; repr. New York, 1977), p. 40. On Linnaeus and his general understanding of nature, I have found the following especially useful: E. Ehnmark, "Linnaeus and the Problem of Immortality," in *Kungl. Humanistiska Vetenskapssamfundet I Lund: Arsberattelse Bulletin de la Societé Royale des Lettres de Lund* 1951–52: 63–93; S. Lindroth, "The Two Faces of Linnaeus," in T. Frangsmyr, ed., *Linnaeus: The Man and His Work* (Berkeley and Los Angeles, 1983), pp. 1–62; in the same volume, G. Eriksson, "Lin-

puts it, the fertilization and dissemination of seeds was a real playground for the physico-theologians who wished to sing the praises of the divine architect, and for Linnaeus in particular the act of fertilization, through pistils and stamens, was a kind of sacrament around which he built his system of botanical classification.[78] In several long descriptions, he outlines the entire evolution of the plant kingdom and then turns to the animal kingdom, through each of their three basic phases: propagation, preservation, and destruction.[79]

What was significant theologically about *The Oeconomy of Nature* was its creative attempt to address the problem of theodicy and God's continual providence over all his creatures. When one fathoms the entire system of creation, the entire chain of being from the lowest to the highest forms, one understands that what might appear evil at first blush ultimately serves a higher purpose and might not be evil at all: "Let us not imagine, when those rapacious animals sometimes do us mischief, that the Creator planned the order of nature according to our private principles of oecomony . . . whereas the stupendous oeconomy of the Diety is one throughout the globe, and if Providence does not always calculate exactly according to our way of reckoning, we ought to consider this affair in the same light, as when different seamen wait for a fair wind, every one, with respect to the part he is bound to, who we plainly see cannot all be satisfied.[80]

Linnaeus shows how even stinking carcasses serve a higher purpose; how

naeus the Botanist," pp. 63–109, and T. Frangsmyr, "Linnaeus as a Geologist," pp. 110–55; the aforementioned essay of Lepenies, and in the same volume edited by Weinstock, V. Heywood, "Linnaeus: The Conflict between Science and Scholasticism," pp. 1–16; F. N. Egerton, "Changing Concepts of the Balance of Nature," *Quarterly Review of Biology* 48 (1973): 322–50; P. R. Sloan, "The Buffon-Linnaeus Controversy," *Isis* 67 (1976): 356–75; idem, "John Locke, John Ray, and the Problem of the Natural System," *Journal of the History of Biology* 5 (1972): 1–54; J. L. Larson, *Reason and Experience: The Representation of Natural Order in the Work of Carl Von Linne* (Berkeley, 1971); A. O. Lovejoy, *The Great Chain of Being: A Study in the History of an Idea* (New York, 1960); and W. F. Bynum, "The Great Chain of Being after Forty Years: An Appraisal," *History of Science* 13 (1975): 1–28.

78. Lindroth, "Two Faces," p. 20, referring to Linnaeus's famous work *De sexu plantarum* of 1760.

79. Linnaeus, *Oeconomy of Nature,* pp. 63–120.

80. Ibid., pp. 120–21.

insects "at once promote their own good, and that of other animals"; and how "wild beasts and ravenous birds, though they seem to disturb our private oeconomy," ultimately serve a higher good. The conclusion is clear from the overwhelming evidence nature itself presents:

> From a partial consideration of things, we are very apt to criticize what we ought to admire; to look upon as useless what perhaps we should own to be of infinite advantage to us, did we see a little farther; to be peevish where we ought to give thanks; and at the same time to ridicule those, who employ their time and thoughts in examining what we were, i.e. some of us most assuredly were, created and appointed to study. In short we are too apt to treat the Almighty worse than a rational man would treat a good mechanic; whose works he would either thoroughly examine, or be asked to find any fault with them. This is the effect of a partial consideration of nature; but he who has candour of mind and leisure to look farther, will be inclined to cry out: How wondrous is this scene![81]

Such lofty religious reflections, directly linking the human mandate to examine nature with a verification of God's ultimate goodness and providential design, undoubtedly affected Levison deeply. He had discovered in Linnaeus's popular writings a genuine resource for demonstrating the critical priestly role of the naturalist in confirming God's existence and continual involvement in his creation. In a chapter entitled "On the Righteousness of the [God's] Administration," Levison opens by declaring that good and evil are subjective categories and immediately offers examples quite familiar to Linnaeus's readers. He cites the dramatic example of rotting carcasses, the intricate interplay between eaters and eaten that insures the proper balance of nature. Levison is convinced that the perfection of the whole depends upon the existence of various degrees of imperfection of the parts—that, in the language of Lovejoy,[82] God loves abundance and variety more than peace and concord among his creatures. This is best illustrated by the complaints of farmers about insects and other creatures that ravage their fields. Levison relates the specific example of birds who de-

81. Ibid., pp. 121–27; the quotation is from p. 127.
82. Lovejoy, *Great Chain of Being*, p. 221.

voured the grain of American farmers. The latter "became 'wise' by destroying all the birds from the land," rewarding anyone who hunted them. However, "God created this fowl in order that they eat the worms that destroy the grass of the field so that when another year had passed, the worms increased to such an extent that they ate the entire grass of the field." The farmers were obliged to order new seed from England because of their foolish action in breaking the ecological chain.[83]

Levison's account of this well-known eighteenth-century example of human ecological abuse recalls Linnaeus's reference: "When the little crows were driven out of Virginia, and at the expense of several tons of gold, the inhabitants would willingly have bought them back at double the price."[84] And elsewhere: "Nature has appointed the Qiscula to watch over the Dermestes pisorum, these being extirpated in North America by shooting, the peas have been totally ruined."[85]

Levison's strong conclusion follows: "The great error of human beings is that they think that God created everything for them but He actually created for Himself, for the thing itself. Nevertheless, man is great and rules over everything while the rest of the creatures don't injure him as most people conceive." Then Levison offers his most impressive evidence, unquestionably borrowed from Linnaeus, whom he cites by name. He points out the discovery of sexuality in plants, adding parenthetically that the author of the *Zohar* had first noticed this fact. But "it is even more wonderful" what the recent naturalists have discovered regarding the pollination of female plants by the male through its "fine dust." Levison then relates Linnaeus's experiments with the fig plant, illustrating how each plant is germinated by its special and appropriate mate.[86]

In the following chapter on providence, Levison reiterates his point that evil and good are felt subjectively by the perceiver, "so that what one thinks good will be imagined as bad by another."[87] And in his final chapters on immortality,

---

83. *Yesodei ha-Torah,* chap. 19, pp. 71a–73b.

84. *Of the Use of Curiosity,* in *Miscellaneous Tracts,* p. 176.

85. C. Linnaeus, *Select Dissertations from the Amoenitates Academicae,* trans. F. J. Brand (London, 1781; repr. New York, 1977), p. 161.

86. *Yesodei ha-Torah,* p. 74a.

87. Ibid., p. 74b.

on angels and demons, and on the revival of the dead—topics that would appear to be hopelessly out of keeping with contemporary sensibilities—Levison reinterprets them in a language befitting modern science, while underscoring the continued credibility of kabbalistic sapience. He refers more than once to the "ladder" of creation, by which one can recognize the perfectability of creation:

> If we distinguish the existence of inanimate objects from that of speaking ones, we shall see how they evolve *[ne'etakim]* from one level to the next. Man himself evolves from the mineral to the vegetable and to the animal until [he attains] the ability to speak. . . . And if we look at the rest of the creatures, we shall see how they evolve from level to level because the faculty of natural speech does not evolve from the mineral to the speaker without an intermediate stage . . . for after the mineral the vegetable will follow (in the order of general nature) . . . and from the vegetable to the quality of animal . . . until we arrive at the voice whose form is actually the form of man . . . and according to this order and natural ladder you shall see how evolution proceeds from the mineral to man in a wondrous progression, the more substances diminish, the greater the intelligences.[88]

This "great chain of being" suggests a natural pattern even in the world beyond man, a world of intelligences, spirits, and angels. If the anatomist can uncover a remarkable web of interactive relations between muscles, organs, and brain, revealing "a vitality that dwells in their midst," "you can imagine a spiritual pattern from all these powers that travel from the brain to every part of the body and back . . . and thus there is no doubt an analogy in this spiritual realm, in the uppermost heights . . . and thus you will understand the words of the kabbalists on the primordial man and similar notions. . . . Therefore, through an examination of the natural order, the existence of angels and the succession of levels can be proven." Even the demonic spirit need not be ruled out in the ascending and descending natural ladder, "as long as there is no proof that denies it nor does its existence contradict the perfection of God and the nature of existence."[89]

88. Ibid., p. 93a.
89. Ibid., pp. 94a–b.

As Zamosc had done before him, Levison likened the traditional notion of the soul as the seat of intelligence from birth to the theory of preformation, made popular by recent scholars through their microscopic observations. The seed, in which the entire tree can be observed in miniature, might be paralleled in the human realm by the fetus. Perhaps, he suggested, the current theory of natural science confirmed the ancient Platonic and kabbalistic views that "the soul of the first human being is included in all human souls" or that "the intelligences are already placed in the soul as seeds are placed in bodies." Levison acknowledges an alternative view whereby the soul acquires its intelligence only after birth, but he prefers the first notion and substantiates it with an account of a child prodigy in music whom he had heard in London.[90]

The greatest and final challenge Levison faced in reconciling a traditional concept with modern science concerned the notion of the revival of the dead, a doctrine even Maimonides found difficult to accept. In this case, he again employs Linnaeus's insights to suggest the possibility that resuscitating life cannot be dismissed out of hand. Levison recounts the cycle of the silkworm and its remarkable metamorphosis, probably drawing on the well-known treatise of Linnaeus on the subject, relating the five stages of the silkworm's life divided by four intervals of sleep. He concludes: "Thus our eyes see that its death is the beginning of its self-transformation so that its end is better than its beginning, and from this, one can judge the matter of the death of man."[91]

In noticing the profound influence that Linnaeus and physico-theology left on this Jewish disciple who had clearly absorbed the latter from his exposure to the scientific ambiance of Sweden and Great Britain, we should add parenthetically that Levison is selective in his citations from the writing of his Swedish mentor. As many of Linnaeus's interpreters have pointed out, Linnaeus was ultimately more famous as a system builder and taxonomist of nature. Indeed, he considered such works as the *Oeconomia* and *De curiositate* mere oratorical exercises, sermons on God's omnipotence that were of less scientific value than his *Systema naturae*. With a certain neoscholastic or Cartesian-like rigidity and

90. Ibid., pp. 95b–97a; and see n. 32 above.

91. Ibid., pp. 99b–100b, and Linnaeus, *Dissertation on the Silk Worm*, in *Select Dissertations*, pp. 437–56.

dogmaticism, he insisted on a rather arbitrary and artificial method of labeling all natural phenomena, becoming a kind of "botanical legislator" and incurring the wrath of several critics, most notably George-Louis Leclerc Buffon. Buffon's Lockean critique of Linnaeus's a priori deductive statements about natural phenomena, and the Frenchman's preference for a chain of successive individual existences, were surely more to Levison's taste. Linnaeus had been unable to resolve the tension between the demands of empiricism and the demands of order. Levison had opted for the first and ignored the second in his own construction of Jewish theology based on Locke and Linnaeus.[92]

In consciously choosing the Linnaeus of the *Oeconomia* as his model, Levison advanced those notions that promoted traditional Jewish principles, not only Maimonidean but kabbalistic as well. His new Linnean sensibility was not without cost, however. In the system of divine nemesis Linnaeus had constructed, all plants and animals fulfill the function of revenge and compensation, creating the balanced order of nature so visible to the trained observer. Linnaeus assumed that this notion applied to human beings as well. Thus all human actions find their just retribution in this world and all human crimes are inevitably punished in the here-and-now. Linnaeus provides numerous examples in *Nemesis divina,* a work Levison may have noticed, to verify empirically what one scholar likens to the work of "a specimen hunting biologist."[93] The net effect of this effort, to be sure, was to offer an apparent empirical solution to the problem of theodicy and to demonstrate on the basis of the senses the providential and purposeful design of creation. On the other hand, Levison and Linnaeus had only "proven" a just retribution in this world. It is not coincidental that Levison offers no discussion of heaven and hell in his treatise. While angels and demons are conceivable by analogy with the natural order, the subject of the afterlife is beyond the purview of sensationalist experimental science and therefore constitutes a mere belief unworthy of a serious scientific explication. Furthermore, if divine providence can be demonstrated as a phenomenon of this world equivalent to the maintenance of the dramatic equilibrium of nature, why resort to such a metaphysical notion of divine spiritual retribution in the first place? By virtue

92. Linnaeus as taxonomist is treated by Sloan, Larson, and Lindroth; see n. 77 above.
93. Lepenies, "Linnaeus's *Nemesis Divina,*" p. 109.

of their considerable modification of the notion of traditional providence, one might be tempted to see the positions of both Linnaeus and Levison as approaching that of Charles Darwin, who eventually substituted "the principle of natural selection for Linnaeus' pious belief in Providence as the direct source of species and the adaptations discoverable in the order of nature," or even Adam Smith's "invisible hand" of political economy.[94] One wonders whether any of Levison's Hebrew readers came to appreciate the full import of his borrowings from Linnaeus. As the rabbinic statement goes, his loss might eventually have canceled his profit *(Yaẓah sekharo be-hefsedo).*

Throughout his commentary on Maimonides, Levison presents himself consistently as an authentic defender of the Jewish faith, ready to take on all atheists and heretics and those who deny any of the principles of Judaism. He thunders against Spinoza on two occasions, even mentioning him by name, and finds his pantheism reprehensible.[95] He vigorously defends the integrity of the kabbalah against the allegation that it was the source of Spinozism. He mentions a group of Christians, and even a Jew, who held the latter position.[96] He is most likely referring to Johann George Wachter's *Der Spinoẓismus im Judenthumb, oder die von dem heutigen Judenthumb und desen geheimen Kabbala Vergötterte Welt,* published in Amsterdam in 1699, or to his later *Elucidarius cabalisticus sive reconditae Hebraorum philosophiae recensio,* published in Rome in 1706, which aimed to reconcile the kabbalah with Spinozism. The contemporary Jews to whom he refers might be exemplified by either Mendelssohn or Maimon, who are said at least to have recognized that the kabbalah and Spinozism were similar systems.[97]

When presenting proofs for God's existence, Levison rejects the Cartesian position that God can be known simply from innate ideas.[98] More significantly, he devotes considerable attention to defending the traditional notion of creation out of nothing *(creatio ex nihilo)* with four distinct proofs. Most original,

94. Ibid., pp. 112–13.

95. *Yesodei ha-Torah,* pp. 19a–b, 31b.

96. Ibid., p. 19a.

97. See G. Scholem, *Avraham Cohen Herrera: Ba'al Sha'ar Shamayim, Ḥayyav, Yeẓirato ve-Hashpa'ato* (Jerusalem, 1978), pp. 45–79; and Altmann, *Moses Mendelssohn,* pp. 609, 687.

98. *Yesodei ha-Torah,* pp. 19b–20a.

at least from the perspective of Jewish thought, is his argument in favor of the authenticity of Mosaic chronology. Following the lines of defense of orthodox Christianity, Levison attempts to invalidate other ancient chronologies that had come to light in the seventeenth century, suggesting that the age of the earth was significantly longer than the biblical account, thus implying its eternity. He quotes from both *Sinicae historiae* (1658) by the Jesuit Martini Martini, who had presented Chinese history earlier than the flood, and Samuel Bochart's *Geographia sacra*, a staunch defense of biblical chronology.[99] Interestingly enough, the Jesuit's Chinese history had been perceived by some as leading to atheism when presented in connection with Preadamite doctrines of the seventeenth century. Traditionalists such as Isaac Vossius, Daniel Huet, Gherard Voss, and Georg Horn had strongly refuted the notion that the world was older than the Bible had related it to be. Horn, in particular, interpreted Martini as disbelieving the Chinese view and actually mocking the idea of China's antiquity.[100] Levison adopts the same approach: "Thus Martinius Martini wrote that he found in the works of the Chinese that they themselves do not believe in their chronology of the world and they mock it." He concludes that the testimony of all ancient peoples supports the biblical account and indirectly confirms the doctrine of creation out of nothing.[101]

Levison's second proof of creation is the evidence of early forests and animals that preceded human population, according to which the world, as we know it, could not have been eternal but evolved gradually from a state of nothingness. Third, quoting Johann Christoph Wolf's *Biblioteca hebraica,* published in Hamburg between 1715 and 1733, he argues that there is evidence of one original language (Hebrew) whose traces are scattered in all languages, indicating as well the purposeful creation of God. Finally, like Zamosc, he contends that the rejection of the theory of spontaneous generation by Redi and others, and the argument that all generation is ovist, demonstrate that creation had a

99. Ibid., p. 28b.

100. See P. Rossi, *The Dark Abyss of Time: The History of the Earth and the History of Nations from Hooke to Vico,* trans. L. G. Cochrane (Chicago and London, 1984), pp. 140–56. See also A. T. Grafton, "Joseph Scaliger and Historical Chronology: The Rise and Fall of a Discipline," *History and Theory* 14 (1975): 156–85; and F. C. Haber, *The Age of the World* (Baltimore, 1959).

101. *Yesodei ha-Torah,* p. 28b.

beginning and hence the world was not eternal. Thus from his knowledge of the sciences of comparative chronology, archaeology and anthropology, linguistics, and biology, Levison presents an impressive, albeit conventional and unoriginal, arsenal of demonstrations in defense of a traditional understanding of creation.[102]

He also defends the institution of prophecy as described in the Bible, although he reduces its miraculous dimension to the vanishing point: "Prophecy in my eyes is like a sensory perception without the need for a divine sign."[103] Similarly, the revelation of the Torah is authentic, since it was based on the sensory experience of a multitude of witnesses who passed down this historical truth from generation to generation. The argument from Saadia to Mendelssohn is not new, as we have seen, but Levison follows a more individualistic approach with respect to the testimony of miracles the Bible conveys. Such miracles, he contends, are analogous to the miracle of digestion and the remarkable potency of saliva recently discovered by contemporary medicine, or to the miracles of electricity and similar phenomena discovered almost daily. It is clear that Levison defines a miracle as not breaking the regular processes of nature but simply being that part of the natural world presently discovered and understood by contemporary scientists. The implication is that all biblical miracles, even the most unnatural, will be explained eventually by the tools of modern researchers.[104]

Levison's defense of the authenticity of the Jewish tradition is also based on his understanding of medicine and science. Consistently with his earlier definition of faith, he declares that a tradition is valid as long as it cannot be disproved by logic, as long as the story and those who relate the story are reliable, and as long as there are more than one witness. Thus ancient testimonies in medicine and mathematics are still valid to this day, he contends. What he fails to address, however, is the frequency with which ancient scientific theories are overturned in favor of better ones on the basis of these same criteria. Nor does he consider the possibility that standards of verification appropriate to the sciences may be inappropriate when applied to religious faith.[105]

102. Ibid., pp. 29a–30a.
103. Ibid., p. 49a.
104. Ibid., pp. 54b–57a.
105. Ibid., p. 57a.

Finally, Levison tackles the most difficult challenge of all: the purpose of the obligatory commandments of Judaism. His response is three-pronged. The commandments, he argues, teach proper doctrines to the masses who are incapable of understanding them without the support of normative prescriptions. Contra Spinoza, he contends that wise men also require these commandments so that their actions may accompany their lofty thoughts. Finally, the commandments contain "wonderful reasons known to God and who would dare rely on his own opinion and reason regarding the commandments and thus allow himself to break the word of the Torah?" The laws of the Torah, Levison concludes, "arouse in our hearts the recognition of God's existence, providence and ability which is perfection in the virtue of intelligence. . . . Therefore, God gave the laws as a royal edict to His servants and desires their good, so they do not request a reason but follow the commandments in the manner God commanded them, for the reasons were made known to Him, the Blessed One."[106]

In a book that clarifies the difference between knowledge and faith according to Locke, and that demonstrates the one principle of God's existence from the purposeful order of nature verified by the senses, Levison's chapter justifying the commandments, particularly the prescription to follow the commandments blindly without utilizing one's reason, has a hollow ring. And how do the laws of the Torah inculcate the truth of divine existence and providence when Levison had argued consistently that such knowledge was available to human beings through their sensory perceptions, through their own experience and that of witnesses, and through scientific experiments? This chapter stands out from the rest of the book as a feeble attempt to rehearse traditional pieties; they clash with, even contradict, both the spirit and substance of the work's major arguments. To a sensitive reader of Levison's subversive commentary on Maimonides, such platitudes were sure to remain unconvincing. Real knowledge of God, his creation, and providence was available through the Book of Nature, not through the Bible and Talmud. The commandments could not lead a person to know the truth; only a laboratory could accomplish that.

106. Ibid., p. 59a.

EPILOGUE

Having considered Levison's reflections on Judaism and science in the last chapter, it would be tempting to conclude this book by tracing an inevitable progression (or regression) of Jewish thinking on science from the limited toleration of science of the Maharal of Prague at the end of the sixteenth century to its enthusiastic endorsement by Mordechai Schnaber Levison at the end of the eighteenth. Obviously, such a conclusion would be overly simplistic, and unwarranted even on the basis of the limited evidence presented in the preceding chapters. We can safely conclude, however, that Jewish thinking about the new developments in science throughout the period roughly demarcated by the lives of these two thinkers exhibits certain continuities. They include the validation and elevation of the study of the sciences, especially medicine, within the Jewish community and a concomitant devaluation and invalidation of philosophy as defined by the Maimonidean tradition; an attempt to see the new discoveries in science as vindicating and confirming previously discredited rabbinic and especially kabbalistic views, thus preserving the seemingly peaceful coexistence between kabbalah, magic, and science among such thinkers as Delmedigo and Basilea well into the eighteenth century; the repeated usage of the argument for God's existence based on the design of his creation, increasingly augmented and refined by the dramatic accumulation of new information about the natural world; and, most of all, a conscious attempt to disentangle physics from metaphysics, the secular from the sacred, science from theology. In general, Jewish thinkers in early modern Europe, like their Christian counterparts, viewed scientific advances as positive resources to be enlisted in the cause of perpetuating their ancestral faith. In fact, Jewish responses to science not only paralleled those in the Christian community; on occasion Jewish thinkers consciously drew upon Christian arguments in shaping their own: del Bene and Nieto, for example, were influenced by Jesuit and Anglican science, respectively. In the main, Jews erected carefully drawn boundaries between the domains of scientific activity and religious faith so that the two could live peacefully and harmoniously with each other, avoiding the bitter consequences of their comingling—the troubled legacy of the medieval period.

As the case of Levison demonstrates, however, it became increasingly difficult to seal off these areas of discourse hermetically. Leaks and even ruptures could occur when scientific sensibilities began to intrude into the space of traditional faith, as the examples of Delmedigo, Luzzatto, and Levison testify. By the nineteenth century, the intellectual challenge of Darwinism and the increasing secularization of Jewish life revealed the enormous challenges of preserving the tenuous alliance of science and Jewish faith. Traditionalists, to be sure, continued to define the relationship between the two on the basis of these early modern thinkers, or fearfully to reject any relationship out of hand. Most secularists found the discourse between Judaism and science uninteresting and hopelessly irrelevant. For those who continued to deem the dialogue worthwhile, the terms of a fruitful interaction and discussion had been set forth more than two centuries earlier.

This book has examined Jewish reflections on scientific activity in the early modern period, not Jewish scientific activity itself. As we have observed from the outset, actual scientific performance among Jews in early modern Europe was inconsequential, with the possible exception of several luminaries in clinical medicine. Amos Funkenstein, in his recent work on Jewish historiography, offers this appraisal of Jewish achievement in science: "The truth of the matter is that we rather ought to ask why the Jewish participation in it [science] was minimal and insignificant. . . . Perhaps it was because they were remote from some centers of science, such as England and France; but they were present in Holland and Italy. A strong contributing factor was, without doubt, the absence of a sense of the relative autonomy of such pursuits as legitimate or even God-willed."[1]

Funkenstein is certainly wrong to view Judaism as less tolerant or enthusiastic than Christianity in validating the autonomous pursuit of the sciences, as the evidence I have presented demonstrates. But he is right to point out that the achievements of Jewish practitioners of science in this era are unimpressive in comparison with those of more recent times.[2]

Judah del Bene in the seventeenth century sensed that Christians had a clear advantage over Jews in their leisure to pursue independent study and in the institutional support provided for that purpose.[3] As we have seen, he was probably referring to the Church, especially Jesuit support for scientific study. By his day, the churches throughout Europe generally controlled, staffed, and supervised universities and other institutions of higher learning. To this obvious difference between Jewish and Christian institutional structures, we might add the growing support of royal courts and the increasingly specialized function of individuals with scientific expertise who were employed by them. The most significant vehicle for fostering scientific knowledge was the scientific academies and societies emerging throughout Europe, which served as reference groups for scientists, as clearinghouses for scientific data, and as goads for collective research. These organizations gave science a new social legitimation and shaped a new class of professional scientists.[4]

For the most part, the support of churches, courts, and especially scientific

1. A. Funkenstein, *Perceptions of Jewish History* (Berkeley, 1993), pp. 216–17.

2. On the later period, see Y. M. Rabkin, "Jews and the Professionalization of Science," paper presented at the conference "The Interaction of Scientific and Jewish Cultures," June 2–5, 1990, to be published in the proceedings of the conference.

3. See chap. 6 above.

4. The subject is well summarized by R. Emerson in "The Organization of Science and Its Pursuit in Early Modern Europe," in R. C. Olby et al., *Companion to the History of Modern Science* (London, 1990), pp. 960–79. See also the classic work of M. Ornstein, *The Role of Scientific Societies in the Seventeenth Century* (Chicago, 1938); and J. E. McClellan, *Science Reorganized: Scientific Societies in the Eighteenth Century* (New York, 1985); J. Ben David, *The Scientist's Role in Society: A Comparative Study* (Englewood Cliffs, 1971). For additional bibliography, consult Emerson, "Organization," as well as chap. 3, n. 56 above.

academies was unavailable to Jews. As I have suggested above, Jewish graduates of Padua, along with university-trained converso physicians, were able to
establish informal social and professional links resembling to some extent a scientific society.[5] But medicine was their only common interest, and their informal
ties were surely a far cry from the scientific societies lavishly supported by private and state interests. Despite the obvious impediments to sharing knowledge
and working in concert, these physicians, especially the conversos, still saw
themselves as a distinct professional group and were aware of one another's
achievements.[6] Isaac Lampronti's attempt to produce an academic journal and
eventually an encyclopedia of rabbinic knowledge might also suggest an incipient attempt to organize Jewish learning along the lines of the new scientific
organizations. But lacking the endorsement of the Ferrarese Jewish community, Lampronti's journal was aborted.[7] Since only a few medical schools—at
Padua, Leiden, and elsewhere—were open to Jews, their participation in science
usually was restricted to medicine and the related life sciences. Delmedigo's
encounter with Galileo and Gans's with Brahe are exceptions that prove the
rule. Jews generally had little opportunity to "do" science other than medicine
in early modern Europe. Only through their medical education and practice, as
well as their reading, could they keep abreast of the latest discoveries in other
scientific disciplines. They remained outside the scientific laboratory because of
social, not religious constraints.

In closing this book about a community of Jewish thinkers attempting to
make religious sense out of the enthralling and liberating moment of scientific
discovery in Western civilization, I cannot fail to note the irony that our own
era often views science from a markedly different perspective. For some of us,
scientific achievement has become synonymous with frightening technologies
of power and domination, oppression, and even terror. The calamity of Adorno's
enlightened "administered world," where control over nature inexorably leads to
domination over other human beings and even to the eradication of all individu-

5. See chap. 3 above.
6. See esp. chap. 10 above.
7. See chap. 9 above.

372

ality, seems unbearable in the context of recent Jewish memory.[8] In the dialectic of these two antithetical perceptions of science and human rationality—one ultimately liberating, the other ultimately oppressive—the thinkers studied in this book may find a more receptive hearing. They attempted creatively to balance the confidence of human achievement and mastery of nature with the acknowledgment of human finitude and the wonder of the unknowable. In a culture where human pretense to knowledge and truth has been shattered by gas chambers and atomic weapons, the lonely world of the survivors and their successors appears a bit closer in spirit to this group of thinkers, who strove to accommodate the new science with their religious beliefs, to balance the insatiable quest for human knowledge and power with the ethical and epistemological implications of human contingency and finitude.

For a historian who seeks to depict the past with objectivity and integrity, this preliminary reconstruction of some early modern Jewish dialogues with science is a sufficient reward. Nevertheless, I would be the first to admit that some readers with postmodern sensibilities, both captivated and horrified by the advances and defeats that scientific technologies have engendered for modern civilization, may find even greater value in the modest reflections of these early modern Jews on science, on the mysteries of the natural world they inhabited, and on their specific human predicament.

8. I have in mind Horkheimer's and Adorno's provocative reading of the Enlightenment. See M. Horkheimer and T. W. Adorno, *The Dialectic of Enlightenment,* trans. J. Cumming (1944; New York, 1969). See also R. Bernstein, "The Rage against Reason," in E. McMullin, *Construction and Constraint: The Shaping of Scientific Rationality,* (Notre Dame, 1988), pp. 189–221. For a recent example of the continued attack on science for its essential amorality and lack of spiritual values, see B. Appleyard, *Understanding the Present: Science and the Soul of Modern Man* (New York, 1993), and the critical review of it by T. Ferris in the *New York Review of Books,* May 13, 1993: 17–19.

BIBLIOGRAPHIC ESSAY

THE STUDY OF NATURE IN ANCIENT JUDAISM

I originally intended to begin this book with an overview of attitudes to the natural world in ancient Judaism, which would have
preceded my survey of the medieval period in chapter 1. Having
reviewed much of the literature on the subject, however, I have
resisted the temptation to summarize a vast body of material in
an area that has not been fully studied and that falls outside my
primary area of expertise. The cultures of Hellenistic and rabbinic Judaism, sprawling over centuries and subject to variegated
social and intellectual influences in Palestine, Babylonia, and
elsewhere, are notoriously difficult to reconstruct historically.
Their materials, ranging from the Dead Sea scrolls to the Apoc-
rypha, Pseudepigrapha, and Hellenistic and Talmudic literatures,
with their complex redactional problems, are extremely slippery
to situate within a specific historical context. Moreover, a systematic study of attitudes toward nature would have to focus on
materials emanating from circles generally thought to be outside
or on the periphery of "official" rabbinic Judaism, materials such
as mystical literature, magical handbooks, amulets, and magic
bowls. To what extent such materials reflect the interests of "low"
and "high" culture and the flow of ideas and values between the
two is a question that remains to be addressed. Finally, there is
the problem of studying attitudes toward nature in their entirety,
that is, the organic relations among such diverse fields as astron-

omy and astrology, geography, biology and botany, medicine and magic. To the ancient and medieval minds, these disciplines were scarcely differentiated, nor was there a clear distinction between the religious, magical, and "scientific" objectives of the person seeking to understand them. Yet modern scholarship, despite its awareness of the interrelatedness of these subjects, more often than not has treated them in isolation. Thus, for example, there exist distinct surveys of rabbinic medicine, astronomy, astrology, zoology, and especially magic, but they contain little analysis of the links between them or the overarching theological attitudes reinforcing this linkage.

For the purposes of this book, I wish merely to suggest that medieval and early modern Jews viewed the ancient legacy of classical Judaism as a primary source of inspiration in understanding and mastering nature and in legitimating and authorizing these pursuits as authentically Jewish. Indeed, their historical awareness of the antecedents of their preoccupations with nature is confirmed by recent scholarship on ancient Judaism, notwithstanding its still undigested and incomplete character.

What follows is an attempt to offer bibliographical support for three assumptions about Jewish attitudes toward nature in the ancient world:

1. Despite their widely diverging positions, the overwhelming sentiment of the rabbis toward the natural world was positive. Many were fascinated by the operations of nature, tried to understand and master them, and saw natural knowledge as a prerequisite for knowing and appreciating God.

2. Notwithstanding a minority position that saw God as the exclusive healer of human illness, the rabbis endorsed the knowledge and practice of medicine and demanded that the ill person seek out medical expertise. The rabbis included medical and naturalistic knowledge among their self-proclaimed skills and fully integrated them with their ritualistic and legal ones. Thus the connection between rabbinic knowledge and medicine, including the notion of medicine being a special Jewish skill, is of ancient origin.

3. The rabbis not only endorsed the mastery of naturalistic knowledge; they were open to improving nature, to mastering its forces, and even replicating it. Despite the emphatic biblical proscriptions against a wide range of magical practices, individual rabbis either ignored, camouflaged, rationalized, or even

endorsed the pursuit of magic among Jews. Some rabbis viewed their own personas as connected with "wonder working." Others complained about magic and its dangers but disregarded those who practiced it. And outside the "official" circles of rabbinic leadership, a belief in the efficacy of magic and its operations to heal the sick, to ward off enemies and dangers, both real and imagined, to enhance friendships, and much more, seems to have been deeply ingrained within Jewish societies in Palestine and in the diaspora in both the ancient and early medieval periods.

In short, medieval and early modern Jews who pointed out that their own naturalistic interests were no more than "the custom of our forefathers" were not far off the mark. Whether or not the rabbis and their constituencies were engaged in "scientific pursuits" in the manner of their later ancestors, they clearly reflected on nature and engaged in understanding and mastering its forces. From the vantage point of the rabbis and their followers, to be a Jew was to view natural study in all its various manifestations as a positive resource of spirituality and human power. Jews living in the period described in this book plainly understood this fact and used it regularly and creatively to endorse and to further their intense efforts to study and master the natural world and to fuse these efforts with the scientific pursuits of their non-Jewish contemporaries. Following the order of these three basic assumptions, I offer the following representative (but not exhaustive) bibliography.

ON APPRECIATING NATURE

I know of no systematic presentation of ancient Jewish attitudes toward nature in general. Much information may be gleaned from the standard studies of the "sciences" in biblical and rabbinic Judaism: Y. L. Lewysohn, *Die Zoologie des Talmuds* (Frankfurt am Main, 1858); F. Rosner, *Medicine in the Bible and the Talmud* (New York, 1971); F. Rosner, trans. and ed., *Julius Preuss's Biblical and Talmudic Medicine* (New York and London, 1978); I. Low, *Die Flora der Juden,* 4 vols. (Vienna, 1926–34); S. Lieberman, "The Natural Sciences of the Rabbis," in *Hellenism in Jewish Palestine* (New York, 1950; repr. 1963), pp. 180–93; S. Gandz, *Studies in Hebrew Mathematics and Astronomy* (New York, 1970); W. H. Feldman,

Rabbinic Mathematics and Astronomy (London, 1931); J. H. Charlesworth, "Jewish Astrology in the Talmud, Pseudepigrapha, and Dead Sea Scrolls, and Early Palestinian Synagogues," *Harvard Theological Review* 70 (1977): 183–200. See also L. Ginzberg, *Legends of the Jews,* 7 vols. (Philadelphia, 1909–38), 1:26–42. One might also consider rabbinic interpretations of such biblical verses as Gen. 1:28 (explored systematically in J. Cohen, *Be Fruitful and Multiply* (Ithaca and London, 1990), Amos 5:8, Isa. 40:26, Ps. 19:3, and Job 38–41; and the rabbinic benedictions on witnessing unusual natural events; but compare the unsympathetic view of nature in Avot 3:9. See also S. Pines and Z. Harvey's study of *Midrash Tehilim* 8, 6, entitled "To See the Stars and Constellations" (in Hebrew), *Jerusalem Studies in Jewish Thought* 3 (1984): 507–11.

ON IMPROVING NATURE: THE STUDY OF MEDICINE IN ANCIENT JUDAISM

The standard study is the aforementioned work of Preuss translated by Rosner, *Julius Preuss's Biblical and Talmudic Medicine.* Additional material may be found in H. Friedenwald, *The Jews and Medicine,* 2 vols. (Baltimore, 1944; repr. New York, 1962); E. Carmoly, *Histoire des médecins juifs anciens et modernes* (Brussels, 1944); M. Steinschneider, "Jüdische Aerzte," *Zeitschrift für hebraische Bibliographie* 17 (1914): 63–96, 121–68; 18 (1918): 25–57; and S. R. Kagan, *Jewish Medicine* (Boston, 1952). See also S. Muntner, "Medicine," in *Encyclopedia Judaica,* 11:1178–1205. On the rabbis' medical interest in Babylonia, see J. Neusner, *The Wonder-Working Lawyers of Talmudic Babylonia* (New York and London, 1987), pp. 54–70. On medicine in the halakha after the Talmud, see Y. Z. Cahana, "Medicine in the Halakhic Literature after the Codification of the Talmud" (in Hebrew), *Sinai* 14 (1950): 62–79, 221–41. A good collection of primary sources on medicine in rabbinic Judaism from antiquity to modern times is found in the booklet compiled by M. Friedman for Jacob Katz's master's seminar "The Approach of Judaism to Rational Activity" (in Hebrew) at the Hebrew University (Jerusalem, 1967).

More recent scholarship has focused on the earliest medical compendium, *Sefer ha-Refu'ot,* attributed to Asaf ha-Rofe and variously dated from the first centuries of the common era to the early tenth century, before the time of

Shabbatai Donnolo (see chap. 1 above). A fine recent overview of the subject is E. Lieber, "Asaf's Book of Medicines: A Hebrew Encyclopedia of Greek and Jewish Medicine, possibly compiled in Byzantium on an Indian Model," in J. Scarborough, ed., "Symposium on Byzantine Medicine," *Dumbarton Oaks Papers* 38 (1984): 233–49. Lieber refers to a substantial part of Asaf's work (vols. 3–6) published by S. Muntner in *Koroth* between 1965 and 1972. See also A. Melzer, *Asaph the Physician: The Man and His Book* (Ann Arbor, 1980); A. Bar Sela and H. E. Hoff, "Asaf on Anatomy and Physiology," *Journal of the History of Medicine* 20 (1965): 358–89; and L. Venetianer, *Asaf Judaeus, der alteste medizinische Schriftsteller in hebraeischer Sprache,* 3 parts (Budapest, 1915–17). See also by Leiber, "The Covenant which Asaf . . . and Yohanan . . . made with Their Pupils," *S. Muntner Memorial Volume,* ed. J. O. Liebowitz (Jerusalem, 1983), pp. 83–87; and idem, "A Medieval Hebrew Presage of the Circulation of the Blood, Derived from the Talmudic Precepts for Animal Slaughter," *Koroth* 9 (1985): 157–63. See also S. Newmyer, "Asaph's 'Book of Remedies': Greek Science and Jewish Apologetics," *Sudhoff's Archiv* 76 (1992): 28–36.

Medieval and early modern Jews underscored the antiquity of Jewish medicine by referring to a *Book of Remedies* composed by Solomon but later suppressed by Hezekiah, a work with obvious magical overtones. See Mishnah Pesaḥim 4:9; B.T. Berakhot 10b; Pesaḥim 56a; and Maimonides on Mishnah Pesaḥim 4:9. See also D. Halperin, "The Book of Remedies, the Canonization of the Solomonic Writing, and the Riddle of Pseudo-Eusebius," *Jewish Quarterly Review,* n.s. 72 (1982): 269–72. A tradition of the Jewish origins of medicine beginning with Noah which later intermingles with that of the *Book of Remedies* is found in the introduction to *Sefer Asaf.* This parallels Josephus's description of the Solomonic origins of medicine. See Ginzberg, *Legends of the Jews,* 1:173–74; J. Blum, "The Legendary Origins of Medicine: Medico-historical Apologetics in Judeo-Christian Sources," *Bulletin of the History of Medicine* (forthcoming); and Philip Alexander's discussion of Solomon and magic in his "Incantations and Books of Magic" in the revised and expanded version of E. Schürer, *The History of the Jewish People in the Age of Jesus Christ (175* B.C.–A.D. *135),* ed. G. Vermes, F. Millar, and M. Goodman, vol. 3, pt. 1, sec. 32, vii (Edinburgh, 1986), pp. 375–78.

E. Leiber has regularly discussed recent work on the history of ancient Jewish medicine in the *Newsletter of the Society for Ancient Medicine and Pharmacy* (since vol. 17 [1989]). See also the many articles on the subject from *Koroth,* especially vol. 9 (1985, 1988), which contains the proceedings of the Second and Third International Symposia on Medicine in the Bible and Talmud.

ON TRANSFORMING AND REPLICATING NATURE:
THE PLACE OF MAGIC IN ANCIENT JUDAISM

The study of Jewish magical theory and practice has engaged the serious attention of a large number of contemporary scholars. Three useful recent surveys of this scholarly literature include Alexander, "Incantations," in Schürer, *History of the Jewish People,* 3:342–79; P. Schäfer, "Jewish Magic Literature in Late Antiquity and Early Middle Ages," *Journal of Jewish Studies* 41 (1990): 75–91; and the introduction to L. Schiffman and M. Swartz, *Hebrew and Aramaic Incantation Texts from the Cairo Genizah* (Sheffield, 1992), pp. 11–62. Each of these works, as well as others cited below, documents the wide diffusion of magic within ancient Judaism, notwithstanding strong condemnations by some religious authorities. Like non-Jews, ancient Jews usually failed to differentiate between medicine and magic, doctor and magician. A primary function of magical amulets, bowls, and incantations was to ward off the supposed evil spirits inflicting disease.

Earlier studies of magic in Judaism focused primarily on traces of magical practice found in Hellenistic and rabbinic literature, as well as in several magical handbooks of recipes written in Hebrew and Aramaic. See, for example, the classic works of L. Blau, *Das altjüdische Zauberwesen* (Budapest, 1897–98) and J. Trachtenberg, *Jewish Magic and Superstition: A Study in Folk Religion* (New York, 1939; repr. 1970), the latter dealing with medieval as well as ancient magic. See also E. E. Urbach, *The Sages: Their Concepts and Beliefs* (Jerusalem, 1975), pp. 97–123; S. Lieberman, *Greek in Jewish Palestine* (New York, 1942), pp. 97–114; J. Neusner, *A History of the Jews in Babylonia,* vol. 2 (Leiden, 1966), pp. 147–50; 3 (Leiden, 1968), pp. 110–26; 4 (Leiden, 1969), pp. 330–62; and 5 (Leiden, 1970), pp. 174–96, 217–43; Y. Bazak, "The Laws of Magic and the Laws of Planting Gourds" (in Hebrew), *Bar Ilan University Annual* 6 (1968): 156–66; J. N. Lightstone, *The Commerce of the Sacred: Mediation of the Divine among Jews in the Graeco-Roman Diaspora* (Chico, Calif., 1984), pp. 17–56; M. Margalioth, *Sefer ha-Razim* (Jerusalem, 1966); and J. Goldin, "The Magic of Magic and Superstition," in *Aspects of Religious Propoganda in Judaism and Early Christianity*, ed. E. S. Florenza (Notre Dame, 1976), pp. 115–47.

More recently, a group of scholars have begun to study systematically the Hebrew and Aramaic inscriptions on amulets, bowls, and Genizah fragments, documenting the wide diffusion of magical beliefs and practices, especially outside the "official" rabbinic leadership. The close connection between ancient Jewish magic and mysticism has also been carefully explored. In addition to the aforementioned work of Schiffman and Swartz, see J. Naveh and S. Shaked, *Amulets and Magic Bowls: Aramaic Incantations of Late Antiquity* (Jerusalem and Leiden, 1985); J. Naveh and S. Shaked, *Aramaic and Hebrew Incantations of Late Antiquity* (Jerusalem, 1992); and J. Naveh, *Al Ḥeres ve-Gomah: Ketubot Aramiyot ve-Ivriyot Bimai Bayit Sheni, Ha-Mishnah ve-ha-Talmud* (Jerusalem, 1992), pp. 145–76. See also J. Gager, *Curse Tablets and Binding Spells From the Ancient World* (Oxford, New York, 1992). Much magical material can be found in the *Synopse zur Hekhalot-Literatur*, ed. P. Schäfer et al. (Tübingen, 1981) and in his *Übersetzung der Hekhalot-Literatur* (Tübingen, 1987–91). Schäfer summarizes his main conclusions in *The Hidden and Manifest God: Some Major Themes in Early Jewish Mysticism* (Albany, 1992), esp. pp. 150–66. See also I. Grünwald, *Apocalyptic and Merkavah Mysticism* (Leiden, 1980).

There has been considerable discussion of the definition of magic in ancient Judaism and within its larger cultural surroundings, particularly of its relation to religious ritual and miracle. A useful survey of the major anthropological approaches is J. Middleton, "Theories of Magic," in *Encyclopedia of Religion* (New York, 1990), 9:81–89. See also A. Segal, "Hellenistic Magic: Some Questions of Definition," *Studies in Gnosticism and Hellenistic Religions Presented to Gilles Quispel on the Occasion of His Sixty-fifth Birthday*, ed. R. van dan Broek and M. J. Vermaseren (Leiden, 1981), pp. 349–75. The essays by H. Penner, J. Neusner, and S. Garrett in J. Neusner, E. S. Frerichs, and P. V. McCracken Flesher, *Religion, Science, and Magic in Concert and Conflict* (Oxford and New York, 1989) focus on the problem of defining ancient magic. These essays underscore Garrett's (and Segal's) conclusion about the futility of precise definitions of magic: "Usages of the labels depends on the culturally governed behavioral norms of the persons involved, their relative social locations, and the complex particularities of the given situation" (p. 144). While Penner intelligently discusses the difficulties of

distinguishing rational from ritual behavior and the need for a broader definition of rationality when approaching ancient beliefs and rituals, there is little
discussion in his essay, or in any of the others, of the relation among magic, science, and religion. I was unable to find any extended discussion of the possible
connections between magical and "scientific" activity in ancient Judaism—as
one might find, for example, in Greek, Roman, or medieval culture—other than
the mere mention of the links between magic and medicine. Compare G. Luck,
Arcana Mundi: Magic and the Occult in the Greek and Roman Worlds (Baltimore and
London, 1985; repr. 1987); G. E. R. Lloyd, *Magic, Reason, and Experience* (Cambridge, 1979); B. Hansen, "Science and Magic," in D. C. Lindberg, ed., *Science
in the Middle Ages* (Chicago, 1978), pp. 483–506; V. I. J. Flint, *The Rise of Magic
in Early Medieval Europe* (Princeton, 1991); and chap. 1 above.

One possible link between magic and science in ancient Judaism might be
located in Jewish aspirations to create life, either animal or human, called *Hilkhot
Yeẓirah* in rabbinic literature and often associated with the ancient Jewish treatise on cosmogony, *Sefer Yeẓirah*. See G. Scholem, "The Idea of the Golem," in
his *On the Kabbalah and Its Symbolism* (New York, 1965), pp. 158–204; M. Idel,
Golem: Jewish Magical and Mystical Traditions on the Artificial Anthropoid (Albany,
1990), esp. part 1. Abraham Yagel in the sixteenth century perceived this link
clearly and exploited it to legitimate his own interest in contemporary magic
and science. See D. B. Ruderman, *Kabbalah, Magic, and Science: The Cultural
Universe of a Sixteenth-Century Jewish Physician* (Cambridge, Mass., 1988), chap. 7
and the rabbinic sources discussed there.

INDEX

Abendana, Jacob, 321

Aboab, Jacob, 222

Abravanel, Isaac, 151, 242, 309

Adorno, Theodor, 372–73

Agrippa, Henry Cornelius, 139, 143, 174

Aḥuz Letter [*Mikhtav Aḥuz*]. *See* Delmedigo,
Joseph

air-pump, 332–38

Akiva ben Mahalal, 146

Alashkar, Moses, 142

alchemy. *See* Paracelsians

al-Constantini, Solomon, 27

Aldabi, Meir ben Isaac, 44–45, 254

Alemanno, Yohanan, 132, 139

al-Ghazzali, Abu Ḥamid, 22

Almosnino, Moses, 71. *See also* Peurbach,
George

Altmann, Alexander, 133

Amsterdam, 137, 247, 281, 302, 317

Anatoli, Jacob, 332

ancient Judaism, and the study of nature,
375–82

Anglicans, 312–17, 330, 370. *See also*
Catholics; Christianity; Protestants

Anglo, Sidney, 143

anti-Semitism, 12. *See also* Christianity

Apfelbaum, Abba, 201

Apology for Raymond Sebond. See Montaigne,
Michel de

Arama, Isaac, 200

Ari Nohem. See Modena, Leone

Aristotle, 20, 36, 37–39, 40, 41, 47, 49, 50,
52, 72, 74, 77, 87, 91, 95, 107, 135, 137,
140, 143, 144, 159, 164, 167, 168, 173,
188–91, 218, 220–24, 234, 244, 248, 251,
253, 263, 267, 277, 314, 324, 333, 341

Asaf, the physican, 40, 378–79

Aselli, Gaspere, 249

Ashkenazi, Eliezer, 83, 85, 151, 189

Ashkenazi, Ḥakham Ẓevi, 272, 317, 326

Ashkenazic Jews: and rationalism, 55–60;
and science, 21, 45–47, 54–99. *See also*
Kupfer, Ephraim; eastern Europe, Jews
of; central Europe, Jews of

astrology, 16; its study by medieval Jews,
23–29; in the thought of Abraham Bar
Ḥiyya, 24–27, 35; in the thought of
Abraham ibn Ezra, 27–29; critique of
Moses Maimonides, 26, 29

astronomy, study of, 209; in eastern
Europe, 11; in the Middle Ages, 19–
20; in Gersonides' thought, 41–44; in
Maimonides' thought, 30–32

atomism, 134–36, 164, 267, 342

Averroes (Ibn Roschd), 41–42, 140

Avicenna, 107, 140, 234, 244, 249, 252, 253,
274, 303

Baccetto, Lorenzo, 253

Bacharach, Ḥayyim Ya'ir, 138

Bacon, Francis, 211, 253, 323

Bacon, Roger, 143

Baḥya ibn Pakuda. *See* ibn Pakuda, Baḥya

Bar Ḥiyya, Abraham, 20, 29, 47, 48, 70, 254; and astrology, 24–27

Baraita of R. Samuel, 24

Barcelona, 24, 36

Baron, Salo W., 56–57, 129

Bartholinus, Thomas, 249

Barzilai, Judah ben, 24

Barzilay, Isaac, 129–31, 133, 136–46, 185–87, 201, 202, 206, 209

Basilea, Solomon, 121, 213–28, 243, 263, 264, 267, 271, 272, 341, 357, 369

Bayle, Peter, 284

Bedersi, Jedaiah ben Abraham ha-Penimi, 214–15, 218, 220

Ben Israel, Menasseh, 133, 136, 137, 146, 282, 284, 309

Ben Sasson, Ḥayyim Hillel, 56–57, 59, 60, 63–68, 95; and his response to Jacob Katz, 63–68

Ben Sira, on the physician, 297

Benatelli, Luigi Maria, 225–26

Benayahu, Meir, 117

Berger, David, 37, 46

Bettan, Israel, 200–203, 206

Binah le-Ittim. See Figo, Azariah

Bivago, Abraham, 84, 140

Bodin, Jean, 143

Bonfil, Robert, 9, 72, 86, 136, 187, 189, 196

Book of the Khazars. See Ha-Levi, Judah

Bouwsma, William J., 177

Boyle, Robert, 253, 314, 315, 319, 322, 323, 333, 336–338, 344, 351, 356, 357

Brahe, Tycho, 77, 83, 136, 263, 341, 372

Brahoslav, Jan, 65

Breuer, Mordecai, 82, 87

Briel, Judah, 226, 257, 261–68, 271

Broyard, Anatole, 2

Brudzewo, Albertus de, 71. *See also* Peurbach, George

Bruno, Giordano, 131, 136

Buber, Martin, 65

Buffon, George-Louis Leclerc, 364

Burton, Robert, 143

Calvin, John, 65, 96, 98

Cambridge Platonists, 319

Cantarini family, 113

Cantarini, Isaac ha-Cohen, 105, 113, 254, 257–59, 282

Capsali, Elijah, 151

Cardoso, Abraham, 121, 225, 326

Cardoso, Isaac, 121, 243–44, 279, 284

Cardoso family, 113

Carrion, Santob de, 172

Cases, Joseph, 220, 257

Castro, Americo, 278, 289, 291, 292

Catholics: and science, 5, 13, 98, 193–94, 196–98, 370; and relations with Jews, 157, 162, 187, 196

central Europe, Jews of: interest in science, 54–99. *See also* eastern Europe, Jews of

Charron, Pierre, 174

Chemical Philosophy. *See* Paracelsians

Christina, queen of Sweden. *See* Sweden

Christianity: and science, 5, 13, 96–98, 193–94, 196–98, 312–17, 370, 371; and preaching, 199; and relations with Jews, 12, 60–61, 157, 196, 327–29; Jewish polemics against, 36, 60–62, 224–28, 236, 242–43. *See also* Protestants; Catholics; Anglicans

Cicero, 173

Clarke, Samuel, 315, 317, 320–22, 324, 327, 329–30

Cohen, Judah ben Solomon, 44

Cohen, Tobias, 83, 105, 110–13, 117, 156, 183, 194, 197, 198, 229–55, 266, 272, 334, 341
Collège de Guyenne, 276, 277
Comenius, J. A., 65
Conegliano, Israel, 105
Conegliano, Solomon, 105, 111–12, 230–31, 238, 259
Conegliano family, 114
Conversos, 7–10; in Amsterdam, 9; and medicine, 11, 104, 105, 109, 122, 273–309; and heterodoxy, 12, 276–85; and biblical criticism, 282–85
Copernicus, Nicolaus, 54, 70, 78, 83, 95, 124, 132, 135, 159, 162, 179, 180, 231, 239, 240, 262, 266–68, 324, 341, 350, 351
Cordovero, Moses, 59, 139, 323
Counter-Reformation and missionizing to Jews, 12
Cracow, 11, 67–72, 100, 229, 230; University of, 54, 68, 71, 98
Crescas, Ḥasdai, 50, 159, 173
Crete, 141, 162, 196
Croll, Oswall, 66
Curtius, Joachim, 302
Czech Brethren. See Unitas Fratrum

Dan, Joseph, 46
Darwin, Charles, 365, 370
Davidson, Herbert, 70
Davis, Joseph, 57–58, 87, 91–92
de Castro, Benedict, 217, 295, 299–308
de Castro, Isaac Orobio, 276, 279, 280, 282, 284, 285
de Castro, Jacob, 277
de Castro, Rodrigo, 294–99, 302, 303, 305, 308

de Castro family, 113
de Jonah, Emanuel, 93
De la Divina Providencia. See Nieto, David
de Pomis, David, 309
de Prado, Juan, 280
de'Rossi, Azariah, 33, 83, 84, 120, 141, 186, 242, 269–71, 283; and his debate with the Maharal, 80–82
Dee, John, 66
Delacrut, Mattathias. See also Peurbach, George
del Bene, Judah Assael, 162, 185–98, 212, 370, 371
Delmedigo, Elijah, 125
Delmedigo, Joseph, 84, 105, 110–11, 117–53, 155, 156, 175, 193, 194, 197, 198, 213, 227, 229, 231, 254, 350, 369, 370, 372
Delmedigo family, 113
demons, 143, 148, 151. See also magic
den Spiegel, Adriaan Van, 249
Derham, William, 357–58
Descartes, René, 16, 250, 267, 279, 293, 313, 314, 324, 342, 351, 363, 365
Dioscorides. See Mattioli, Pietro Andrea; Lusitanus, Amatus
doctors, Jewish: image of, 2; in Converso community, 11, 273–309; in ancient Judaism, 378–80; in medieval Europe, 51–52; in eastern and central Europe, 92–94; as students at Padua, 100–117, 229–55; and use of medical analogies, 206–08; ancients and moderns, 220, 244–55; and their diagnostic ability, 286–89
Dodoens, Rembert, 249, 253, 304
Donnolo, Shabbatai, 23–24
Duchesne, Joseph (Quercetanus), 234
Duhem, Pierre, 16
Duties of the Heart. See ibn Pakuda, Baḥya

early modern period: and Jewish culture,
6–9; and Western culture, 6–7
eastern Europe, Jews of, 8; interest in
science, 11, 54–99; and Italy, 58–59
Ebreo, Leone, 132, 137, 161, 309
Elazar ben Arakh, 140
Elbaum, Jacob, 58–60, 68, 92
Emden, Jacob, 60, 67, 272
England, 311–17, 325
Enriquez, Henrique Jorge, 294
enthusiasm, 314, 315
Ephraim of Lunshitz, 192
Esh ha-Dat. *See* Nieto, David
Ettmüller, Michael, 248, 250–54
Evans, R. J. W., 66–67
Eybeshitz, Jonathan, 60, 200, 272

Falaquera, Shem Tov ben Joseph, 44
Fano, Ezra, 120
Fano, Menaḥem Azariah da, 120
Faur, José, 277–78
Feldhay, Rivka, 197
Feldman, Seymour, 41
Felix, Gabriel, 111, 230. *See also* Cohen,
Tobias
Felix family, 114
Ferrara, 185, 256–59, 307, 372
fever, 234, 249–52
Fiametta, Joseph, 216
Ficino, Marsilio, 143
Figo, Azariah, 102, 121, 185, 186, 198–212
Firkovich, Abraham, 148–50, 152
Fishman, David, 69, 70–71, 77, 86, 93–94
Flagellum calumniantium. *See* de Castro,
Benedict
Fludd, Roger, 247
Formigini, Solomon, 215

Fortis, Isaac, 93
Frances, Emanuel, 120, 182, 215–17
Frances, Jacob, 120, 182, 215–17, 224,
226, 227
Franco, Solomon, 27
Freudenthal, Gad, 42, 51–52
Friedenwald, Harry, 290, 301, 302, 306, 307
Funkenstein, Amos, 370–71

Galen, 193, 206–07, 234, 244, 248, 250, 252,
274, 303
Galenti, Yedidiah, 122–23
Galilei, Galileo, 16, 124, 132, 134, 136, 162,
165, 175, 204, 211, 334, 336, 343, 372
Gans, David, 63–68, 76, 77, 82–87, 96, 198,
254, 263, 341, 372
Gassendi, Pierre, 212, 253, 267, 324
Geiger, Abraham, 128–30, 133, 137, 146, 147
150, 152
gene pool, Jewish, 1–2
Gerondi, Nissim, 269, 271
Gershom ben Solomon of Arles, 44, 74
Gersonides (Gerson ben Levi), 10, 15,
41–44, 47, 50, 53, 143, 159, 222
ghetto, 9, 213, 222, 232
Gilman, Stephan, 278, 291–93
Goitein, S. D., 19
Goldenberg, S. L., 148
golem, 139–40, 382
Gomez, Antonio Enriques, 279
Gordon, Aaron, 94
Graetz, Heinrich, 128, 147, 154
Graupe, Heinz Mosche, 345, 351
Gries, Ze'ev, 9
Guericke, Otto von, 333, 336, 337, 351
Guide of the Perplexed. See Maimoni-
des, Moses
Guillén, Diego Gracia, 293–94

Gumpertz, Aaron Solomon, 334–35, 338, 339, 341, 343–44, 350, 351

ha-Cohen, Abraham, of Zante, 112, 117
ha-Cohen, Joseph, 86
Ḥagiz, Moses, 224, 243, 325–26
ha-Ḥazan, Isaac, 147, 148
Haleluyah, Mahalel, 216
Ha-Levi, Joseph b. Isaac, 87, 90–91
Ha-Levi, Judah, 28, 29, 30, 33–35, 37–40, 47, 61–62, 79, 95, 189, 210, 211, 242, 321, 332, 357; and astrology, 28, 34; and magic, 34–35
Hamburg, 295–308, 334, 348
Ḥamiẓ, Joseph ben Judah, 100–102, 105, 116, 118, 119, 121, 122, 126, 127, 138, 152, 201, 202, 206, 213
Hanson, Bert, 49
Hartmann, Johann, 249
Harvey, William, 231, 247, 250, 253
Haskalah, 148–52, 338–40
Ḥayon, Nehemiah, 225–26, 316, 325–30
Ḥayyat, Judah, 140
Ḥayyim ben Beẓalel, 63
Heller, Yom Tov Lipmann, 77, 87, 90–92
Herrera, Abraham, 133, 136, 137, 323
Hevelius, Johannes, 350
hidden miracles, 37
Hilkhot Yeẓirah. See golem
Hippias, 157–59, 168–73, 177, 178, 180, 181
Hippocrates, 107, 234, 244, 252, 274, 303
Hobbes, Thomas, 313, 314, 318
Hoernigk, Ludovicus von, 301–02
Horn, George. *See* Martini, Martini
Horowitz, Abraham, 87
Horowitz, Elliott, 9
Huarte, Juan de San Juan, 285–89, 291–94, 303

Hunter, John, 346–47

ibn Ezra, Abraham, 10, 15, 27–29, 35, 47, 53, 70, 140, 215, 218, 219, 309; and astrology, 27–29
ibn Gabbai, Meir, 140
ibn Gabirol, Solomon, 140
ibn Motot, Samuel, 27
ibn Pakuda, Baḥya, 21–23, 29, 47, 85, 193, 332, 350
ibn Sarsa, Samuel, 27
ibn Shaprut, Shem Tov, 27
ibn Sid, Isaac, 20
ibn Tibbon, Judah, 23
ibn Wakar, 27
Idel, Moshe, 8, 132–33, 136, 137
Inquisition. *See* Conversos; Spain
Isidore of Seville, 48
Iskandrandi, Jacob, 150
Islam: Jewish culture under, 17–18; Jewish medicine in, 19
Israel, Jonathan, 8
Israeli, Isaac, 254
Isserles, Moses, 11, 56–58, 64, 67–78, 80, 82–84, 87, 89, 94, 98, 191, 192, 341; and Maimonides, 74–76
Italy, 11, 17, 18, 23–24; and eastern European Jewry, 58–59, 90; Jewish intellectual groupings in, 119–21

Jacob, Margaret, 312
Jesuits. *See* Catholics
Jewish law. *See* rabbis
Johanan ben Nuri, 223
Judah the Pious and nature, 46–47

Kabbalah, 7, 8, 20, 36, 47, 88, 89, 202, 362, 363, 365; and magic, 40–41, 48–49, 131–

33, 369; and the Maharal, 98; and science, 118–52, 213–28, 264, 369; in Joseph Delmedigo's writing, 125–52; correlations with ancient philosophy, 126–27, 130–33; in Rodrigo de Castro's writing, 298–99

Kaplan, Lawrence, 56, 59, 87, 88–90

Kaplan, Yosef, 273–75, 279–80

Karaites, 131, 135, 146–50, 152

Karo, Joseph, 233

Katz, Jacob, 60–64, 67, 95, 338–39

Kepler, Johann, 77, 132, 136, 223

Kimḥi, Joseph, 242, 309

Kissot le-Veit David. See Del Bene, Judah Assael

Kleinberger, Aharon, 65

Kopelman, Jacob, 87

Kulka, Otto Dov, 65–68, 95

Kupfer, Ephraim, 55–60, 68

Lampronti, Isaac, 105, 121, 256–72, 341, 342, 372

Langermann, Y. Tzvi, 28, 36, 45, 71–72

La Peyrère, Isaac, 172, 184, 276, 280–81, 284, 285, 366

Law of the Lord Is Perfect. See Naḥmanides, Moses

Lazzarelli, Ludovico, 139

Leibes, Yehudah, 8, 132

Leiden, University of, 103, 247, 249, 303, 372

Levi, Joseph, 134–35

Levison, Mordechai Schnaber, 332, 335–36, 338–40, 343, 345–70

Levita, Elijah, 141

Limborch, Philip van, 280

Linnaeus, Carl, 350, 357–65

Lipsius, Justus, 158, 173, 174, 177. *See also* stoicism

Lisker, Chaim, 87

Locke, John, 344, 354–57, 364

London. *See* England

Loria family, 114

Luria, Isaac, 7, 8, 59, 92, 123, 126, 127, 131, 136

Luria, Solomon, 70, 72–76. *See also* Isserles, Moses

Lusitanus, Amatus, 234, 273, 278, 297, 306–08

Lustro, Solomon, 112, 117

Luther, Martin, 96–98, 301

Luzzatto, Moses Ḥayyim, 120

Luzzatto, Simone, 119, 120, 123, 135, 150, 153–84, 186, 190–92, 194, 197, 198, 279, 370

Ma'aseh Bereshit, 122, 223–24

Ma'aseh Merkavah, 223–24

Ma'aseh Tuviyyah. See Cohen, Tobias

Machiavelli, Niccolò, 174, 178

magic, 16, 17, 20, 48–49, 148, 369, 376–77; in ancient Judiasm, 380–82; in Judah Ha-Levi's thought, 34–35; in Naḥmanides' thought, 38–40; Christian versus Jewish, 48–49; in Prague, 66–67. *See also* demons

Magnus, Albertus, 143

Maharal of Prague (Judah Loew ben Beẓalel), 11, 61, 63–67, 70, 76–92, 94–98, 100, 181, 192, 212, 242, 263, 264, 283, 343, 357, 369; on miracles, 78–80; his debate with Azariah de'Rossi, 80–82; and nominalism, 95–98

Maharsha (Samuel Eliezer ben Judah Ha-Levi Edels), 63

Maier, Michael, 66

Maimon, Solomon, 348, 365

Maimonides, Abraham, 32–33, 80

Maimonides, Moses, 10, 15, 16, 29–33, 36, 37, 39–42, 44, 47, 53, 69, 70, 77–78, 81–

84, 87–89, 120, 122, 123, 145, 152, 182–84,
191, 214, 215, 218–22, 241, 242, 254, 262,
264, 266, 268–71, 277, 278, 283, 309,
332, 346, 348, 350, 352, 363, 365, 368; his
critique of astrology, 26, 29; on rabbinic
knowledge of astronomy, 30–32, 80; and
nominalism, 49–50; and Isserles, 74–76;
and kabbalah, 142
Maisel, Mordecai, 66
Malpighi, Marcello, 265
Manfredi, Eustachio, 223
Manoaḥ Hendl b. Shmarya, 87
Maravall, José Antonio, 293–94
Marini, Shabbatai, 112, 117
Marini, Solomon, 111
Marranos. See Conversos
Martini, Martini, 366
Marupk, David, 94
Maskilim. See Haskalah
Mateh Dan. See Nieto, David
Mattioli, Pietro Andrea, 307–08
Maurogonato family, 114
Maʒref la-Ḥokhmah. See Delmedigo, Joseph
medical schools. See universities
medicus politicus. See de Castro, Rodrigo
Melamed, Abraham, 174
Mendelssohn, Moses, 161, 331, 332, 339,
340, 348, 349, 365, 367
Mersenne, Marin, 212, 267, 324, 334
Messer Leon, Judah, 258–59
Messianism. See Ẓevi, Shabbatai
Michael, Ḥayyim, 147
Middle Ages, Jewish attitudes toward
nature in, 14–53
Miesis, Judah Leib, 147–48
mitigated skepticism. See skepticism
Modena, Aaron Berakhia of, 120
Modena. Leone, 101, 118–153, 155, 156, 159,
174, 182, 183, 186, 194, 198, 201, 206, 213

Montaigne, Michel de, 174, 178–80, 277–80
Montalto, Elijah, 122–24, 127, 273, 285,
306, 309
Montpellier, University of, 50, 51, 276
Morgagni, G. Battista, 253
Morpurgo, Samson, 120, 213–28, 243–
44, 272
Morpurgo family, 113
Moscato, Judah, 140, 200, 321
Mussafia, Benjamin, 102, 217, 308, 309
Musschenbroeck, Pieter van, 351, 357
mysticism, Jewish. See kabbalah

Naḥmanides, Moses, 35–42, 47, 79, 95, 139;
and hidden miracles, 37, 79; on Aristotle,
38–39; on magic, 38–40
Neher, André, 76–77, 82, 83, 87
Neḥmad ve-Naʿim. See Gans, David
Neoplatonism, 133–36, 160. See also Cam-
bridge Platonists; Plato
New Christians. See Conversos
Newton, Isaac, 132, 310, 314, 315, 317, 322,
323, 325, 350, 351
Nieto, David, 105, 121, 182, 241, 243–44,
264, 266, 267, 310–31, 334, 341, 342, 357
nominalism, 44, 49–50, 96–99, 160
Nordeskjold, Auguste, 348

Oberman, Heiko, 97
Ozment, Steven, 98

Padua, University of, 11–12, 50, 93, 118,
124, 135, 138, 155, 206, 214, 227, 230–32,
237, 249, 252–54, 257, 259, 264, 299, 311,
372; and the Jews, 100–117; curriculum
of medical school, 107–09
Paḥad Yiẓḥak. See Lampronti, Isaac
Paracelsians, 162, 175, 244–49, 255, 267,
274, 280, 297, 301, 324

Pardo family, 113

Petuchowski, Jacob, 310, 323, 325

Peurbach, George, 69, 71–72, 84

Philo, 154, 183

philosophy: and Jewish culture, 11, 17–18, 90–91; and science, 11, 15–16, 47–48; in eastern Europe, 55–60. *See also* Aristotle; Plato; Neoplatonism; Socrates

physico-theology, 332, 357–65

Pico della Mirandola, Giovanni Francisco, 159, 173, 181

Pistorius, Johann, 66

plastic nature, 319–20

Plato, 164, 172, 175, 187, 189–91, 223, 304, 363. *See also* Neoplatonism; Cambridge Platonists

Poland. *See* eastern Europe, Jews of; Cracow

Popkin, Richard, 280–81

Portaleone, Abraham, 121

Prague, 11, 57, 58, 65–67, 77, 86, 90, 91, 95, 96, 98, 100. *See also* Rudolf II

Pre-Adamism. *See* La Peyrère, Isaac

preformation, 342–43, 363

printing and Jewish culture, 9, 10. *See also* Cohen, Tobias

Protestants and science, 5, 13, 96–98, 197, 312–17. *See also* Calvin, John; Luther, Martin; Anglicans

Provençal, David, 111, 258

Provence, 17, 18, 20, 41, 44

prudenza, 168–71, 190

Ptolemy, 159, 179, 180, 240, 263

Pyrrhonism. *See* skepticism

Pythagoras, 160, 191

rabbis: and religious authority, 12, 256–72; on nature, 17, 375–82; and their scien-tific knowledge, 30–32. *See also* ancient Judaism

Rabinowicz, Harry, 201

ragione di stato. See Machiavelli, Niccolò

Rashba (Solomon ibn Adret), 73

Ray, John, 357

Recanati, Menahem, 88

Redi, Francesco, 265, 267, 271, 366

Reformation, and Jewish culture, 63, 65–66, 96–99. *See also* Brahoslav, Jan; Unitas Fratrum; Protestants; Christianity

Reiner, Elhanan, 9

Reuchlin, Johannes, 139, 301

Rhazes, 107, 303

Ribash (Isaac ben Sheshet Perfet), 73, 74

Ricius, Paulus, 298, 299

Rivkes, Moses, 61–62

Rosales, Jacob, 308

Ross, Tamar, 78–80, 95–96

Rudolf II of Prague, 66–67; and his obser-vatory, 83

Saadia Gaon, 126, 140, 144, 242, 350, 357, 367

Sabbatianism. *See* Zevi, Shabbatai

Sanchez, Francisco, 172, 174, 276–80

Saperstein, Marc, 199

Sardi, Samuel, 200

Sarmento, Jacob de Castro, 330–31

Sarug, Israel, 126

Sasportas, Jacob, 243

Schaefer, David Lewis, 178–80

Schaffer, Simon, 337, 356

Schoeps, Hans Joachim, 345, 346, 348, 351

Scholem, Gershom, 59, 132, 214, 217

Schudt, Johann Jacob, 102, 301

scientific societies and Jews, 115–16, 371–72

Sefer Elim. See Delmedigo, Joseph

Sefer ha-Zohar, 40–41, 48, 125, 150, 342, 361. *See also* kabbalah

Sefer Yeẓirah, 140, 341–42

Sennert, Daniel, 248, 253, 304

Septimus, Bernard, 154, 182–84

Sermoneta, Joseph, 187, 196

sermons and science, 198–212

Sextus Empiricus, 173, 176, 181

Shalom, Abraham, 142–44

Shapin, Steven, 337, 356

Shi'ur Komah, 73

Simeon ben Samuel, 57

Simon, Richard, 280, 284

Siraisi, Nancy, 252–53

skepticism, 153–84, 190–91, 212, 266, 276–80

Snow, C. P., 1

Socrate. See Luzzatto, Simone

Socrates, 161, 163–67, 171–72, 175, 176, 178–81, 184, 187–91, 349

Solomon, 34, 163, 171, 299, 304, 309, 379

Spain, 17, 18, 20, 44, 289, 292. *See also* Conversos

Spinoza, Benedict, 172, 182–85, 276, 280–85, 313, 317–18, 365; and kabbalah, 365

spiritual sciences, 36–40

Stancaro, Francesco, 68

stoicism, in Simone Luzzatto's thought, 157–58, 160, 173, 177–80

Strauss, Leo, 183, 284

Sweden, 300, 348, 349, 363

Sylvius de la Boe, 247–48, 250, 252, 253, 304

Ta'alumot Ḥokhmah. See Delmedigo, Joseph

Tacitus, Cornelius, 158, 174, 188–90

Ta-Shema, Israel, 45, 46, 58–60

Teller, Issachar, 237, 254

Themistius, 140

Timon, 170–71, 175–76, 181, 190

Toland, John, 218, 314, 330

Torat ha-Olah. See Isserles, Moses

Torricelli, Evangelista, 334–37, 344, 351

Toulouse, University of, 276, 277, 279, 280

Tov Elem, Joseph, 27

translators, Jewish, 18, 52

Troki, Isaac, 63, 242

Twersky, Isadore, 30

universities, Jewish entrance into, 11, 49–50, 102–17. *See also* Padua, University of; Cracow, University of; Leiden, University of; Toulouse, University of

Unitas Fratrum, 65, 67, 98

Van Helmont, Joan Baptista, 246–47, 253

Vega, Thomas Rodericus a, 297, 306

Venice, 106, 123, 153, 155, 157, 160–63, 173, 175, 184, 185, 200, 201, 203, 222, 229, 231, 232, 279

Vives, Juan Luis, 278

Wallich, Abraham, 237, 254

Wallich family, 113

Wars of the Lord. See Gersonides

Willis, Thomas, 247–48, 250–51, 253, 254

Winkler, Jacob, 94

Winkler family, 114

Wolf, Johann Christoph, 366

Yaffe, Mordecai, 56, 77, 87–90, 350

Yagel, Abraham, 121, 133, 139, 143, 151, 175

Yates, Frances, 131, 132

Yerushalmi, Yosef, 203, 279

Yoḥanan ben Zakkai, 140

Yoḥanan the Grammarian, 140

Yosha, Nissim, 133, 136

Zacuto, Abraham, 20
Zacuto, Moses, 120, 138, 217–19, 227
Zacutus Lusitanus, 234, 273, 300, 302–03, 306–09
Ẓahalon, Jacob, 198, 232–35, 243, 244, 249, 254
Zamosc, Israel ben Moses Ha-Levi of,

332–34, 336, 338, 339, 341–43, 350, 363, 366
Ẓemaḥ, Jacob, 174
Zeraḥ ben Nathan, 149, 156
Ẓevi, Shabbatai, 7–9, 12, 92, 118, 215, 217, 224–25, 231, 242–43, 247, 272, 299, 300, 316, 326
Zinberg, Israel, 128, 147–48, 201
Zunz, Leopold, 147